RJ 45 ILL

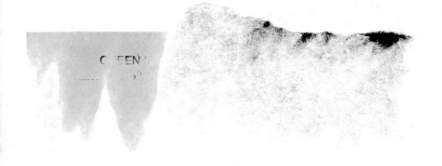

# Common Symptoms of Disease in Children

*The Normal Child*, 9th edition 1987
Churchill Livingstone
Translated into Greek, Spanish, French, Italian, Japanese and
Farsi

*Development of the Infant and Young Child,*
*Normal and Abnormal*, 9th edition 1987
Churchill Livingstone
Translated into Japanese, French, Polish, Spanish and Italian

*Lessons from Childhood: Some Aspects of the*
*Early Life of Unusual Men and Women* with
C. M. Illingworth, 1968
Churchill Livingstone
Translated into Japanese

*Babies and Young Children: Feeding,*
*Management and Care* with C. M. Illingworth,
8th edition 1988
Churchill Livingstone
Translated into Polish

*Treatment of the Child at Home: A Guide for*
*Family Doctors*, 1971
Blackwell Scientific Publications
Translated into Greek

*Basic Development Screening*, 4th edition 1988
Blackwell Scientific Publications
Translated into Greek, Italian, Japanese and Spanish

*The Child at School: A Paediatrician's*
*Manual for Teachers*, 1975
Blackwell Scientific Publications
Translated into Italian

*Your Child's Development in the First Five Years*, 1981
Churchill Livingstone
Translated into Spanish

*Infections and Immunisation of Your Child*, 1981
Churchill Livingstone
Translated into Spanish

# Common Symptoms of Disease in Children

### R. S. ILLINGWORTH

DSc, MD, FRCP, DPH, DCH

*Emeritus Professor of Child Health*
*The University of Sheffield*
*Formerly Paediatrician to the*
*Children's Hospital, Sheffield*

## NINTH EDITION

OXFORD

## BLACKWELL SCIENTIFIC PUBLICATIONS

LONDON EDINBURGH BOSTON
PARIS BERLIN VIENNA MELBOURNE

©1967, 1969, 1971, 1973, 1975,
1979, 1982, 1984, 1988 by
Blackwell Scientific Publications
Editorial offices:
Osney Mead, Oxford OX2 OEL
25 John Street, London WC1N 2BL
23 Ainslie Place, Edinburgh EH3 6AJ
3 Cambridge Center, Cambridge,
   Massachusetts 02142, USA
54 University Street, Carlton
   Victoria 3053, Australia

First published 1967 -
Second edition 1969
Third edition 1971
Fourth edition 1973
Reprinted 1974
Fifth edition 1975
Sixth edition 1979
Reprinted 1980
Seventh edition 1982
Eighth edition 1984
Ninth edition 1988
Reprinted 1991

Translated into Spanish,
Greek, German, Italian
and Portuguese

Photoset by
Enset (Photosetting),
Midsomer Norton, Bath, Avon
Printed and bound
in Great Britain
by Biddles of Guildford

DISTRIBUTORS

Marston Book Services Ltd
PO Box 87
Oxford OX2 0DT
(*Orders*: Tel. 0865 791155
   Fax: 0865 791927
   Telex: 837515)

USA
Mosby-Year Book, Inc.
11830 Westline Industrial Drive
St Louis, Missouri 63146
(*Orders*: Tel. (800) 633-6699)

Canada
Mosby-Year Book, Inc.
5240 Finch Avenue East
Scarborough, Ontario
(*Orders*: Tel. (416) 298-1588)

Australia
Blackwell Scientific Publications
(Australia) Pty Ltd
54 University Street
Carlton, Victoria 3053
(*Orders*: Tel. (03) 347-0300)

British Library
Cataloguing in Publication Data

Illingworth, Ronald S.
   Common symptoms of disease in
   children—9th edn
   1. Children—Diseases—Diagnosis
   2. Symptomatology
   I. Title
   618.92'0072      RJ50

ISBN 0-632-01912-3

# Contents

# Preface to the Ninth Edition

This is an extensive revision. Many sections have been completely rewritten, and many scores of additions and alterations have been made. Once more I have grappled with the impossible, by trying not only to give non-disease before disease, but also to give the common before the rare and conditions mainly in the newborn before conditions seen mainly in older children.

I have avoided classifications, because they so commonly lead to one giving the rare conditions first. A well-known textbook of paediatrics arranges the cause of symptoms in alphabetical order—and the first cause of pallor given is albinism.

I have tried, often without success, to omit lists or to cut them down to a minimum. Colleagues with whom I discussed this advised me not to cut out introductory lists. At least I have abbreviated many of them. I have tried always to include a brief summary of all conditions mentioned, however rare; but for the sake of brevity all summaries have been kept as short as possible. The selection of rare syndromes is eminently suitable for criticism: many hundreds could be added; but it would be difficult to find any which cannot be found in the books listed at the end. Because of the nature of this book, I have taken particular care to make the index comprehensive and, partly to avoid duplication, I have included cross-references throughout.

I have always found it difficult to decide what references to omit, and what to add, at the same time keeping references to a minimum. In this edition I have added 280 new references.

*My aim, as in previous editions, is to help the student and doctor to consider possible clinical diagnoses on the basis of a child's presenting symptoms.* I assume that all clinical diagnoses are based on the history (the symptoms), the physical signs, special investigations, where relevant, and the interpretation of all these. Once one has thought of a possible disease or syndrome, it is easy to read about it in any relevant textbook, and I have listed relevant books at the end, and relevant references after each section. Standard textbooks do not, for the most part, help one to think of the possible diagnoses on the basis of the child's symptoms—and children usually present with symptoms. For instance, when revising my section on dyspnoea, I looked at a variety of textbooks to determine whether I had omitted any condition which I should mention; but the word dyspnoea, or its synonym, was not in the index of 20 textbooks—on general paediatrics, the respiratory system, paediatric cardiology (five books), neonatal paediatrics, or paediatric emergencies. Three other books included the word in the index: one of these gave beriberi as the only cause, and another gave only two causes—choanal atresia and pulmonary stenosis. Schaffer's book on the newborn gave a discussion on the symptoms.

Of two paediatric textbooks said by the authors to be intended for medical students, one (in the index) listed 137 conditions and the other listed 450 conditions which, in both cases, I have yet to see in over 50 years of postgraduate experience; but they did not include such symptoms (or their synonyms) as wheezing, acute abdominal pain, failure to thrive, epistaxis, encopresis, clumsiness, torticollis, appetite or sleep problems, neonatal convulsions, fever of unknown origin, stuttering or the side effects of drugs.

Reviewers have again appeared to think that the title of the book is 'Symptoms of Common Diseases'—and criticized me for giving rare conditions. But the title is 'Common Symptoms of Disease'—and rarities had to be mentioned. I have also been criticized for not discussing the pathology of the diseases mentioned, the special investigations and the treatment (and even the effectiveness of treatment). These would be irrelevant to my aim and would cover several complete volumes. I have mentioned special investigations only on rare occasions when I thought that it was particularly relevant to the discussion.

I have tried, from my own experience, to include pitfalls in diagnosis, the diagnostic snares, the mistakes to avoid. Throughout I have paid special attention to a very common snare—the side effects of drugs. This is important, for *well over 90 per cent of all the symptoms in this book could be merely drug side effects*. When discussing the causes of a symptom I have tried to shorten some long lists of drugs by arranging them in groups—such as antibiotics, anticonvulsants, cytotoxic drugs, non-steroidal anti-inflammatory drugs, and tranquillizing or sedative drugs. The alphabetical list of named drugs on pp. 370–82 remains unchanged apart from many additions and the naming of the groups above. I have taken particular care to make this list comprehensive because of its great importance for diagnosis. It was impossible to separate common reactions from rare ones.

R. S. Illingworth

# Preface to the First Edition

When I was talking to my 13-year-old child about my attempt to write a book concerning the common symptoms of disease in children, mentioning the difficulties which I was encountering, and the fact that no one, to my knowledge, has attempted it, she said 'Isn't that all the more reason why you should do it?' I replied that it may well be that the reason why others have not done it is the fact that they have more sense than to try.

I have attempted to write a precis of the common symptoms of disease in children because I felt that the family doctor, when faced with a symptom in a child whom he is examining, would find it useful when in difficulty to refer quickly to conditions which have to be considered. The textbooks, general or specialist, for the most part do not deal with symptoms. For instance, I referred to a large textbook of otorhinolaryngology for information about stridor, but the word was not in the index. It is likely to take a family doctor a long time to find a textbook which discusses the very common cyanotic or apnoeic attacks of the newborn. The great majority of the symptoms which I have discussed in this book are not in fact mentioned in the index of the majority of textbooks, and many of the symptoms are not mentioned in the index of any of them. This is not intended to be a criticism of textbooks. Discussion of symptoms would have greatly lengthened them, and inevitably have caused repetition.

In consequence I have discussed about 100 common symptoms of disease in childhood. I have made no attempt to provide a complete list of all the possible causes of a symptom, but I have tried to pick out the important causes, making it clear which I think are the most common ones, and which I consider to be rare.

Though classifications are useful for memorizing, and though they look neat and tidy, I have avoided them almost completely, because of their inherent weakness in not giving the common conditions first.

Where a symptom may be psychological or organic I have included it, but where a symptom is entirely psychological I have omitted it, because I have discussed psychological problems in my books *The*

*Normal Child in His First Five Years** and *The Child at School*†. I have, however, included a section concerning psychological manifestations of organic disease, and the somatic manifestations of psychological symptoms.

The book is confined to the subject of diagnosis. I have named common investigations which need to be carried out in order to elucidate the problem—but again have made no effort to name them all. (In a recent article on jaundice in the newborn, the author listed 75 special investigations which should be carried out.) I have not described the normal values of the investigations, nor the methods of performing them; but I have named the investigations in order that the family doctor would known some of the tests which are necessary to establish the diagnosis, and would then know when to refer the child to a special centre for study. I thought, furthermore, that knowledge of the necessary tests would help him in his talks with the parents. I have made a special point of emphasizing the conditions which do require such special investigations.

There is inevitably a certain overlap between signs and symptoms and I have allowed myself a little licence in interpreting the word 'symptoms'. For instance, I have included a short section on enlargement of the spleen. Admittedly an adult experiences discomfort when his spleen is felt. My reason for including it, however, was the frequency of splenic enlargement in children and therefore its importance in the diagnosis of so many different diseases.

I have assumed that the family doctor has basic medical knowledge. I have also had to assume that the family doctor does not want or need profound knowledge on any subject. My notes may well, therefore, be criticized for being superficial. They are deliberately made so, because I did not feel that the family doctor would want more. But I have throughout assumed that, having looked through a section of this book to read about a particular symptom, he would then refer to one of the recognized textbooks for more information. To this end I have listed principal sources of further knowledge. For instance, as a general source of information on a paediatric problem I have recommended *Nelson's Textbook of Pediatrics*.

*The normal child*, Ninth Edition, 1987. London, Churchill Livingstone.
†*The child at school: a paediatrician's manual for teachers*, 1975. Oxford, Blackwell Scientific Publications.

In my opinion no one should attempt to make a diagnosis in a sick child without knowing what drugs he has already received. The side effects of drugs are so frequent and far-reaching, and the number of drugs taken, whether prescribed by a doctor or otherwise, is so great, that it is essential to know what medicines have been given. I have mentioned the side effects of drugs in the relevant sections, and summarized them in a special section.

At the risk of repetition, I have inserted a brief section about commonly held misbeliefs in paediatric diagnosis—incluidng such a misbelief as the idea that convulsions are caused by teething. I am aware of the fact that there is a small amount of repetition in different sections. I decided to retain this for the convenience of the reader.

I hope that family doctors will find this book useful in General Practice. I believe that students will find this book useful for the purposes of revision. It would not serve as a basic textbook for them, but I believe that it would be useful in conjunction with one of the standard textbooks.

It is certain that many will think of causes of which I have not thought, or of symptoms which should have been included. I should greatly welcome comments and suggestions so that the book can be improved if another edition is required.

I wish to thank my friends Dr Peter Wyon, Family Doctor, of Thirsk, Yorks, Dr Frank Harris, Lecturer in Child Health, the University of Sheffield, and my wife, Dr Cynthia Illingworth, for reading every word of the script and for their most useful criticisms: and to my secretaries, Miss D. Bain, Miss J. Grundy and Mrs D. Ackroyd, for typing the drafts of this book.

# Failure to Thrive

All those who are concerned with the care of children are repeatedly faced with the problem of the child who refuses to gain weight in the approved manner. It is surprisingly difficult to obtain a composite picture of this problem in the standard texts. In this chapter I have attempted to put together the main conditions which have to be considered when a child's weight gain is below the average. *In the first place one must decide whether or not there is anything wrong with the child.*

All children are different. Some are small and some are big, some are thin and some are fat. Though nutrition has much to do with this, it is not the only factor. Many factors are unknown. It is difficult and usually impossible to draw the line between normal and abnormal. A child may be kilograms below the average weight, and centimetres below the average in height, and yet be normal. It is far more important that the child should be full of energy, free from lassitude and abounding in *joie de vivre*, than that he should be average in weight and height. It is more healthy to be below the average weight than above it . All that one can say is that the further away from the average is the child's weight and height, the less likely he is to be 'normal'.

When a child is smaller than average, his appetite is likely to be correspondingly less than that of others, so that the parents become worried and try to persuade him to eat. The inevitable result is food refusal—termed by mothers 'poor appetite'.

Mothers are often worried about the normal slowing down of weight gain in the second half of the first year. This is associated with a reduction in appetite, which may cause food forcing and so food refusal. Children take all they need if given a chance and it is never necessary to try to make them eat. A well child's poor appetite is almost always due to food forcing.

## Normal physical growth and variations

Tables 1 and 2 show the average weight and height of boys and girls in the first 10 years.

*Failure to Thrive*

Table 1. Average weight of boys and girls

*Boys*

| Age in years | CENTILES | | | | | |
|---|---|---|---|---|---|---|
| | 10 | | 50 | | 90 | |
| | lb | kg | lb | kg | lb | kg |
| 0 | 6.17 | 2.8 | 7.72 | 3.5 | 9.04 | 4.1 |
| 0.25 | 11.05 | 5.01 | 13.07 | 5.93 | 15.41 | 6.99 |
| 0.5 | 14.99 | 6.8 | 17.42 | 7.9 | 20.28 | 9.2 |
| 0.75 | 17.59 | 7.98 | 20.28 | 9.2 | 23.43 | 10.63 |
| 1.0 | 19.40 | 8.8 | 22.49 | 10.2 | 25.79 | 11.7 |
| 2 | 24.25 | 11.0 | 28.0 | 12.7 | 32.19 | 14.6 |
| 3 | 28.00 | 12.7 | 32.41 | 14.7 | 37.26 | 16.9 |
| 4 | 31.52 | 14.3 | 36.60 | 16.6 | 42.11 | 19.1 |
| 5 | 34.61 | 15.7 | 40.72 | 18.5 | 47.4 | 21.5 |
| 6 | 38.14 | 17.3 | 45.20 | 20.5 | 52.91 | 24.0 |
| 7 | 41.89 | 19.0 | 49.82 | 22.6 | 59.29 | 26.9 |
| 8 | 46.03 | 20.9 | 55.11 | 25.0 | 66.13 | 30.0 |
| 9 | 50.48 | 22.9 | 60.62 | 27.5 | 73.63 | 33.4 |
| 10 | 55.56 | 25.2 | 66.68 | 30.3 | 82.23 | 37.3 |

*Girls*

| Age in years | CENTILES | | | | | |
|---|---|---|---|---|---|---|
| | 10 | | 50 | | 90 | |
| | lb | kg | lb | kg | lb | kg |
| 0 | 6.28 | 2.85 | 7.50 | 3.4 | 8.71 | 3.95 |
| 0.25 | 10.6 | 4.81 | 12.26 | 5.56 | 14.13 | 6.41 |
| 0.5 | 14.2 | 6.44 | 15.21 | 6.9 | 18.72 | 8.49 |
| 0.75 | 16.71 | 7.58 | 19.22 | 8.72 | 22.09 | 10.02 |
| 1.0 | 18.52 | 8.4 | 21.38 | 9.7 | 24.69 | 11.2 |
| 2 | 22.93 | 10.4 | 26.89 | 12.2 | 31.09 | 14.1 |
| 3 | 27.11 | 12.3 | 31.52 | 14.3 | 36.15 | 16.4 |
| 4 | 31.09 | 14.1 | 35.93 | 16.3 | 41.44 | 18.8 |
| 5 | 35.05 | 15.9 | 40.34 | 18.3 | 47.17 | 21.4 |
| 6 | 38.8 | 17.6 | 44.97 | 20.4 | 53.79 | 24.4 |
| 7 | 42.33 | 19.2 | 49.82 | 22.6 | 61.07 | 27.7 |
| 8 | 46.29 | 21.0 | 55.34 | 25.1 | 68.78 | 31.2 |
| 9 | 50.7 | 23.0 | 61.07 | 27.7 | 78.04 | 35.4 |
| 10 | 55.34 | 25.1 | 68.56 | 31.1 | 90.39 | 41.0 |

Table 2. Average height of boys and girls

*Boys*

| Age in years | CENTILES | | | | | |
| | 10 | | 50 | | 90 | |
| | in | cm | in | cm | in | cm |
|---|---|---|---|---|---|---|
| 0 | 20.2 | 51.4 | 21.3 | 54.0 | 22.3 | 56.6 |
| 1 | 28.7 | 72.8 | 30.0 | 76.3 | 31.4 | 79.7 |
| 2 | 32.6 | 82.7 | 34.2 | 86.9 | 35.9 | 91.1 |
| 3 | 35.1 | 89.3 | 37.1 | 94.2 | 39.0 | 99.1 |
| 4 | 37.8 | 96.1 | 40.0 | 101.6 | 42.1 | 107.1 |
| 5 | 40.2 | 102.2 | 42.6 | 108.3 | 45.0 | 114.4 |
| 6 | 42.5 | 108.0 | 45.1 | 114.6 | 47.7 | 121.2 |
| 7 | 44.7 | 113.5 | 47.4 | 120.5 | 50.2 | 127.5 |
| 8 | 46.8 | 118.8 | 49.7 | 126.2 | 52.6 | 133.5 |
| 9 | 48.8 | 124.0 | 51.8 | 131.6 | 54.8 | 139.3 |
| 10 | 50.7 | 128.8 | 53.9 | 136.8 | 57.0 | 144.8 |

*Girls*

| Age in years | CENTILES | | | | | |
| | 10 | | 50 | | 90 | |
| | in | cm | in | cm | in | cm |
|---|---|---|---|---|---|---|
| 0 | 19.8 | 50.4 | 20.9 | 53.0 | 21.9 | 55.9 |
| 1 | 27.9 | 70.8 | 29.2 | 74.2 | 30.6 | 77.7 |
| 2 | 32.0 | 81.3 | 33.7 | 85.6 | 35.4 | 89.8 |
| 3 | 34.7 | 88.1 | 36.6 | 93.0 | 38.5 | 97.9 |
| 4 | 37.4 | 94.9 | 39.5 | 100.4 | 41.7 | 105.9 |
| 5 | 39.8 | 101.1 | 42.4 | 107.2 | 44.6 | 113.2 |
| 6 | 42.0 | 106.8 | 44.5 | 113.4 | 47.2 | 120.0 |
| 7 | 44.2 | 112.4 | 47.0 | 119.3 | 49.7 | 126.3 |
| 8 | 46.3 | 117.6 | 49.2 | 125.0 | 52.1 | 132.4 |
| 9 | 48.4 | 122.9 | 51.4 | 130.6 | 54.4 | 138.3 |
| 10 | 50.5 | 128.3 | 53.7 | 136.4 | 56.9 | 144.5 |

Tanner, Whitehouse & Takaishi [30].

4

Mothers are liable to be worried if a child is smaller than usual. After the first year it may be useful to attempt to predict the child's eventual height. Prediction can be only approximate because of the many variables, but it may help a parent's understanding and allay anxiety. Table 3, based on the work of Tanner, shows the eventual height likely to be reached by a child in relation to his present height. An example of the value of such a table is as follows. A child of 3 years was referred because of her small size, being 34 in (86 cm) high. Her mother was 5 ft

Table 3. Height in childhood in relation to expected adult height

| Expected adult height | 5ft | 150 cm | 5 ft 6 in | 165cm | 6 ft | 180 cm |
|---|---|---|---|---|---|---|
| Height of boys Age in years | in | cm | in | cm | in | cm |
| 1 | 25.8 | 65.5 | 28.3 | 72.0 | 30.9 | 78.6 |
| 2 | 29.4 | 74.7 | 32.1 | 81.7 | 35.3 | 89.6 |
| 3 | 31.8 | 80.8 | 35.1 | 89.2 | 38.1 | 97.0 |
| 4 | 34.4 | 87.3 | 37.8 | 96.1 | 41.2 | 104.7 |
| 5 | 36.6 | 93.0 | 40.3 | 102.3 | 43.9 | 111.6 |
| 6 | 38.7 | 98.4 | 42.7 | 108.4 | 46.4 | 118.4 |
| 7 | 40.7 | 103.5 | 44.8 | 113.9 | 48.9 | 124.2 |
| 8 | 42.6 | 108.2 | 46.9 | 119.0 | 51.1 | 129.9 |
| 9 | 44.6 | 113.2 | 49.0 | 124.4 | 53.4 | 135.7 |
| 10 | 46.2 | 117.4 | 50.8 | 129.1 | 55.5 | 140.9 |
| Height in girls Age in years | in | cm | in | cm | in | cm |
| 1 | 27.0 | 68.5 | 28.3 | 72.0 | 32.4 | 82.2 |
| 2 | 31.1 | 79.2 | 34.3 | 87.1 | 37.4 | 95.0 |
| 3 | 33.9 | 86.0 | 37.2 | 94.5 | 40.6 | 103.1 |
| 4 | 36.5 | 92.8 | 40.2 | 102.1 | 43.9 | 111.4 |
| 5 | 39.0 | 99.1 | 43.0 | 109.1 | 46.6 | 119.0 |
| 6 | 41.3 | 104.8 | 45.4 | 115.3 | 48.9 | 125.9 |
| 7 | 43.5 | 110.5 | 47.8 | 121.5 | 52.2 | 132.6 |
| 8 | 45.6 | 115.7 | 50.1 | 127.3 | 54.6 | 138.8 |
| 9 | 47.6 | 120.9 | 52.2 | 133.0 | 57.1 | 145.1 |
| 10 | 49.5 | 125.7 | 54.4 | 138.3 | 59.4 | 150.9 |

As a rough guide, the height on the second birthday is half the expected adult height. Calculated from Tanner et al. [30]. Example—7-year-old girl, height 43.5 inches. Probably eventual height is 5 feet.

(150 cm) tall and was relieved to hear that the girl could be expected to reach a similar height.

When an apparently well child is unusually small for his age, the two most likely causes are genetic factors (the child taking after his parent) or low birth weight. When a parent is unusually small, not only in height and weight but also in physical build, the child may be correspondingly small. There is often a familial pattern of growth, such as a tendency for slower than usual growth in the early months.

The smaller the child is at birth, especially if he was small for dates, the smaller he is likely to be in later years [11]. His low birth weight may have been due to preterm delivery (of which one cause is multiple pregnancy) or to intra-uterine growth retardation caused by malnutrition, placental insufficiency, hypertension, kidney disease, infections such as rubella (or malaria in tropical countries), or drugs (notably nicotine, alcohol and other drugs of addiction).

Apart from the above essentially prenatal factors, the most likely causes for an apparently well child being unusually small are adverse socio-economic circumstances. They include poverty, malnutrition, emotional deprivation and child abuse (non-accidental injury). The above should all be seriously considered, on the basis of the history and examination, before costly and time-consuming investigations for 'failure to thrive' are instigated [20]. The presence of disease or the possibility of child abuse will be strongly suggested by serial measurements on the centile chart, showing a falling off in the normal rate of growth.

A well child's unusually small size may be due to previous defective growth as a result of disease, now cured. Experimental work on animals has shown that, if growth is retarded in early life, the growth remains defective in spite of adequate nutrition. Many human infants who suffer major surgical procedures in the early weeks, and who were excessively small in weight in that period, are small in later years [5]. The longer the growth retardation persists before the cause is corrected, the greater the subsequent growth deficit. Children operated on for ligation of a patent ductus arteriosus, and who were far below the average in size at the time of the operation, did not usually catch up to the average height after the ligation [33]. It seems that there is a 'critical period' in physical growth, after which a normal diet will not restore the child to an average size.

For organic causes of an unusually small height see p. 21.

*Classification of causes of failure to thrive*

Defective intake
  Insufficient breast milk
  Formula-fed babies—inadequate quantity, incorrectly prepared feeds
  Emotional deprivation—prolonged crying
  Child abuse
Protein calorie malnutrition
Anorexia nervosa
Vitamin deficiency on synthetic diets
Chronic infection—urinary tract, tuberculosis, malaria (in the tropics)
Defective absorption—fat, carbohydrate, protein
                      —Hirschsprung's disease
                      —allergy to cow's milk
Increased loss—diarrhoea, vomiting, excessive perspiration, inadequate fluid intake in hot climates
(Rare) Metabolic diseases, especially those associated with polyuria—hypophosphatasia, storage diseases, organic acidaemias, Leigh's syndrome, Di George syndrome, Wolman's syndrome
Organ diseases
  Brain—severe mental subnormality, cerebral tumour, subdural effusion
  Heart—congenital heart disease
  Chest—severe asthma, bronchiectasis
  Pancreas—cystic fibrosis, diabetes mellitus
  Liver—severe liver disease
  Kidney—renal insufficiency
Chromosome and various dysmorphic syndromes
Other prenatal factors—addictive drugs: fetal alcohol syndrome

## Defective intake

A breast-fed baby is more likely to suffer from underfeeding than an artificially fed baby, because the mother cannot know how much milk she has without weighing him. Mothers think that the leaking of milk from the breast (lactorrhoea) signifies that there is an abundance of milk, though it signifies nothing more than the draught reflex, or the unusually easy escape of milk from the breast. Many doctors think that if a baby is contented he must be obtaining sufficient milk from the breast. This is far from the truth. Many young babies are content to starve and do not cry, even though receiving a totally inadequate amount of milk.

The most accurate way of establishing the diagnosis of defective intake by a breast-fed baby is the test feed—weighing the baby before and after every feed in the day, expressing milk fully after each feed and measuring it, and then adding up the total. If expression is not carried out, the result is seriously misleading, for all that one is then measuring is the milk which the baby has taken from the breast, but not the milk available in the breast. If a baby sucks badly or is drowsy or irritable or if the nipple is a difficult one for him, he may not obtain the available milk. Breast milk alone after the age of about 6 months may be nutritionally inadequate.

A small preterm baby may fail to gain weight on human milk, but thrive on a cow's milk preparation. A common cause of the failure of a preterm baby to gain weight is inadequate intake: it is often forgotten that whereas a full term baby usually needs 2½ oz of milk per lb per day (150 ml per kg), a preterm baby after two weeks usually needs 3 oz per lb per day (188 ml per kg) and 4 oz per lb per day (250 ml per kg) after 4 weeks: but overfeeding may cause vomiting and loss of weight. Some causes of failure to thrive have been ascribed to *chloride deficiency* in breast milk [10] or in artificial feeds [8]. The symptoms include poor appetite and weight gain, with hypokalaemic metabolic acidosis.

A bottle-fed baby may be underfed either because of starvation, or because of errors in the constitution of the feeds. When investigating the method of feeding, one asks how much milk powder and water the mother is putting into each feed, and how many feeds she is giving per day. It is futile to accept a mother's statement that she is giving the baby 'five oz of Cow & Gate' at each feed. She may be making the feed up too dilute, so that the baby is underfed. Sometimes mothers wrongly ascribe their baby's loose stools, wind or other symptoms to *overfeeding* and therefore reduce the feeds and cause underfeeding. After early infancy, underfeeding may be due to parental food fads or ignorance.

When a baby is seriously underweight, one commonly finds that the quantity which the mother states that she is giving is inadequate, but that when the baby is admitted to the ward he is ravenously hungry, has a far bigger than average weight gain, and has been half starved. I have known such babies gain as much as 25 oz a week (709 g) when given as much as they want. *It is important to accept with scepticism the mother's story of the quantity given. When a child is failing to thrive, and no obvious cause can be found, one should suspect underfeeding, whatever the mother says.* This must be eliminated before one embarks on complex laboratory investigations.

An important cause of defective intake of food is *emotional deprivation*. One often sees older babies who refuse to gain weight in hospital, in the absence of evidence of disease, but gain weight normally when the mother is admitted to the hospital to be with the child, or when she takes him home. An important cause of failure to thrive is excessive crying. There are many possible causes of this (p. 292). Continual crying not only uses up energy, but also leads to loss of fluid through the lungs and so to defective weight gain. It may tire the baby, so that when food is offered he does not take it well.

*Child abuse* (non-accidental injury) is an example of severe emotional deprivation. It may take the form of emotional cruelty, deliberate starvation, the deprivation of fluid, physical trauma (broken bones, bruises, subdural effusion, the infliction of burns, injury to the mouth or viscera), sexual abuse, or the administration of poison, salt or overdose of drugs. As child abuse is almost always denied by the parents, diagnosis can be difficult. Factors which should arouse suspicion are repeated injuries, complaints about the child's bad behaviour or constant crying, delay in seeking advice, an implausible story which does not fit the clinical findings, previous injury, a history that a parent suffered abuse in childhood, a history of injury to siblings, burns or poisonings, frequent attendances at the hospital, or failure to thrive. Risk factors include low birth weight, nursing in an intensive care unit causing separation of mother and baby, poverty, unemployment, bad social conditions, or maternal illness. Any fracture under the age of 2 years should arouse the suspicion of child abuse. Features suggestive of non-accidental injury include multiple fractures, fractures of ribs, spiral or oblique fractures of long bones with subperiosteal new bone [35]. Other suggestive signs include bruises around the neck or in places not normally involved in the usual falls, small round cigarette burns, a torn alveolar frenum, haemorrhages in the optic fundus, bruises of different ages and evidence of old fractures as indicted by a skeletal survey. Radiological changes may indicate that the date of the fracture could not correspond with the mother's story. Emotional deprivation may cause functional pituitary growth hormone deficiency with poly-dipsia, abdominal distension and dwarfism [22]. It is sometimes found that a child whose failure to thrive was due to parental neglect or cruelty may also fail to progress satisfactorily in hospital, but promptly improves when placed in a good loving foster home.

*Infection.* Acute infections, even when frequent, do not usually cause defective weight gain, because children have a compensatory increase of appetite after a febrile illness and make up lost ground, but a severe chronic infection such as bronchiectasis or urinary tract infection may well cause defective weight gain.

*Congenital cytomegalovirus or toxoplasma infection* may lead to failure to thrive. There may he hepatosplenomegaly and purpura with retinal changes. Chronic malaria, ankylostomiasis or tuberculosis in developing countries may cause defective growth partly because of associated defective intake.

*Synthetic diets.* Failure to thrive may be related to synthetic diets [18] for phenylketonuria, galactosaemia or hypercalcaemia. Sores may develop around the external nares, lips, at the outer canthus of the eyes, or on the buttocks. These children respond immediately to Ketovite tablets and syrup. A frequent cause of failure to thrive, especially in the case of immigrant children, is *'fad' or vegetarian diets.*

*Protein calorie malnutrition,* manifestations of which are often precipitated by infection, is of importance in many developing countries.

## Defective absorption

When considering the cause of failure to thrive due to defective absorption, we must think of defective absorption of fat, carbohydrate and protein.

### Defective absorption of fat (steatorrhoea)

There are many causes of steatorrhoea. In an analysis of 266 cases of steatorrhoea in children, Anderson & Burke [1] found that 52 per cent were due to cystic fibrosis, 35 per cent to coeliac disease, and 13 per cent to other causes, of which the main ones were giardiasis, chronic intestinal infection, anomalies of the alimentary tract, and certain diseases of the liver and pancreas.

The commonest cause of steatorrhoea is *cystic fibrosis*. It occurs in approximately one in every 2400 children. There are four main modes of presentation—meconium ileus in the newborn baby, failure to thrive, steatorrhoea, and chronic or recurrent chest disease. Meconium ileus (p. 72) presents as intestinal obstruction in the newborn. Failure to thrive is seen at any age in young children from infancy onwards. Bulky, offensive or loose stools may be noticed by the mother at any stage, but this is relatively unusual. In many cases of coeliac disease or cystic fibrosis, the mother has not noticed anything unusual about the stools. One should always investigate for cystic fibrosis when a child has asthma, chronic wheezing, chronic pulmonary infection such as bronchiectasis or persistent radiological abnormality in the lung such as pulmonary collapse. Two other signs may draw attention to the possibility of cystic fibrosis—unexplained generalized oedema or prolapse of the rectum: there are other causes of both of these conditions, but both are sometimes early features of steatorrhoea and in particular cystic fibrosis. Other features sometimes found are cirrhosis of the liver, portal hypertension, gastro-oesophageal reflux, nasal polypi, pancreatitis, hypoprothrombinaemia, recurrent arthritis, hypertrophic pulmonary osteoarthropathy, haemoptysis, sinus infection, abdominal pain and later development of diabetes. Sterility in males is usual. Delayed puberty may occur. Cystic fibrosis is sometimes accompanied by coeliac disease [7], asthma, diabetes and aspergillosis.

*Coeliac disease* (gluten enteropathy) is the second most common cause of steatorrhoea. The majority of cases are due to sensitivity to gluten, but a few may be confused with milk allergy. There may be associated carbohydrate intolerance which confuses the diagnosis because it may be responsible for an unsatisfactory response to exclusion of gluten. There is a genetic factor, and there may be a familial association between coeliac disease and ulcerative colitis [19].

The symptoms of coeliac disease commence when cereals are introduced to the diet, so that the age of onset is variable. The usual initial symptom is vomiting. Other symptoms are undue irritability, sometimes constipation, loss of appetite and failure to thrive. In any advanced case there is wasting of the buttocks with a protuberant abdomen (as in other forms of steatorrhoea). The appetite in coeliac disease tends to be poor, while that in cystic fibrosis tends to be unusually good, but in the absence of chronic pulmonary infection one cannot distinguish the two conditions on clinial grounds. It is most important that the diagnosis should be properly established by laboratory means: it is bad practice to rely on the response to treatment, because once one has embarked on a special diet it is difficult to discontinue it because of fear of harming the baby. In severe cases 6 to 8 weeks may elapse before improvement occurs.

Steatorrhoea may result from *chronic intestinal infection,* particularly *giardiasis* or *salmonella.* Though rare in England, giardiasis is common in many developing countries. Some feel that giardiasis is secondary to other conditions, and not the principal cause of the steatorrhoea.

Certain *congenital anomalies of the alimentary tract* may cause steatorrhoea. They include *malrotation, stenosis, gastrocolic fistula, intestinal lymphangiectasia and intestinal reduplication* [16]. *Crohn's disease* (regional ileitis) may cause failure to thrive due to defective absorption of protein and fat. There may be no other symptom or sign pointing to that condition. The early symptoms may be entirely non-specific [2]; they include lethargy, abdominal pain, loss of weight, defective physical growth and then perhaps diarrhoea. Common symptoms are abdominal pain, fever, diarrhoea, weight loss or defective growth. Less common are arthritis, anorectal disease including fistula or erythema nodosum [21].

Steatorrhoea may be associated with *pancreatic insufficiency and chronic neutropenia.*

Steatorrhoea may be found in cases of *carbohydrate intolerance, protein-losing enteropathy, tuberculosis of mesentery, biliary atresia, cirrhosis of the liver and ulcerative colitis.* It is found in the rare *abetalipoproteinaemia* in which there is ataxia, absence of betalipo-proteins in the serum, reduced serum lipoids and a crenated appearance of the red cells (acanthocytosis). Retinal changes occur in the later stages. Steatorrhoea may occur in *vitamin E deficiency* (p. 208). It has been ascribed to *food allergy* [23]. There is a rare form of familial steatorrhoea with mental retardation and *calcification of the basal ganglia* [3]. A cause which is rare in childhood is *Whipple's disease,* in which there is steatorrhoea, polyarthralgia, fever, weight loss and lymphadenopathy. Steatorrhoea may be a feature of *acquired agamma-globulinaemia.*

Steatorrhoea may result from the administration of certain *drugs*—kanamycin, mercaptopurine, methotrexate, neomycin and PAS.

*Carbohydrate intolerance and malabsorption*

*Carbohydrate intolerance* may be primary (genetic) or secondary to coeliac disease, cystic fibrosis, sprue, gastro-enteritis or giardiasis. It should be seriously considered whenever one is faced with the problem of a child with failure to thrive and loose stools. The stools are tested for reducing substances by the Clinitest, and if that is positive, the sugar is identified by paper chromatography. Only the fluid part of freshly collected stools should be tested, and the child should have been on a normal diet.

*Lactose intolerance* presents usually with diarrhoea, vomiting, lactosuria and failure to thrive. Symptoms begin as soon as the baby is put to the breast. The child promptly improves when lactose is excluded from the diet.

In *alactasia* there is diarrhoea due to unabsorbed disaccharides, because of defective absorption of lactose. The child improves when sucrose is given and lactose is excluded. The Clinitest on the stools is positive.

*Maltose or sucrose intolerance* are rather less common. Diarrhoea and failure to thrive are the usual features.

In *fructosaemia and fructose intolerance* there is vomiting, failure to thrive, lassitude, perspiration, trembling, palpitation and fits, with hepatic enlargement and sometimes jaundice. Some of the symptoms are the result of hypoglycaemia. The symptoms begin when the child eats sugar, sweets, fruit, honey or certain vegetables. There are no symptoms when the baby is breast feeding. There may be albumin and fructose in the urine and abnormal aminoaciduria. There may be a particular aversion to sweet food. Older children experience vomiting and abdominal pain 20 to 30 min after eating sugar-containing substances. There is usually no diarrhoea. Fits on eating sugar-containing foods suggest the diagnosis. The Clinitest on the stools is positive.

*Amylase deficiency* is associated with diarrhoea.

*Galactosaemia* usually presents in the newborn baby with vomiting, purpura, weight loss and jaundice with hepatic enlargement as soon as he receives breast milk. Cataracts and mental deficiency soon develop. Galactose is found in the urine. The Clinitest or Benedict test is positive. The Clinistix may also be positive, because the damaged renal tubule allows glucose to leak through.

Udani *et al.* [31] described a high calorie form of malnutrition due to *carbohydrate deficiency*: there was polyuria, failure to thrive, abdominal distension, irritability, constipation, and an excessive appetite. The polyuria was thought to be due to the high solute load.

## Defective protein absorption

This may be due to chronic diarrhoea from any cause, such as ulcerative colitis. It may be due to deficiency of trypsinogen; this presents with oedema due to hypoproteinaemia. Enterokinase deficiency is associated with hypoproteinaemia and oedema.

The so-called exudative enteropathy is a condition in which there is generalized oedema due to protein loss in the stools. It may result from ulcerative colitis, regional ileitis or other conditions.

Silverman, Roy & Cozzetto [28] listed 21 causes of protein-losing enteropathy in their list of 70 diseases causing malabsorption. I have purposely listed only a few.

## Allergy to cow's milk or soya

Otherwise unexplained failure to thrive may be due to *allergy to cow's milk or soya* [9, 17, 23, 34]. Symptoms ascribed to food allergy include rashes, angioneurotic oedema, anaphylaxis; respiratory symptoms—rhinitis, wheezing, stridor; unexplained crying and colic; alimentary symptoms—abdominal pain or distension, constipation, vomiting, diarrhoea, steatorrhoea, colitis and melaena [15]; migraine (p. 101), failure to thrive and over-activity. Occult bleeding from the bowel may result from pasteurized or other heat-treated cow's milk given to babies under the age of about 4 months [6]. Sometimes the presenting symptom is a failure to recover fully after gastro-enteritis. There may be secondary lactose intolerance. The clinical diagnosis may be confused by additional sensitivity to egg or soya, and by the fact that the symptoms may develop 24 hrs or more after challenge [17].

*Hirschsprung's disease*

Defective absorption and failure to thrive may result from Hirschsprung's disease. There will be a history of severe constipation from birth, often with abdominal distension, and a story that no stool was passed in the first 24 to 36 hrs. On the other hand the symptom of constipation may not be impressive, and the diagnosis may be missed because of attacks of severe diarrhoea and vomiting. These suggest enterocolitis, when in fact the cause is Hirschsprung's disease. On rectal examination it is found that the rectum is empty. Swenson, Sherman & Fisher [29] analysed 501 cases. Ninety-four per cent had not passed meconium in the first 24 hrs; 94 per cent were constipated; 87 per cent had abdominal distension; 64 per cent had vomited; 26 per cent had diarrhoea; 3 per cent presented with perforation in the newborn period. In a study of 26 infants with Hirschsprung's disease [14], 21 were male; 4 had Down's syndrome and 5 had congenital heart disease or other anomalies. Fifteen presented with vomiting, 9 of these with biliary vomiting. Eleven had passed meconium within 24 hrs and 15 within 48 hrs. It can present later than the newborn period [4].

A closely similar condition, neuronal intestinal dysplasia, presenting with similar symptoms, and diagnosed only by enzyme and histological examination of a biopsy specimen from the rectosigmoid, was described by Schärli & Meier-Ruge [25].

**Increased loss of nutriments and fluid**

Excess loss of fluid in perspiration may result from *over-clothing* or an *excessively hot environment*. It leads to constipation and failure to gain weight adequately. In hot climates I have seen infants who were given quantities of fluid suitable for the British climate, but unsuitable for the country in question. They were being given 2½ oz per lb (150 ml per kg) per day, which is the usual quantity in England, but insufficient in a country such as Egypt, where there is a greater fluid loss through perspiration. The loss of fluid through the lungs resulting from excessive crying has already been mentioned.

Chronic vomiting or diarrhoea will prevent an adequate weight gain. A cause which is readily missed is *oesophageal reflux*, causing vomiting.

## Some metabolic causes of failure to thrive (rare)

When a baby or toddler who is failing to thrive in spite of adequate food intake is found to be grossly constipated, one should think of one of the conditions associated with polyuria, notably renal acidosis, hypercalcaemia and, particularly in a boy, nephrogenic diabetes insipidus.

*Renal tubular acidosis* is an uncommon but important condition of infancy. It is important because appropriate treatment will enable the baby to gain weight normally, and failure to diagnose it is likely to lead to the child's death. It is manifested by vomiting and failure to thrive, often with polyuria. It is due to failure of the renal tubules to reabsorb bicarbonate.

*Idiopathic hypercalcaemia* presents with similar symptoms. There is polyuria with resulting constipation. In severe cases there is a characteristic facies and a systolic cardiac murmur. The diagnosis is made by estimation of the serum calcium, though this level usually falls to normal after infancy. Proper treatment may prevent mental deterioration and should enable the child to thrive normally.

*Nephrogenic diabetes insipidus* is another condition with symptoms like those of renal acidosis. Tests are needed to distinguish it from diabetes insipidus due to pituitary deficiency, and investigation in hospital is essential.

*Adrenocortical hyperplasia* with salt loss may cause vomiting, diarrhoea and failure to thrive. The diagnosis would be suggested when a girl is found to have a large clitoris or a boy has a large penis—though the enlargement of the penis may not be obvious. The presence of hypospadias in an infant who is not thriving would suggest the likelihood that the child is a girl with virilization due to adrenocortical hyperplasia. Pigmentation of the nipples and scrotum is a useful sign in affected boys. The buccal smear should establish the nuclear sex. It is urgent to make the diagnosis, for many affected babies die in early infancy without the diagnosis being made, whereas they would have survived with proper treatment.

*Hypophosphatasia.* Children with this rare condition fail to thrive, have rickets, other bone deficiencies, and sometimes vomiting, constipation and convulsions.

In the *De Toni–Fanconi syndrome* there may be polyuria, abnormal aminoaciduria, glycosuria and rickets.

*Conn's syndrome* consists of polyuria, polydipsia, alkalosis, hypertension, hypokalaemia, albuminuria and low specific gravity urine.

*Bartter's syndrome* consists of polyuria, polydipsia, alkalosis, weakness, hyperaldosteronism, short stature and a craving for salt.

*Cystinosis* is associated with polyuria, polydipsia, defects in growth, photophobia and constipation.

*Wolman's syndrome* is an autosomal recessive cholesterol storage disease, manifested by abdominal distension, hepatosplenomegaly, diarrhoea, vomiting, anaemia, mental subnormality, jaundice, and low-grade fever. The diagnosis may be established by bone marrow examination. There may be calcification of the adrenals. Death usually occurs in the first year.

Other causes are *organic acidurias, storage diseases* and *Leigh's syndrome* (subacute necrotizing encephalomyelopathy), in which there are failure to thrive, vomiting, ptosis, extra-ocular palsies, ataxia and progressive deterioration. For *Di George syndrome*, see p. 237.

## Organ disease involving the brain, heart, chest, kidney, liver or pancreas

A variety of diseases of the brain, heart, chest, kidney, liver and pancreas may be responsible for the failure of the infant to thrive. *Certain brain diseases*, other than mental deficiency, are associated with defective physical growth. *Mentally handicapped children*, especially when they also have cerebral palsy, are commonly malnourished, partly because they are unable to chew until much later than a normal child. As a result they have to be fed on semi-liquid feeds, and defective intake of necessary foodstuffs may result. It is easy to miss the age at which they learn to chew, and if they are not given solids at the time when they have recently learnt to chew, they will be diffident about taking them later, refusing them or vomiting. This depends on the so-called 'sensitive' or 'critical' period [12]. Defective physical growth in mentally handicapped children may be due to the underlying brain defect.

A *craniopharyngeal cyst* or *craniopharyngioma* may cause defective physical growth. The usual presenting symptom is that of increased intracranial pressure; but other cases present as visual disturbance, defective physical growth or diabetes insipidus. Unilateral failing vision is an important presentation; unilateral optic atrophy or papilloedema would suggest the diagnosis. I have seen children with craniopharyngioma whose only symptom was defective weight gain.

Other *neoplasms in the region of the hypothalamus and third ventricle, including the diencephalic syndrome,* are associated with failure to thrive. Affected children are emaciated, notably alert, and have a normal or increased appetite. The onset is usually in the first year. Growth is at first accelerated, but loss of weight then follows. There may be signs of autonomic disturbance, such as profuse sweating, and there may be nystagmus. There are usually no abnormal neurological signs and there is no papilloedema. The important feature in many is a high CSF protein.

A *chronic subdural effusion* may be associated with failure to thrive. This could be explained by vomiting, reduced appetite or non-accidental injury.

*Congenital heart disease,* such as a patent ductus arteriosus, atrial or ventricular septal defect, or Fallot's tetralogy, is liable to be associated with stunting of growth. The reasons for this are not altogether clear. I have seen several examples of severe food refusal resulting from food forcing, which in turn resulted from the parents' anxiety about slow weight gain and smallness of size. It is important that the cause of the stunting of growth should be recognized, partly because it may be remedied surgically, and partly because the parents may then avoid food forcing.

*Bronchiectasis, asthma and other chronic pulmonary conditions* are likely to be associated with defective weight gain. Most children with severe asthma are small in height and below the average weight. This is aggravated by prolonged corticosteroid treatment. Tuberculosis in England is now a rare cause of failure to thrive.

*Renal insufficiency* should be remembered when an infant or child is not thriving. It may be due to renal dysplasia, posterior urethral valves, polycystic kidneys, hydronephrosis or chronic pyelo-nephritis. The importance of the specific gravity is commonly forgotten. A fixed low specific gravity suggests renal insufficiency or other cause of polyuria. The blood pressure should be recorded.

It should not be difficult to diagnose *cirrhosis of the liver,* a rare cause of failure to thrive. One cause of cirrhosis of the liver is cystic fibrosis. Other causes include hepatolenticular degeneration, diagnosed largely by the estimation of serum copper oxidase, tyrosinosis, which is associated with renal tubular defects and rickets, and alpha-1-antitrypsin deficiency.

## Miscellaneous conditions

A variety of *chromosomal abnormalities* and the rubella syndrome are associated with failure to thrive. The *fetal alcohol syndrome* [13, 36], due to maternal alcoholism in pregnancy, is characterized by a typical facies, with a flat bridge of nose, an upturned nose, maxillary hypoplasia, prominent forehead, short small palpebral fissures, small eyes, facial hirsutism, sometimes cleft palate, restricted joint movements, congenital heart disease, tremors and mental subnormality, with defective physical growth.

Acquired immune deficiency syndrome (AIDS) due to the human immunodeficiency virus (HIV) in children [24, 26, 27, 32], occurring particularly in children of drug addicts and in those with haemophilia, is characterized by low birth weight (in congenital cases), chronic diarrhoea, eczema, alopecia, failure to thrive, lymphadenopathy, hepatosplenomegaly, interstitial pneumonia, stomatitis, candida and repeated infections, delayed motor and mental development, parotitis and thrombocytopenia. There may be progressive deterioration alone or in association with neurological signs including spasticity.

## Conclusion

Failure to thrive is a common problem, and it is often difficult to decide whether full investigation is required. Many children are subjected to extensive and costly special investigations, which clinical judgement, simple clinical observation and a little thought would have made unnecessary.

The doctor will be guided by the child's weight progress on the centile chart. Provided that the family doctor has satisfied himself that the unduly small infant or small child is not small merely because he takes after one of his parents, or because he was an unusually small baby at birth, and that the problem is not merely one of defective intake, he should have the problem investigated by an expert. The hospital doctor will be guided by the child's progress in hospital. The problem of failure to thrive is one of the most difficult and yet one of the most common problems facing the paediatric physician. It is important to make the diagnosis in order that the appropriate treatment can be given. Failure to do so may mean that the child will not survive or that his growth will remain permanently defective.

## References

1 Anderson C, Burke V. *Paediatric gastroenterology.* Oxford: Blackwell Scientific Publications, 1975.
2 Chong SKF, Bartram C, Campbell CA *et al.* Chronic inflammatory bowel disease in childhood. *Br Med J* 1982; **1:** 101.
3 Cockel R, Hill EE, Rushton DI, Smith B, Hawkins CF. Familial steatorrhoea with calcification of the basal ganglia and mental retardation. *QJ Med* 1973; **42:** 441.
4 Doig CM. Childhood constipation and late-presenting Hirschsprung's disease. *J Roy Soc Med* 1984; **73** (suppl. 3): 3.
5 Eid EE. A follow up study of physical growth following failure to thrive with special reference to a critical period in the first year of life. *Acta Paediatr Scand* 1971; **60:** 39.
6 Fomon SJ, Ziegler EE, Nelson SE, Edwards BB. Cow's milk feeding in infancy, gastrointestinal blood loss and iron nutritional status. *J Pediatr* 1981; **98:** 540.
7 Goodchild MC, Nelson R, Anderson CM. Cystic fibrosis and coeliac disease. *Arch Dis Child* 1973; **48:** 684 (see also p. 692).
8 Grossman H, Duggan E, McCammon S, Welchert E, Hellerstein S. The dietary chloride deficiency syndrome. *Pediatrics* 1980; **66:** 366.
9 Hill DJ, Davidson GP, Cameron DJS, Barnes GL. The spectrum of cow's milk allergy in childhood. *Acta Paediatr Scand* 1979; **68:** 847.
10 Hill ID, Bowie MD. Chloride deficiency syndrome due to chloride deficiency breast milk. *Arch Dis Child* 1983; **58:** 224.
11 Illingworth RS. *The normal child.* London: Churchill Livingstone, 9th edn, 1987.
12 Illingworth RS, Lister J. The critical or sensitive period with special reference to certain feeding problems in infants and children. *J Pediatr* 1964; **65:** 839.
13 Iosub S, Fuchs M, Bingol N, Gromisch DS. Fetal alcohol syndrome revisited. *Pediatrics* 1981; **68:** 475.
14 Klein MD, Coran AG, Wesley JR, Drongowski RA. Hirschsprung's disease in the newborn. *J Pediatr Surg* 1984; **19:** 370.
15 *Lancet.* Leading article. Infantile bloody diarrhoea and cow's milk allergy. 1984; **1:** 1158.
16 Leslie JWM, Matheson WJ. Failure to thrive in early infancy due to abnormalities of rotation of the mid gut. *Clin Pediatr Phila* 1965; **4:** 681.
17 McCarty EP, Frick OL. Food sensitivity: keys to diagnosis. *J Pediatr* 1983; **102:** 645.

18  Mann TP, Wilson M, Clayton BE. A deficiency state arising in infants on synthetic foods. *Arch Dis Child* 1965; **40**: 364.
19  Mayberry JF, Smart HL, Toghill PJ. Familial association between coeliac disease and ulcerative colitis. *J Roy Soc Med* 1986; **79**: 204.
20  Mitchell WG, Gorrell RW, Greenberg RA. Failure to thrive: a study in a primary care setting. *Pediatrics* 1980; **65**: 971.
21  O'Donoghue DP, Dawson AM. Crohn's disease in childhood. *Arch Dis Child* 1977; **52**: 613.
22  Raynes PHW, Rudd BT. Emotional deprivation in three siblings associated with functional pituitary growth hormone deficiency. *Australian Paediatr J* 1973; **9**: 79.
23  Royal College of Physicians and British Nutrition Foundation. Food intolerance and food aversion. *J Roy Coll Phys* 1984; **18**: 83.
24  Rubinstein A. Acquired immunodeficiency syndrome in infants. *Am J Dis Child* 1983; **137**: 825.
25  Schärli AF, Meier-Ruge W. Localised and disseminated forms of neuronal intestinal dysplasia mimicking Hirschsprung's disease. *J Pediatr Surg* 1981; **16**: 164.
26  Scott GB, Buck BE, Leterman JG, *et al.* Acquired immunodeficiency syndrome in infants. *New Engl J Med* 1984; **310**: 76.
27  Shannon AM, Ammann AJ. Acquired immune deficiency syndrome in childhood. *J Pediatr* 1985; **106**: 332.
28  Silverman A, Roy CC, Cozzetto FJ. *Pediatric clinical gastroenterology*. St Louis: Mosby, 1971.
29  Swenson O, Sherman JO, Fisher JH. Diagnosis of congenital megacolon. An analysis of 501 patients. *J Pediatr Surg* 1973; **8**: 587.
30  Tanner JM, Whitehouse RH, Takaishi M. Standard from birth to maturity for height, weight, height velocity and weight velocity. *Arch Dis Child* 1966; **41**: 613.
31  Udani PM, Parekh UC, Shah BP, *et al.* Carbohydrate malnutrition (carbo-hydrate deprivation syndrome). *Indian Pediatrics* 1972; **9**: 311.
32  Ultmann MH, Belman AL, Ruff HA, *et al.* Developmental abnormalities in infants and children with acquired immune deficiency syndrome (AIDS) and AIDS related complex. *Dev Med Child Neurol* 1985; **27**: 563.
33  Umansky R, Hauck AJ. Factors in growth of children and patent ductus arteriosus. *Pediatrics* 1962; **30**: 540.
34  Walker-Smith JA. Food allergy and bowel disease. *J Roy Soc Med* 1985; **78**: 3.
35  Worlock P, Stower M, Barbor P. Pattern of fractures in accidental and non-accidental injury in children; a comparative study. *Br Med J* 1986; **2**: 100.
36  Wright JT, Barrison IG, Lewis IG, *et al.* Alcohol consumption, pregnancy and low birth weight. *Lancet* 1983; **1**: 663. Leading article 683.

# Shortness of Stature

Short stature can be defined as a height below the third centile on the Tanner Whitehouse Chart [12, 16]. Most of the causes of 'failure to thrive', reviewed in the previous section, are relevant to shortness of stature. The subject has been reviewed by Langer [7], who listed 112 causes, Smith [13], Schaff-Blass and colleagues [10] and Smail [12].

Without attempting to give a complete list, I have divided the causes as follows:

Prenatal

    Genetic and familial

    Low birth weight, especially small for dates

    Intrauterine growth retardation

    Drugs in pregnancy: nicotine, alcohol, other addictions

    Chromosome defects. Turner. Ullrich Noonan. Down's syndrome

    Dysmorphic and other rare syndromes. Bone dysplasias. Prader–Willi, Bloom, Rubenstein–Taybi, Rothmund Thomson, Schwartz–Jampel

    Endocrine—pituitary dysfunction, growth hormone deficiency, Aarskog and Laron syndrome, craniopharyngioma. Hypothyroidism. Diabetes. Cushing's syndrome. Pseudohypoparathyroidism

    Metabolic diseases—phenylketonuria (unsatisfactorily controlled). Mucopolysaccharidoses. Storage diseases.

Postnatal

    Socioeconomic. Malnutrition

    Chronic disease—heart, chest, kidney, pancreas, gastro-intestinal tract. Chronic infection. Coeliac disease

    Obesity (later stages)

    Trauma to epiphyses

    Drugs—corticosteroids, neurostimulants

Unusual smallness of stature is not usually due to organic disease. The commonest causes are *genetic*, including familial, *low birth weight* or *socio-economic factors*. In a Newcastle study [9], of 82 children whose height was below the third centile, 84 per cent had no organic disease. Factors included low birth weight, smallness of parents, low parental IQ and social class and large size of family. A third had suffered *emotional deprivation*. *Child abuse* is an important cause. In developing countries *malnutrition and infection* are important factors. A *low birth weight* is a major cause. Numerous studies [4, 5] have shown that the smaller the child is at birth, especially if he were small for dates, the smaller he is likely to be in childhood and adolescence. All the causes of intra-uterine growth retardation are relevant [4].

*Alcohol, benzodiazepines, nicotine and other drugs of addiction* may cause defective growth *in utero* and in later childhood, sometimes in association with congenital heart disease or other anomalies [14].

### Chromosomal and dismorphic conditions

*Turner's syndrome* in girls is diagnosed in infancy by the finding of oedema of the lower limbs, short length, often with webbing of the neck, pigmented naevi, coarctation of the aorta, a low hair-line at the back of the neck, cubitus valgus and a short fourth metacarpal. The child remains small in height: there may be osteoporosis, and there is a risk of gonadal neoplasm [1]. There is failure of development of secondary sexual characteristics. It is easy to diagnose cubitus valgus when it is non-existent. Usually, when the upper arms are fully extended and touching, the forearms cannot without difficulty be brought parallel, whereas they can in Turner's syndrome (and some normal people). The short fourth metacarpal is demonstrated by placing a ruler or firm card across the outer knuckles: normally the ruler will not touch all three knuckles. If there is a short fourth metacarpal, the card touches the third and fifth metacarpals, acting as a bridge over the fourth. There are variants of Turner's syndrome which in the older child are less easy to diagnose; the height may be normal, apart from the absence of breast enlargement. When a young girl is unusually small in height and there is no obvious disease, Turner's syndrome is a possibility to be considered even if the mother is also unusually small: nevertheless, the most likely explanation of a girl's unusually small height, when the mother is small, is merely the familial factor.

The *Ulrich–Noonan syndrome* closely resembles Turner's syndrome. It is an autosomal dominant condition, with congenital heart disease, short stature, undescended testes, a low hair-line, cubitus valgus, webbing of the neck, naevi, lymphoedema and facial anomalies. Whereas in Turner's syndrome the commonest cardio-vascular defect is coarctation of the aorta, in the Noonan syndrome pulmonary stenosis with or without an atrial septal defect is more common. Chromosomal findings are normal.

### Dysmorphic and other rare syndromes

The *Prader–Willi syndrome* [8, 18] is diagnosed by a characteristic facies, low birth weight, often breech delivery, sucking difficulties in early infancy, undescended testes, hypoplastic scrotum or labia, hypogonadism, hypotonia in the early months, with the development of excessive appetite and obesity in the second or third year. There is smallness of hands and feet, dwarfism, mental subnormality and sometimes areflexia. There may be diabetes in later years [15]. Chromosomal changes have been described in several cases [8]; they include deletion of the long arm of chromosome 15.

In the *Rubenstein–Taybi syndrome* [2], there are broad thumbs and toes, mental subnormality, anti-mongoloid slant of eyes, unde-scended testes and small stature. In the rare *Schwartz–Jampel syndrome* (p. 41) there is dwarfism and muscle stiffness [11], some-times with a risk of hyperpyrexia.

For three rare syndromes which include dwarfism and telangiec-tasia (Bloom, Cockayne, Rothmund–Thomson), see p. 364.

There are many *chondrodystrophies*, mostly short-limbed, associ-ated with dwarfism. Warkany's book [17] lists 72 of them. They include various forms of *rickets, achondroplasia* and *punctate epi-physeal dysplasia. Achondroplasia* should be readily diagnosed by the shortness of the humerus and femur, with a large head and depressed bridge of nose. When the child puts his hands down by his side, they do not reach as far as those of a normal child. There are several rare allied conditions. One is *punctate epiphyseal dysplasia*, commonly due to the mother taking warfarin during pregnancy; there is a cataract, the appearance of achondroplasia, limited extension of some joints and characteristic X-ray changes.

### Endocrine disorders

*Hypopituitarism* is rare in children. The child is usually dwarfed but often fat. An X-ray of the skull may show evidence of a craniopharyngioma. *Growth hormone deficiency* may be genetic or due to a craniopharyngioma, or damage to the hypothalamus or emotional deprivation. Isolated growth hormone deficiency occurs in *Aarskog's syndrome* [6] of short stature, genital anomalies and unusual facies sometimes with hypertelorism. *Laron's syndrome* resembles hypopituitarism. There is defective growth in height, which does not respond to human growth hormone.

A child with *thyroid deficiency* is small due to delayed skeletal maturation. He retains the infantile proportions of a larger upper than lower segment (pubis to heel). One should think of this condition when a child stops growing before puberty. When an older child develops thyroid deficiency the facies may not be characteristic at least for several months.

*Pseudo-hypoparathyroidism* is a rare condition in which there is shortness of stature, short fingers and often mental subnormality or fits. The middle finger may be shorter than the index finger.

For *Cushing's syndromes*, see pp. 30 and 343.

Growth delay is said sometimes to precede the usual manifestations of *diabetes mellitus* [3]. It also occurs when control of diabetes is unsatisfactory. Growth delay may be an early manifestation of coeliac disease.

*Obesity.* The obese child is normally tall for his age at first, because of secondary adrenocortical over-activity, but this is followed by premature closure of the epiphyses, so that the child is then small for his age. For obesity in the young child associated with smallness of stature, see p. 30.

*Other metabolic diseases.* Other metabolic diseases associated with small stature include *storage diseases, mucopolysaccharidoses,* and inadequately controlled phenylketonuria.

*Drugs.* Corticosteroid drugs taken over a long period of time cause severe stunting of growth. Neurostimulant drugs, notably methylphenidate or amphetamines, prescribed by some for the attention-deficit disorder, cause defective growth in height.

*Trauma* to the epiphyses by accident or surgery retards growth.

### References

1 Brook CGD. Turner syndrome. *Arch Dis Child* 1986; **61:** 305.
2 Gillies DRN, Roussounis SH. Rubenstein–Taybi syndrome. Further evidence of a genetic aetiology. *Dev Med Child Neurol* 1985; **27:** 751.

3 Hoskins PJ, Leslie RD, Pyke DA. Height at diagnosis of diabetes in children: a study of identical twins. *Brit Med J* 1985; **1**: 278.

4 Illingworth RS. *The normal child*. London: Churchill Livingstone, 9th edn, 1987.

5 Illsley R, Mitchell RG. *Low birthweight*. London: John Wiley, 1984.

6 Kodama M, Fujimoto S, Namikawa T, Matsuda I. Aarskog's syndrome. *Eur J Pediatr* 1981; **135**: 273.

7 Langer LO. Short stature. *Clin Pediatr Phila* 1969; **8**: 142.

8 Matsuo N, *et al*. Prader–Willi syndrome. *Acta Paediatr Japonica* 1981; **23**: 283.

9 Parkin JM. Short stature. *Br Med J* 1976; **2**: 1139.

10 Schaff-Blass E, Burstein S, Rosenfield DRL. Diagnosis and treatment of short stature. *J Pediatr* 1984; **104**: 801.

11 Seay AR, Ziter FA. Malignant hyperpyrexia in a patient with the Schwartz–Jampel syndrome. *J Pediatr* 1978; **93**: 83.

12 Smail P. Short stature. *Brit Med J* 1984; **2**: 1371.

13 Smith DW. Compendium on shortness of stature. *J Pediatr* 1976; **70**: 463–519.

14 Smithells RW, Smith IJ. Alcohol and the fetus. *Arch Dis Child* 1984; **59**: 1113.

15 Stephenson JBP. Prader–Willi syndrome: neonatal presentation and later development. *Dev Med Child Neurol* 1980; **22**: 792.

16 Tanner JM, Whitehouse RH, Takaishi M. Standard from birth to maturity for height, weight, height velocity and weight velocity. *Arch Dis Child* 1966; **41**: 613.

17 Warkany J. *Congenital malformations*. Chicago: Year Book Publications, 1971.

18 Zellweger HZ. Prader–Willi syndrome. *JAMA* 1984; **251**: 1835.

# Loss of Weight

When a child loses weight, other than in the course of an acute infection, one always feels concern. There are many possible causes, some of them serious.

In considering a mother's complaint that her child has lost weight, the first essential is to determine the evidence for her statement. It may be just that the mother is worried about him. Usually she has no figures to support her claim, but she may say that his clothes no longer fit because they are now too big for him. He may have been weighed

on different scales—perhaps one time in clothes and one time
without—and the mother had not thought of the possibility that the
scales were inaccurate. When the weight of a baby is to be compared
one day with that on another, it is essential that it should be recorded
on each occasion at the same time in relation to feeds. It would not be
profitable to weigh the baby before a feed one day and to compare this
with his weight after a feed on another day. He should always be
weighed unclothed.

Loss of weight, other than that during an ordinary acute infection
such as gastroenteritis, may be due to any of the following conditions,
amongst others:

> Overheating (in the case of a baby)
> Emotional causes. Child abuse. Anorexia nervosa. Self-
>    induced vomiting (older child)
> Conditions causing persistent vomiting
> Conditions causing diarrhoea
> Conditions associated with polyuria—diabetes mellitus,
>    diabetes insipidus, hypercalcaemia, renal
>    acidosis, renal failure
> Malabsorption
>    Fats, carbohydrates, protein
>    Hirschsprung's disease
>    Beriberi in the tropics
> Regional ileitis (Crohn's disease)
> Infections—urinary tract, tuberculosis, partial lung collapse,
>    other
> Asthma
> Drugs
> Rare—thyrotoxicosis, Addison's disease, malignant disease,
>    muscular dystrophy, lipodystrophy

In the section 'Failure to thrive' it was stated that an infant separated
from his moher may fail to gain weight or may lose weight. Worries
about home or school may cause an older child to lose weight. I have
seen anorexia nervosa in older children who have been teased on
account of obesity. Other children may lose weight because of
repeated *self-induced vomiting*. This may be associated with childhood
anorexia nervosa (p. 67).

*Persistent vomiting,* such as that due to hiatus hernia, or *persistent diarrhoea,* as in ulcerative colitis, may cause loss of weight. In *regional ileitis* (p. 11), failure to thrive may precede the development of diarrhoea.

A useful test which should be carried out when there is unexplained loss of weight is estimation of the specific gravity of the urine. A fixed low specific gravity would lead to investigation for one of the causes of *polyuria,* such as renal failure, nephrogenic diabetes insipidus or hypercalcaemia. The other causes of polyuria have been described in the section entitled 'Failure to thrive'.

Loss of weight may be due to *malabsorption,* including cystic fibrosis and coeliac disease. In the case of carbohydrate intolerance there is usually some diarrhoea.

A chronic *urinary tract infection* may present as loss of weight with lassitude. No examination of a child who has lost weight is complete without microscopy and culture of a clean specimen of urine. In the same way no examination would be complete without a tuberculin test unless the child has previously been given BCG.

Lassitude and loss of weight following what appeared to be a simple upper respiratory tract infection may be due to *partial collapse of the lung.* This may be suspected because of physical signs, but an X-ray is needed for confirmation.

Most children with *severe asthma* are underweight and some lose weight.

Certain *drugs* may cause loss of weight. When one institutes treatment for hypothyroidism loss of weight is common. Loss of weight may be a side effect of sulthiame or a stimulant drug given for over-activity.

*Thyrotoxicosis* and *Addison's disease* are rare in children, but the signs are the same as those in adults and can hardly be missed.

*Malignant disease,* whether cerebral, intrathoracic, intra-abdominal or elsewhere, may be the cause of loss of weight.

There is general muscle wasting in the later states of *muscular dystrophy.*

Generalized *lipodystrophy* is a rare cause of loss of weight [1]. The child will be well, and it can be seen that the appearance of emaciation and the weight loss are due to loss of fatty tissue only.

## Conclusion

Loss of weight is one of the important symptoms of childhood which demands full investigation, exept where the cause is obvious, such as gastroenteritis or diabetes mellitus. Hospital laboratory facilities are usually necessary for the elucidation of this symptom.

## Reference

1  Stern LM, Penfold JL, Jureidini K. Partial and total lipodystrophy. *Records of the Adelaide Children's Hospital* 1982; **3**: 48.

# Excessive Height

The following are the usual causes of excessive height:
> Familial
> Rare
>> Cerebral gigantism
>> Additional Y chromosome, Klinefelter's syndrome
>> Marfan's syndrome, homocystinuria
>> Weaver's syndrome, eosinophilic adenoma of the piturity

The commonest reason for excessive height is genetic, the child taking after one of the parents. Obese children are usually tall for their age (until the epiphyses fuse). Children with sexual precocity or adrenocortical hyperplasia are tall for their age.

*Cerebral gigantism* is rare [3]. It is associated with large size at birth, large head, hands and feet, excessive growth in the first four years, hypertelorism, an antimongoloid slant of the eyes, mental subnormality, fits and clumsiness. There is an association with Wilms' tumour, parotid or ovarian tumour and neurofibromatosis.

*Weaver's syndrome* is characterized by excessive growth, large ears, large hands and thumb, protruberant lower lip, hypertelorism, limited knee and elbow extension, kyphosis and mental subnormality. The X-ray shows height and bone age much in advance of chronological age [1, 2].

An *additional Y chromosome* is often associated with tallness.

*Marfan's syndrome* of arachnodactyly, dislocation of the lens and congenital heart disease is associated with excessive height.

### References

1  Ardinger HH, Hanson JW, Harrod M, *et al.* Further delineation of Weaver's syndrome. *J Pediatr* 1986; **108:** 228.
2  Dawood AA, Machado GT, Winship WS. Weaver's syndrome—primordial excessive growth. *South African Med J* 1985; **67:** 646.
3  Dodge PR, Holmes SJ, Sotos JF. Cerebral gigantism. *Develop Med Child Neurol* 1983; **25:** 248.

# Obesity

The commonest type of obesity is the so-called *simple obesity*—a misnomer, because the cause of obesity is far from simple. It is of multifactorial origin [2, 3]. In summary, the following are the most important factors:

*Imbalance between intake and output.* Most fat children have developed the sweet-eating habit, and are commonly seen to be eating potato crisps, sweets, lollipops and icecreams, and taking frequent sugar-containing drinks. In infancy they may have been given an excess of carbohydrates. The mother may regard the child as 'delicate' and plan his diet accordingly. The child follows the example of his parents and siblings in overeating. Socio-economic factors are relevant, for obesity is more common in the lower social classes, presumably due to the nature of the diet. The obesity of the Prader–Willi syndrome is largely due to the excessive eating. Children, like adults, tend to eat when bored, depressed or worried.

Reduced output of energy may be due to personality or to a physical handicap which causes relative inactivity—such as Duchenne muscular dystrophy, Werdnig–Hoffman syndrome, Down's syndrome or cerebral palsy of the spastic type.

*Genetic factors.* Apart from the common family history of obesity (only partly explained by the familial liking of good food and plenty of it), there are many hereditary diseases and syndromes associated with obesity. They include the *Laurence–Moon–Biedl syndrome* of polydactyly, retinitis pigmentosa, hypogonadism and mental subnormality; the *Prader–Willi syndrome* (p. 23): *Carpenter's syndrome* of acrocephaly, brachysyndactyly, polydactyly, mental subnormality and hypogonadism; the *Summitt syndrome* of acrocephaly, syndactyly and genu valgum; the *Cohen syndrome* of hypotonia, mental subnormality, hyperextensible joints and characteristic facies: and the Klinefelter (p. 346) and Turner (p. 340) syndromes.

*Endocrine and metabolic factors.* These include hypopituitarism (including *Frohlich's syndrome* of adipososkeletogenitodystrophy with glycosuria and polydipsia—so rare that I have never seen a case), Cushing's syndrome, insulinoma and pseudohypoparathyroidism. Some degree of obesity may occur in hypothyroidism. In *Cushing's syndrome* there is a characteristic distribution of fat, involving mainly the trunk (buffalo hump) and face, with relatively normal limbs, a plethoric face, deep voice, hypertrichosis, purple striae and often hypertension.

The other important metabolic factor is the metabolism of brown fat [1].

Most young fat children are tall in the early years, because of secondary adrenocortical activity, but the epiphyses fuse early, so that growth ceases and the child is then likely to be small for his age. If a young fat child is small for his age, one should consider the following rare conditions: Cushing's syndrome, Prader–Willi syndrome, Turner's syndrome, hypothyroidism, pseudohypoparathyroidism, or pituitary disease. Prolonged corticosteroid therapy may be a cause.

*Drugs* which increase the appetite and cause excessive weight gain include clonazepam and sodium valproate.

## References

1 Himms-Hagen J. Thermogenesis in brown adipose tissue as an energy buffer: implications for obesity. *N Engl J Med* 1984; **311:** 1549.

2 Illingworth RS. *The normal child.* London: Churchill Livingstone. 9th edn, 1987.

3 Taitz LS. *The obese child.* Oxford: Blackwell Scientific Publications, 1983.

# Unexplained Fever

In this section I shall refer to the problem of prolonged temperature elevation whose cause has not been determined by taking the history and examining the child—there being no abnormal physical signs apart from the fever and the appearance of illness. It is assumed that the physical examination has included the inspection of the eardrum for otitis media. The problem is a fairly common one, and it is one which may be extremely difficult to solve even with the fullest laboratory assistance.

Pyrexia of unknown origin should be defined as fever for at least 3 weeks, exceeding 38·3°C on several occasions, defying diagnosis after a week of intensive investigation [12]. Most cases prove to be atypical manifestations of common diseases rather than exotic conditions [5]. When faced with a child with pyrexia of unknown origin, common conditions are more likely than rare ones. Pizzo, Smith & Lovejoy [14] in a study of 100 such children in Boston, found that 52 per cent had infection, 20 per cent collagen vascular diseases and 6 per cent neoplasms. They found that in 18 per cent of their cases the temperature eventually settled to normal without a diagnosis having been made.

The following conditions should be considered, not necessarily in the order of likelihood:

    Normal variation

    Dehydration, overheating. Ectodermal dysplasia. Polyuria

    Malingering. Munchausen syndrome. Child abuse

    Infections

    Absorption of blood. The effect of trauma and surgical procedures. CNS haemorrhage

    Juvenile chronic arthritis (pre-arthritic stage)

    The effect of drugs and poisons

Rare causes:

    Collagen diseases

    Reticuloses and malignant disease

    Sarcoid

    Chronic granulomatous disease. Kawasaki disease

Alimentary conditions
   ulcerative colitis
   regional ileitis (p.11)
Liver disease
Subdural effusion
Agammaglobulinaemia. Hyperimmunoglobulinaemia
Familial dysautonomia

## Normal variations

Excitement or exertion may cause a slight rise of temperature. The temperature should not be taken immediately after a hot drink.

An occasional child has a slight persistent elevation of the temperature, or a daily elevation up to 38°C, without discoverable disease. The elevation of temperature is usually discovered after childhood infection. The child appears to be well and is symptom-free. Exhaustive tests fail to reveal any abnormality. Eventually the parent is advised to stop taking the temperature, and on follow-up the child remains well. These cases are worrying and have to be investigated and followed up with the greatest of care, for one never feels confident in concluding that there is no disease. One would be especially uncertain if the child, in addition to the elevation of temperature, does not feel well, is tired, or has an unsatisfactory weight gain. A good non-specific test which helps, and one which is easily carried out in the doctor's surgery, is the ESR. A normal figure does not exclude disease but it does make it less likely. A raised figure means that disease is almost certainly present and must be looked for.

A rectal temperature is commonly a little higher than that in the mouth. The rectal temperature depends on the depth to which the thermometer is inserted.

## The newborn

In the *newborn infant*, fever may be due to dehydration, overheating, phototherapy, absorption of blood, ectodermal dysplasia, familial dysautonomia or withdrawal from the mother's drug of addiction.

The so-called *dehydration fever of the newborn* consists of a sudden rise of temperature a day or two after birth. It is thought to be due to loss of fluid. The temperature rapidly settles when boiled water or other fluid is given.

## Dehydration after the newborn period

A baby may develop a rise of temperature if *overheated*. The most striking example of this occurred during a ward round. A baby was well when I saw him, but an hour later had a temperature of 41°C and was severely dehydrated, because his crib had been in contact with a radiator. The dehydration was such that he had to be given an immediate intravenous infusion.

Because of the absence of sweat glands, the temperature may rise in infants with *ectodermal dysplasia* when overheated. In the congenital anhydrotic type of ectodermal dysplasia, the child seems to be normal at birth. Later there is a dry skin, unexplained fever, sparse hair, delayed or absent dentition or widely-spaced incisors and conical canines, often with a saddle-shaped nose and frontal bossing. In the dominant hydrotic form there are dystrophic nails, hyperkeratosis of the palms and soles, absent or sparse hair at birth, and later hyper-trichosis and pigmentation.

A rise of temperature may result from other conditions causing dehydration, apart from the ordinary infections. These include *nephrogenic diabetes insipidus* and *idiopathic hypercalcaemia*.

## Malingering. Munchausen syndrome. Child abuse

A 10-year-old girl was referred from another hospital on account of high swinging fever of some weeks' duration. She had been exten-sively investigated and no cause had been found. The suddenness of the rise of temperature and the fact that the girl was well when the temperature was markedly raised suggested the diagnosis of malingering. When a nurse turned her back the girl rapidly rubbed the bulb of the thermometer with her bedclothes. Vigorous rubbing of the bulb of the thermometer will raise the mercury from 36 to 40°C in some 5 seconds. It takes longer to raise the temperature to that point by placing it in contact with the average hot water bottle. Vigorous shaking of the inverted thermometer may have a similar result. When in doubt, the urine temperature may be a guide to the diagnosis of malingering.

The Munchausen syndrome by proxy (perhaps correctly 'Münchhausen' syndrome) has been fully reviewed by Meadow [10]. He wrote that it should be considered when:

**1**   An illness is unexplained, prolonged and so extraordinary that it prompts experienced colleagues to remark that they 'have never seen anything like it before'.

**2**   Symptoms and signs are inappropriate and incongruous, or are present only when the mother is present.

**3**   Treatment is ineffective or poorly tolerated.

**4**   The child is alleged to be allergic to a great variety of foods and drugs.

**5**   Mothers are not as worried by the child's illness as the nurses and doctors.

**6**   Mothers are constantly with their ill child in hospital, and are happily at ease in the ward.

**7**   The family has experienced sudden infant deaths.

**8**   The family contains members alleged to have a serious incidence of medical disease.

**9**   The mother has herself had the Munchausen syndrome (true in 20 per cent of Meadow's cases).

The manifestations are protean. They include vomiting, convulsions, wheezing, haematuria, haematemesis and unexplained fever. Unexplained fever in a child having an intravenous infusion was traced to a mother introducing infective substances into the drip tube [3, 7]. Haematuria may be due to the mother adding blood to the child's urine [11]. Haematemesis can be due to a similar practice. I saw a child of 4 years who had been in hospital for a total of 18 months on account of 'haematemesis': the mother's story of coffee ground vomiting was found to be explained by the presence of cocoa in the so-called vomited material. 'Diabetes' may be due to the mother adding sugar to the urine. Warner & Hathaway [18] described 17 children with the syndrome, presenting as bizarre allergy. 'Unexplained fever' may be due to the mother altering the temperature chart.

Meadow [9] described 32 children with fictitious epilepsy, invented by the parents, 21 of them with 'fits' caused by partial suffocation in a pillow. Sixteen had other false symptoms—diarrhoea, haematuria, haematemesis, apnoeic attacks or abdominal pain.

Excessive sleeping may be due to the mother giving the child drugs to get him into hospital (or to kill him). In this case (and others) it is difficult to eliminate *child abuse*. Hypernatraemia has been found to be due to the deliberate addition of salt to a baby's feeds. One has seen children investigated for recurrent coma which occurred each time the mother visited them in hospital. I saw children with overventilation due to salicylate poisoning—despite vigorous denials by the parents that the children could have had access to the drug [13].

## Urinary tract infection

The most common cause of fever in a child without abnormal physical signs is a urinary tract infection. There are usually no symptoms referable to the urinary system, and it is not usual to find either loin tenderness or albumin in the urine (p. 320).

The absence of infection in a specimen of urine does not absolutely exclude infection. The flow of urine from a pyonephrosis may be blocked, the urine examined having come from the other kidney.

## Other infections

*Tuberculosis* can be eliminated by a tuberculin test, though when a child has miliary or meningeal tuberculosis the tuberculin test may be negative on account of anergy, as it may be in measles or severe malnutrition. On ophthalmoscopic examination choroidal tubercles can be found in over 60 per cent of children with miliary tuberculosis [4]. An X-ray of the chest would clinch the diagnosis. Meningeal tuberculosis would be confirmed by lumbar puncture.

In *typhoid and paratyphoid fever* there is almost always enlargement of the spleen, and there are usually rose spots on the abdomen.

*Roseola infantum* can cause confusion for 3 or 4 days. The child has a high temperature without abnormal physical signs, and then the temperature subsides as the erythematous rash develops.

An occasional child may have a raised temperature throughout the incubation period of *measles*. In many other children there is a high temperature for 5 or 6 days, in association with an infection of the upper respiratory tract, before the measles rash appears. Koplik's spots can be seen in the buccal mucosa during the pre-eruptive phase.

*Infectious mononucleosis* (glandular fever) may occasionally present with fever but without other abnormal signs, though there is usually enlargement of the spleen and often lymph node enlargement.

*Acute toxoplasmosis and acute cytomegalovirus infection* resemble glandular fever. Both may be associated with lymphadenopathy, hepatosplenomegaly, thrombocytopenia, choroidoretinitis, fever and jaundice, with atypical mononuclear cells in the blood film.

*Toxocara canis or cati* infection may give no abnormal signs apart from fever. There may be fever, polyarthritis, hepatomegaly, jaundice, rash, epididymitis, fits and abdominal pains. There is usually an eosinophilia.

*Meningococcal septicaemia* may present as fever of unknown origin. It is essential to look for petechial haemorrhages, particularly on the conjunctival surfaces of the eyelids. A joint effusion in conjunction with petechiae would suggest the diagnosis and a blood culture would confirm it.

Certain *closed-off abscesses* may give rise to fever without physical signs, at least for a time. They include particularly the subphrenic or perinephric abscess, a pulmonary abscess or an abscess in a silent area of the brain. The pulmonary abscess can be seen in an X-ray of the chest, but the others may present difficulty. Continued fever following an attack of abdominal pain should suggest the possibility of a subphrenic abscess following the perforation of an appendix. An X-ray or scan may show gas under the diaphragm. A perinephric abscess may present considerable difficulties: it may be preceded by a trauma or a staphylococcal skin infection. There are likely to be rigors, and there may be pain on the affected side, with pain on flexing the spine. There are not usually urinary symptoms; an ultrasound scan may show a bulging psoas shadow; there is usually intermittent but not continuous pyuria.

Fever following or persisting after an operation may be due to a *retained swab*.

A rise in temperature due to the *absorption of blood* (perhaps postoperative) usually lasts only a day or two. Fever may occur in CNS haemorrhage.

A cerebral abscess is usually associated with headache and often with neck stiffness. There is often but not always papilloedema, but there may be no localizing neurological signs. The diagnosis would be suspected if there had been a neighbouring focus of infection, as in the ear or scalp, or if there were bronchiectasis or congenital heart disease. A cerebral abscess may persist undiagnosed for some weeks. The ESR would probably be raised.

A low-grade *osteitis* may cause difficulty in diagnosis. The possibility must be remembered in a child with prolonged low-grade fever and signs of an infection. The routine examination of a child with unexplained fever must include palpation of all the bones for local tenderness, and if there is a suspicion of tenderness (or if there is local pain) or heat, an X-ray should be taken. I have known a low-grade osteitis persist for many months before localizing signs developed. A raised ESR and a polymorphonuclear leucocytosis should suggest the possibility but there may be leucopenia.

*Caffey's disease* in the infant may be manifested by unexplained fever for 3 or 4 weeks before the characteristic swelling of the jaw appears—possibly with tender swelling of the tibia [2].

A child with unexplained fever without abnormal physical signs may have a low grade *septicaemia*. If there is a heart murmur, the possibility of *subacute bacterial endocarditis* should be remembered. There is not necessarily a history of previous heart disease. In a London study [8] of sixty patients with bacterial endocarditis, twenty-one had a history of rheumatic fever, thirteen of congenital heart disease, but eighteen had no previous heart trouble. A particularly careful search for petechiae should be made, and the urine should be examined for excess of red cells in the deposit. In cases of *hydrocephalus* treated with a Spitz–Holter valve, colonization of the valve is a common occurrence, causing septicaemia.

An *apical tooth infection* may cause difficulty in diagnosis. We have seen several examples of such infection in children receiving corticosteroids. The infection was painless and there were no local signs pointing to the root of the tooth. When a child or adult has an unexplained fever (or lassitude), the teeth should be examined. If any tooth is known to be dead, or to have a root filling, an X-ray of the tooth should be taken.

When children have lived in countries in which amoebic infections occur, an *amoebic abscess of liver* should be considered. There may (or may not) be obvious liver enlargement. Screening may show decreased movement of the diaphragm on the affected side. Sigmoidoscopy may show amoebic ulcers and amoebae may be found in the stools.

*Subclinical hepatitis* may cause unexplained fever. A history of exposure to infection together with liver function tests may lead to the correct diagnosis.

*Other infections* include mycoses, psittacosis, and, after holidays in certain countries (e.g. Mediterranean area), malaria or leishmaniasis. When a child (or adult) has been in a country in which malaria or leishmaniasis occur, fever and other symptoms may develop many months after visiting (or living in) that country.

*Juvenile chronic arthritis* is an important cause of prolonged or recurrent unexplained fever (see also p. 279). Schaller & Wedgwood [16] found that episodes of fever occurred in 26 per cent of their cases of rheumatoid arthritis, and that in 10 per cent prolonged fever preceded joint symptoms.

## Drugs

The so-called 'drug fever', which occurs especially with sulphonamides, but occasionally with many other antibiotics, including rifampicin, may cause considerable difficulty in diagnosis. The temperature falls by crisis when the drug is withdrawn. Lipsky & Hirschmann [6] wrote that the fever may be a pharmacological action, the effect of the drug on thermoregulation, a local complication of parenteral administration, or unexplained. It probably has an immunological basis. The fever usually begins after 7 to 10 days of treatment. Other drugs may sometimes cause elevation of temperature. They include acetazolamide, aminophylline, amphetamine, anticonvulsants, antihistamines, atropine group, azathioprine, iodides, metronidazole, nitrofurantoin, non-steroidal anti-inflammatory drugs, penicillamine, salicylates, thiouracil and tranquillizers. Methicillin may cause rigors.

## The reticuloses and collagen diseases

Systemic lupus erythematosus, dermatomyositis and periarteritis nodosa must be considered when there is unexplained fever.

*Systemic lupus* may present with fever, a butterfly rash on the face, arthralgia and thrombocytopenic purpura. There may be polyserositis, hepatosplenomegaly, enlarged lymph nodes, hypertension and albuminuria. Other symptoms include fever, weight loss and abdominal pain. There may be puncta on the palms and fingertips. It may follow the use of a variety of drugs, including antibiotics (especially sulphonamides), anticoagulants, anti-arrhythmic drugs (e.g. propranolol), anticonvulsants, anti-inflammatory drugs, analgesics, chlorpromazine, gold, griseofulvin, isoniazid, methyldopa, PAS, penicillamine, reserpine and thiouracil. Of these drugs, phenytoin is the commonest cause.

Disseminated lupus may occur with maternal auto-immune disease [1].

*Periarteritis nodosa* can present with unexplained fever often with cough, conjunctivitis, abdominal or limb pains, and arthralgia— sometimes resembling rheumatoid arthritis. There is sometimes oedema of hands and feet. One should palpate the skin of the whole body for nodules, which consist of aneurysmal dilatations of the vessel walls.

In *Hodgkin's disease and the reticuloses,* splenic enlargement is usually present. Unless there is obvious lymph node enlargement, permitting biopsy, the diagnosis can be difficult. Fever is common in *leukaemia,* but is less common in Hodgkin's disease: it occurs in 20 per cent of children with Wilms' tumour at some stage. *Sarcoidosis* (p. 281) may cause unexplained fever. *Chronic granulomatous disease* (p. 348) is a rare cause.

The *Kawasaki syndrome* [15] is manifested by fever, often pro- longed, followed by an urticarial or morbilliform rash, pharyngitis, cracked lip, conjunctivitis, uveitis, swelling and oedema of the hands and feet followed by desquamation, pustules on the knees, or lymph- adenopathy, and sometimes by arthritis, urethritis, meningitis, hepatitis, hydrops of the gall bladder, myocarditis, coronary aneurisms or diarrhoea. (For a review see *Acta Paediatr Japonica* 1983; **25**: 79–209).

## Alimentary conditions

*Ulcerative colitis* may be associated with fever, but the presence of diarrhoea with blood and mucus in the stools usually points to the diagnosis. *Regional ileitis* can cause fever with failure to thrive for some weeks before alimentary symptoms develop (p. 11).

## Liver disease

Cirrhosis of the liver, malignant tumours and other conditions of the liver including subclinical hepatitis may be associated with fever.

*Miscellaneous*

A *subdural effusion* in an infant may be accompanied by fever. The fontanelle may be bulging and retinal haemorrhages are likely.

*Agammaglobulinaemia* and *Riley's syndrome* of *familial dysautonomia* may be associated with unexplained fever (p. 46).

Periodic fever has been described with *hyperimmunoglobulinaemia* [17].

## References

1 de Swiet M. Maternal autoimmune disease and the fetus. *Arch Dis Child* 1985; **60**: 794.

2 Greer L, Friedman AC. Periosteal reaction of the femur in an infant with fever. *JAMA* 1981; **245**: 1765.

3 Halsey NA, Frentz JM, Tucker TW, *et al*. Recurrent nosocomial polymicrobic sepsis secondary to child abuse. *Lancet* 1983; **2**: 558.

4 Illingworth RS, Lorber J. Tubercles of the choroid. *Arch Dis Child* 1956; **31**: 467.

5 Jacoby GA, Swartz MN. Fever of undetermined origin. *N Engl J Med* 1973; **289**: 1407.

6 Lipsky BA, Hirschmann JV. Drug fever. *JAMA* 1981; **245**: 851.

7 Liston TE, Levine PL, Anderson C. Polymicrobial bacteremia due to Polle syndrome: the child abuse variant of Munchausen by proxy. *Pediatrics* 1983; **72**: 211.

8 Lowes JA, Williams G, Hamer J, *et al*. Ten years of infective endocarditis at St Bartholomew's Hospital. Analysis of clinical features and treatment in relation to prognosis and mortality. *Lancet* 1980; **1**: 133.

9 Meadow R. Fictitious epilepsy. *Lancet* 1980; **1**: 25.

10 Meadow R. Management of Munchausen syndrome by proxy. *Arch Dis Child* 1985; **60**: 385.

11 Outwater KM, Lipnick RN, Luban NLC, Ravenscroft K, Ruley EJ. Factitious hematuria. *J Pediatr* 1981; **98**: 95.

12 Petersdorf RG, Beeson PB. Fever of unexplained origin; report on 100 cases. *Medicine (Baltimore)* 1961; **40**: 1.

13 Pickering D. Salicylate poisoning. The diagnosis when its possibility is denied by the parents. *Acta Paediatr Uppsala* 1964; **53**: 501.

14 Pizzo PA, Smith DH, Lovejoy FH. Prolonged fever in children: review of 100 cases. *Pediatrics* 1975; **55**: 468.

15 Price J. Kawasaki syndrome. *Br Med J* 1984; **1**: 262.

16 Schaller J, Wedgwood RJ. Juvenile rheumatoid arthritis: a review. *Pediatrics* 1982; **50**: 940.

17 Van der Meer JWM, Vossen JM, Radl J, *et al*. Hyperimmunoglobulinaemia and periodic fever. *Lancet* 1984; **1**: 1087.

18 Warner JO, Hathaway MJ. Allergic form of Meadow's syndrome. *Arch Dis Child* 1984; **59**: 151.

# Hyperpyrexia

McCarthy & Dolan [1], in a study of ninety-three children, found the causes, in order, were pneumonia (16), otitis media (16), meningitis (13), septicaemia (7), pharyngitis (3), dehydration (3), cellulitis (1), unknown (34). They emphasized the high incidence of meningitis in their cases.

*Malignant hyperpyrexia* during anaesthesia is associated with a number of myopathies. There is usually fever, generalized muscle rigidity and severe metabolic acidosis, especially on exposure to halothane. The creatine phosphokinase is usually high.

Hyperpyrexia may occur in the newborn baby as a result of *adrenal or intraventricular haemorrhage.* In older infants and children it may result from *infections of the central nervous system,* including bulbar poliomyelitis, tuberculous meningitis, cerebral haemorrhage or abscess, malaria, heat stroke, dehydration after burns of scalds, or severe liver disease. It may occur in the *Schwartz–Jampel syndrome* (p. 23).

The so-called 'neuroleptic malignant syndrome' of hyperthermia, muscular rigidity, tachycardia, sweating and sometimes dystonic movements may be caused by haloperidol, chlorpromazine and similar drugs. Drugs which may cause hyperpyrexia include amphetamine, antihistamines, atropine, tricyclic antidepressants, and salicylates in an overdose.

Malignant hyperthermia is a feature of *King's syndrome* [2], in which there is a subclinical myopathy, short stature and characteristic face.

## References

1 McCarthy PL, Dolan TF. Hyperpyrexia in children. *Am J Dis Child* 1976; **130:** 849.
2 Steenson AJ, Torkelson RD. King's syndrome with malignant hyperthermia. *Am J Dis Child* 1987; **141:** 271.

# Hypothermia

Hypothermia in an infant, apart from chilling, may be due to a serious infection, such as septicaemia. Other causes are hypothyroidism, malnutrition (especially kwashiorkor), hypoglycaemia, and drugs—phenothiazines and chlormethiazole. It occurs in Menke's kinky hair syndrome (p. 354). The symptoms and signs include lethargy, poor sucking and sclerema. Hypoglycaemic convulsions may result from over-rapid rewarming.

# Lassitude

It is common to hear the complaint that a child seems to be constantly tired or lacking in energy. In this section only chronic lassitude will be discussed. Lassitude of acute onset is likely to be due to an infection, such as measles or tonsillitis. It may be an early symptom of *diabetes mellitus*.

The following are conditions which have to be considered when there is chronic lassitude or lack of energy:

    Developmental feature: puberty
    Familial feature
    Insufficient sleep
    Malnutrition
    Psychological factors, including personality, depression and
        insecurity, school phobia, overventilation
    Hypoglycaemia
    Anaemia
    Infection
        Low grade infection, such as pyelonephritis, tuberculosis
        Persistent haemolytic streptococcal throat infection, or early
            rheumatic fever
        Apical tooth infection

Infectious mononucleosis
Chronic or subclinical hepatitis
Partial collapse of the lung. Cystic fibrosis
Juvenile chronic arthritis
Effect of drugs
Rare
  Myasthenia gravis
  Dermatomyositis, systemic lupus
  Muscular dystrophy, motor neurone disease
  Gilbert's disease
  Hyperammonaemia (p. 223)
  Regional ileitis
  Malignant disease
  Congenital or acquired heart disease
  Bacterial endocarditis, chronic obstruction of the airway
  Gross obesity
  Renal failure
  Endocrine—hypothyroidism, hyperthyroidism, Cushing's
    syndrome. Addison's disease

Apparent lack of energy may be a *developmental feature*. It is common for a child of 2 to 5 to show little inclination to play outside and to seem to become tired easily.

Many mothers become worried when the boy or girl at *puberty* seems to have no energy after having been constantly 'on the go' only a year or two previously. This is a common feature of early puberty. Nevertheless, it is the doctor's responsibility to see that there is not one of the other causes, such as tuberculosis, anaemia or urinary tract infection.

Many children are thought to be lacking in energy and easily tired when the problem is their *personality*, which is usually a familial feature. Some children prefer to read books rather than to play active games out of doors: some prefer their own company and that of their family to that of children in the street. Sometimes children are afraid to go out to play or are worried about so doing, because they are teased by others or are being bullied. A child may seem to his mother to be tired or lacking in energy when he is well and fit but worried about home or school, or feeling insecure. It may be a feature of boredom or depression.

After infancy lassitude may be due to *insufficient sleep*. Children may go to bed too late or stay awake, usually as a result of parental mismanagement.

A child may refuse to play with others and therefore prefer to stay indoors because he is a *'clumsy'* child (p. 209), and cannot keep up with other children. His mother may think that he is tired or lacking in energy. For overventilation see p. 148.

One must never conclude that a child's lassitude is entirely psychological until one has eliminated organic disease, because organic disease may cause behaviour problems. As in the case of unexplained fever, a useful non-specific test is the ESR. If it is normal it does not eliminate organic disease, but if it is raised it makes organic disease almost (not quite) certain.

Lassitude, pallor and irritability before meals may be due to *hypoglycaemia*.

*Low-grade anaemia* is an important organic cause of lack of energy and easy fatigability. If there is any doubt a haemoglobin estimation should be performed.

A common cause of undue fatigue and vague unwellness is a chronic *urinary tract infection*. It is essential to eliminate a *tuberculous infection* by performing a tuberculin test.

One commonly sees children who are well until they develop acute tonsillitis, and are then tired and lacking in energy for 3 or 4 weeks or more. This may be due to a *persistent haemolytic streptococcal infection*, or may represent the onset of an attack of rheumatic fever. It is worth while taking a throat swab and carrying out a therapeutic test with oral penicillin for 10 days, provided that other causes have been eliminated.

Whenever there is unexplained fatigue (or unexplained fever), an *apical tooth infection* should be considered, especially if it is known that there is a dead tooth. An X-ray examination is required.

Another infection seen in a children's hospital out-patient department is *partial collapse of the lung*. The child presents with lassitude and perhaps a slight cough, following a respiratory infection without known pneumonia. The clinical signs may suggest the diagnosis, but an X-ray of the chest is required to establish it.

*Juvenile chronic arthritis* may present as easy fatigability and sometimes with unexplained fever for weeks or months before eventually arthritis becomes manifest (p. 279).

*Drugs* may give rise to the complaint of lassitude. This may be due to drowsiness or to muscle weakness. Muscle weakness may be a side effect of amitriptyline, beta-blockers, carbenoxolone, chloroquine, clonazepam, diuretics, ethosuximide, haloperidol, nalidixic acid, piperazine or streptomycin. Corticosteroids may cause weakness through a form of myopathy.

*Myasthenia gravis* is rare in childhood. The symptoms become more marked towards the end of the day. The first symptom may be ptosis. The child may find it tiring to climb stairs or to walk. There is no atrophy of muscle. The therapeutic test with neostigmine is valuable confirmatory evidence.

*Dermatomyositis* may present as fatigue, muscle pain, fever, weight loss and weakness, especially in the legs. The child is miserable and the muscles may feel stiff. There may be a facial rash with a violaceous hue, periorbital oedema and characteristic 'cigarette paper' lesions on the knuckles, elbows and knees, with telangiectasia around the nail bed, sometimes with oedema of hands and feet. The skin tends to become bound to the underlying tissues at the joints. It occurs at any age including infancy. It is more common in girls than boys. There is commonly a raised creatine phosphokinase. For *systemic lupus* see p. 38.

*Muscular dystrophy* may present as easy fatigability (p. 258). I saw a girl who had been attending a child guidance clinic for 2 years for so-called hysteria, the main symptom being lassitude. A glance at the tongue, which showed wasting and fasciculation, immediately made the diagnosis of motor neurone disease.

# Excessive sweating

Excessive sweating in the absence of fever is rarely due to disease. It may be due to *over-clothing*; even in cold weather I have seen babies with sweat rashes and even 'prickly heat'.

*Sweating around the head* is a common symptom in normal children. The cause is ill-understood: it used to be ascribed to rickets. Sweating hands are often a feature of normal children and adults.

Excessive sweating is rarely due to tuberculosis; to put it another way, night sweats are not a feature of childhood tuberculosis.

For unexplained fever, see p. 31.

In the newborn, excessive sweating may result from the withdrawal from the mother's *drugs of addiction* (see p. 219). In later infancy mercury poisoning, as in Pink disease (now virtually eliminated), may cause excessive sweating. Drugs which may cause it include amitriptyline, amphetamine, antihistamines, ephedrine, haloperidol, imipramine, methylphenidate, pethidine and phenothiazines. Thyroxine overdose in the treatment of hypothyroidism may cause the symptom. *Thyrotoxicosis* may be associated with excessive sweating:

Excessive sweating is one of the symptoms of *Riley's syndrome* of familial dysautonomia in Jewish children (rare). The child does not shed tears. He sweats excessively, has a blotchy rash and exhibits hypotonia and areflexia. There is a characteristic smooth tongue without the normal papillae. The affected newborn baby usually has difficulty in sucking and swallowing, has poor muscle tone, and an absent or poor Moro reflex. The condition is usually associated with mental subnormality. Other features are ataxia, recurrent pneumonia, attacks of vomiting, nasal speech and fits. Riley's syndrome is a genetic condition with an error of catecholamine metabolism.

Attacks of excessive sweating may be associated with fainting, anaemia or pain.

If there are unexplained attacks of excessive sweating not associated with fainting, one should consider *hypoglycaemia*, *phaeochromocytoma* or *neuroblastoma* [1]. Phaeochromocytoma causes attacks of headache, chest or abdominal pain, sweating, polydipsia and polyuria, vomiting, sweating, fits, lassitude, anxiety, tremors, postural hypotension and often, but not always, elevation of blood pressure. In a review of seventy-one cases in adults and children [2] constipation was a feature in 8 per cent of the children. The condition can be confused with thyrotoxicosis or diabetes mellitus.

In the *auriculotemporal syndrome* (Frey's syndrome) [1] there is facial flushing and sweating over the distribution of the auriculotemporal nerve immediately after food or drink.

## References

1  Davis RS, Strunk RC. Auriculotemporal syndrome in childhood. *Am J Dis Child* 1981; **135**: 832.
2  Hume DM. Pheochromocytoma in the adult and child. *Am J Surg* 1960; **99**: 458.

# Enlargement of the Lymph Nodes

The important causes of enlargement of the lymph nodes in children are the following:

Infection

    Local—throat or scalp (cervical nodes), arm infection or immunization (axillary nodes), leg infection, perineal or perianal (inguinal nodes)

    General—eczema with secondary infection, catscratch fever, rubella, infectious mononucleosis, toxoplasmosis, toxocara, cytomegalovirus, syphilis, brucellosis, tularaemia, tuberculosis, atypical mycobacteria, BCG, AIDS (p. 18).

Serum sickness

Immunological diseases—hypergammaglobulinaemia with fever, haemolysis and thrombocytopenia. Farber's disease. Chronic granulomatous disease (p. 348)

Kawasaki disease (p. 39)

Juvenile chronic arthritis

Reticuloses, neoplasms, histiocytosis X, leukaemia

Sarcoidosis

Drugs

The commonest cause of enlargement of the lymph nodes is *infection*. Those in the neck are enlarged if there is infection in the throat, in the skin of the face, the skin behind the ear or scalp. When there is no other obvious source of infection, one must examine the scalp for sore places in association with pediculosis or other infection. Regional lymph nodes may be enlarged as a result of a small and apparently insignificant skin lesion due to primary tuberculosis.

Atypical microbacteria are an important cause of caseating cervical adenitis, especially in Asian immigrants.

In the case of enlargement of the axillary lymph nodes, the cause may lie in BCG *vaccination*.

*Cat scratch fever* is due to a virus infection. Ten to thirty days after infection there is malaise, fever and enlargement of the lymph nodes draining the infected area. Keratitis and encephalitis have sometimes occurred as complications.

*Infectious mononucleosis* may cause a wide variety of symptoms, including lymph node enlargement (not necessarily always), fever, rash, abdominal pain, jaundice, meningism, purpura and sudden hearing loss [3, 4]. There are clinical conditions which closely resemble infectious mononucleosis but in which the usual tests for that infection are persistently negative. *Toxoplasmosis and cytomegalovirus infection* give a similar picture, and can be diagnosed by serological tests.

*Juvenile chronic arthritis* may be associated with lymphadenopathy and hepatosplenomegaly (Still's disease).

*Farber's lipogranulomatosis* [1] consists of adenitis, hoarseness, granulomatous skin lesions, repeated staphylococcal infections (due to a metabolic abnormality of the granulocytes), arthritis, hepatosplenomegaly and hypergammaglobulinaemia. It is an X-linked recessive condition.

*Histiocytosis X* (which includes Hand–Schüller–Christian disease, Letterer–Siwe disease) may include generalized lymphadenopathy, hepatosplenomegaly, rash, bone and pulmonary lesions.

*Sarcoidosis* [2] may cause generalized lymphadenopathy, parotitis, uveitis, rash, bone and pulmonary lesions.

Various *drugs* may cause lymphadenopathy. They include antibiotics, anticonvulsants, meprobamate, non-steroidal anti-inflammatory drugs and thiouracil. Phenytoin may cause not only lymphadenopathy but also hepatosplenomegaly.

**References**

1  Moser HW. Farber's lipogranulomatosis. *Am J Med;* **47:** 869.
2  Pattishall EW, Strope GL, Spinola SM, Denny FW. Childhood sarcoidosis. *J Pediatr* 1986; **108:** 169.

3 Sumaya CV, Ench Y. Epstein Barr virus infectious mononucleosis in children. *Pediatrics* 1985; **75**: 1003.
4 Williams L, Lowery HW, Glaser R. Sudden hearing loss following infectious mononucleosis. *Pediatrics* 1985; **75**: 1020.

# Swelling of the Face

Swelling of the face may be caused by the following:

 Trauma, bites, stings

 Ventilation (newborn resuscitation)

 Subcutaneous emphysema

 General oedema (see also p. 331)

  Angioneurotic oedema

  Allergy to cow's milk or soya (p. 13)

  Serum sickness

 Oedema of eyelids and conjunctiva—rubbing (mainly hay fever), crying, sensitivity to eye drops

 Acute local infections—conjunctivitis, dacryocystitis, chalazion, acute sinusitis, orbital cellulitis, sinus thrombosis, boils, erysipelas, dental abscess, osteitis

 General infections—infectious mononucleosis, measles, Lyme disease, roseola, erythema infectiosum

 Lymphadenitis

 Caffey's infantile cortical hyperostosis

 Anaphylactoid purpura

 Naevus, lymphangioma, tumour

 Melkersson's syndrome

 Drugs

 Parotid swelling

Oedema of the face and neck may follow ventilation of the newborn apnoeic infant.

*Subcutaneous emphysema* may arise from the ethmoid sinus, or from the chest (as in asthma).

*Angioneurotic oedema* may be due to a variety of allergens, hereditary deficiency of $C_1$ esterase inhibitor, or drugs—notably clonidine, cotrimoxazole, disodium cromoglycate, demeclocycline, imipramine, nitrofurantoin, non-steroidal anti-inflammatory drugs, and tartrazine colouring matter. It can result from allergy to cow's milk protein or soya (p. 13).

*Orbital cellulitis* and *sinus thrombosis* are readily confused [5, 6, 9, 11]. In orbital cellulitis there is commonly proptosis, limitation of eye movement, with oedema of the conjunctiva and eyelids. The signs tend to be unilateral and more localized than in cavernous sinus thrombosis. The latter is usually secondary to infection around the orbit, sinus or face, with fever and rigors. There may be raised protein and pleocytosis in the cerebrospinal fluid; cranial nerves 3, 4, 5 and 6 may be affected.

As for acute sinustis, *acute ethmoiditis* is the most important in the young child. The ethmoid sinus is always present at birth; the maxillary sinus is not usually important until after the age of 18 months, and the frontal sinus is not usually liable to infection until 7 or 8 years. In acute ethmoiditis there may be infection of the conjunctiva, photophobia, periorbital oedema or orbital cellulitis, and sometimes local pain or tenderness. It may be complicated by cavernous sinus thrombosis.

*Acute osteitis* should always be considered when there is acute inflammation over bone.

*Erythema infectiosum* ('Fifth disease') due to the parvovirus [10] is manifested by a malar flush, an intensely red 'slapped face' appearance, with a pleomorphic rash (sometimes recurrent) spreading on to the trunk and limbs, with a reticular appearance. There may or may not be an elevation of temperature or febrile aches and pains; frequently there are no general symptoms, but there may be arthralgia, transient hypoplastic anaemia or respiratory symptoms. The incubation period is probably 13 to 18 days.

*Enlargement of the preauricular lymph nodes* is often wrongly thought to be mumps, as is *enlargement of the cervical or submaxillary lymph nodes.*

*Melkersson's syndrome* [8] consists of chronic swelling of the face, peripheral type of facial palsy and furrowed tongue. The facial palsy may precede the other symptoms by several years.

*Drugs* which cause oedema of the face, other than those causing angioneurotic oedema or parotid swelling, include the following:

Aspirin (by far the commonest)

Antibiotics(including cephalosporins, cotrimoxazole and rifampicin)

Anticonvulsants, non-steroidal anti-inflammatory drugs

Tranquillizers, vitamin A excess

## Parotid swelling

By far the commonest cause of acute parotitis is mumps, but it can be due to other viruses, such as parainfluenza [13], Coxsackie or pyogenic organisms [3, 12]. It can ocur as a result of mumps vaccine [7], which may cause purpura, deafness and peripheral neuritis.

It is sometimes a feature of acquired immunodeficiency syndrome (AIDS) (see p. 18).

Parotid swelling, commonly associated with uveitis, may be due to sarcoidosis.

*Recurrent parotitis* is of uncertain cause [4, 12]. It has been ascribed to the Epstein–Barr virus [1], allergy, auto-immune disease, stricture of Stenson's dust—possibly trauma, sialectasis, inspissated mucus or calculus. It can occur at any age from the newborn period onwards, and attacks frequently cease by puberty. The parotitis may or may not be painful, and may involve one side on one occasion and the other at another time. The attacks last from an hour or so to a few weeks, but averaging 3 to 7 days. Sometimes there is slight residual swelling of the gland between attacks. In the attacks the duct orifice may be red and sometimes exudate can be expressed.

*Sjögren's syndrome* (rare) may present as recurrent parotid swelling [2]; it is associated with collagen diseases, xerostomia, keratoconjunctivitis sicca and enlargement of salivary glands. In the *Mikulicz syndrome* there is idiopathic bilateral painless enlargement of the parotid and lachrymal glands, often with dry mouth and eyes; it may be associated with leukaemia or lymphosarcoma.

### Other causes of parotid swelling

I have seen parotid swelling in adults as a form of *malingering*—deliberately blowing (e.g. into a pillow) against obstruction.

*Drugs* may cause swelling of the parotid. They include clonazepam, iodides, isoprenaline, nitrofurantoin and phenylbutazone.

# References

## References

1 Akaboshi I. Recurrent parotitis. *Lancet* 1983; **2**: 1049.
2 Chudwin DS, Daniels TE, Wara DW, *et al.* Spectrum of Sjögren's syndrome in children. *J Pediatr* 1981; **98**: 213.
3 David RB, O'Connell EJ. Suppurative parotitis in children. *Am J Dis Child* 1970; **119**: 332.
4 Friis B, Pedersen FK, Schiodt M, Wiik A, Hoj L, Andersen V. Immunological study in 2 children with recurrent parotitis. *Acta Paediatr Scand* 1983; **72**: 265.
5 Haynes RE, Cramblett HG. Acute ethmoiditis; its relationship to orbital cellulitis. *Am J Dis Child* 1967; **114**: 261.
6 Healy G. Acute sinusitis in childhood. *N Engl J Med* 1981; **304**: 779.
7 Immunisation practices advisory committee. Mumps vaccine. *Ann Int Med* 1980; **92**: 803.
8 Kunstadter RH. Melkersson's syndrome. *Am J Dis Child* 1965; **110**: 559.
9 *Lancet*. Leading article. Orbital cellulitis 1986; **2**: 497.
10 Plummer FA, Hammond GW, Forward K, *et al.* An erythema infectiosum-like illness caused by human parvovirus infection. *N Engl J Med* 1985; **313**: 74. (Editorial p. 111.)
11 Weiss A, Friendly D, Eglin K, Chang M, Gold B. Bilateral periorbital and orbital cellulitis in childhood. *Ophthalmology* 1983; **90**: 195.
12 Wilson WR, Eavey RD, Lang DW. Recurrent parotitis during childhood. *Clin Pediatr (Phila)* 1980; **19**: 235.
13 Yamauchi T, Vollman EC. Epidemic parotitis due to parainfluenza 3 virus. *Pediatr Res* 1979; **13**: 394.

# Anaemia and Pallor

Many children are treated for anaemia in family practice when there is no anaemia at all. The child may be pale because he has been indoors a good deal, is tired, or has an infection, or because he has a pale complexion, taking after a parent in that respect. The sudden development of pallor may be due to a wide variety of illness. Attacks of pallor and a shock-like appearance, occurring every few minutes, may be due to *intussusception,* even though there is no pain or vomiting (p. 113). In mild degrees of anaemia it is impossible to be certain of the diagnosis without a haemoglobin estimation.

Many are unaware of the normal levels of haemoglobin at different ages. The following are the normal figures in grams per cent [5].

|  | Mean | Range |
|---|---|---|
| Cord blood | 17·1 | 13·7–20·5 |
| 7 days | 18·8 | 14·6–23·0 |
| 20 days | 15·9 | 11·3–20·5 |
| 45 days | 12·7 | 9·5–15·9 |
| 75 days | 11·4 | 9·6–13·2 |
| 120 days | 11·9 | 9·9–13·9 |
| 1 year | 12·2 | 10·0–13·0 |
| 5 years | 12·5 | 12–13 |
| 10 years | 13·5 | 13–14 |
| Older | 15 | 14–16 |

The normal range in the young baby depends on the birth weight. A drop from 16·0 g at birth to 8·0 at 6 weeks is normal for a 1·5 kg low-birth-weight baby, but not at 2 weeks, and is not normal for a full term baby.

In the newborn baby, anaemia at birth may represent haemolysis due to blood group incompatibility; but it could be due to bleeding from a placental vessel, feto-maternal transfusion, or in the case of twins, to bleeding of one twin into the other. An important cause is bleeding from the umbilical cord, and on the second to about the fifth day, the most likely cause is blood loss due to haemorrhagic disease of the newborn. Anaemia may arise in the first days as the result of infection.

In later infancy the most likely cause is prematurity. It is the commonest cause of anaemia between 6 and 12 months of age. Another cause is severe maternal anaemia in late pregnancy. From 10 months onwards nutritional anaemia is the most common, due to a poor diet.

A simple classification of the causes of anaemia is as follows:

Blood loss
Nutritional defects
Infection
Haemolysis
Defective red cell production and other serious blood diseases

There is some overlapping between these groups.

**Anaemia due to blood loss**

> Bleeding from placental vessels, or into the placental circulation
> Bleeding of one twin into the other
> Bleeding from the umbilical cord
> Haemorrhagic disease of the newborn. Late vitamin K deficiency
>   Melaena. Haematemesis
> Extensive cephalhaematoma
> Nose bleeds
> Bleeding from the alimentary tract (p. 95)
> Bleeding from the urinary tract
> Blood diseases—haemophilia, etc.
> Trauma

*Bleeding from placental vessels, etc.* This is the second most common cause of anaemia at birth, the most common being haemolytic disease of the newborn. It is due to rupture of the cord, anomalous placental vessels, damage to the placenta by instruments or separation of the placenta. Transplacental haemorrhage may also occur; this consists of bleeding into the maternal circulation. The child is pale and the pallor persists in spite of normal respirations and the administration of oxygen. The child's pulse is rapid, while the child with pallor due to hypoxia has a slow pulse. If the haemoglobin is below 9 g per cent, transfusion is urgent.

*Bleeding of one twin into the other* [6]. One twin is born plethoric, the other anaemic, and intra-uterine brain damage may occur. Both twins may need treatment, the plethoric one needing a replacement transfusion, replacing some blood by plasma, and the other needing the administration of blood.

*Bleeding from the umbilical cord.* Bleeding from the umbilical cord is usually due to contraction of the cord, leaving the ligature slack. Serious bleeding may occur and an urgent transfusion may be required.

*Haemorrhagic disease of the newborn.* When a newborn baby in the first 3 or 4 days vomits blood or passes blood per rectum, it is essential to determine whether it is the mother's blood, swallowed during delivery or from her nipple, or the baby's blood, because, if it is the baby's blood, the appropriate treatment must be given (usually vitamin K) and a careful watch must be kept in order to determine whether a transfusion is necessary. The material should be filtered, and to 5 parts of the supernatant fluid one adds 1 part of $0.25$ N (1 per cent) NaOH. If the colour changes to yellow it is the mother's blood; if it remains pink it is the baby's blood, because the fetal haemoglobin is more resistant to alkali. This condition is a matter of urgency. It is a tragedy to allow an infant to die from melaena neonatorum when his life could readily have been saved by a transfusion. Evidence of Vitamin K deficiency may be delayed until several weeks after birth [1, 3, 7], especially in breast-fed babies. It may present as cerebral haemorrhage or bleeding elsewhere. It is thought that routine administration of Vitamin K to the newborn may not prevent later indications of hypoprothrombinaemia.

Vitamin K deficiency may be latent [7] but it may cause symptoms not only in normal infants, but also in children with cystic fibrosis, biliary atresia or alpha$_1$-antitrypsin deficiency.

It is rare for bleeding into a *cephalhaematoma* to be excessive. If it does occur, it should suggest a blood disease such as haemophilia. It is common for haemophilia to occur without a family history of that condition. A subaponeurotic haemorrhage causes a more diffuse swelling, for the cephalhaematoma, being subperiosteal, is confined by the sutures.

Bleeding from the alimentary tract may be the result of *oesophageal varices* in cirrhosis of the liver, hiatus hernia (indicated by traces of blood in the vomitus), hookworm infection, Meckel's diverticulum (p. 96), reduplication of the intestine, ulcerative colitis, rectal polyp or drugs.

The main cause of alimentary tract bleeding as a result of *drugs* is aspirin. Other drugs include acetazolamide, chlortetracycline, cyto-toxic drugs, non-steroidal anti-inflammatory drugs and thiazides.

Allergy to cow's milk protein may present as bleeding from the alimentary tract (p. 13).

*Haematuria.* Prolonged haematuria may follow an attack of acute nephritis. I have seen severe anaemia develop from this cause.

**Haemolysis**

> Haemolytic disease of the newborn
> > Blood group incompatibility, including ABO incompatibility, vitamin E deficiency
> Acholuric jaundice; spherocytosis; elliptocytosis
> Hereditary non-spherocytic haemolytic anaemia (rare)
> Sickle-cell anaemia, haemoglobinopathies
> Glucose-6-phosphate dehydrogenase deficiency (rare in Britain)
> Pyruvate kinase deficiency (rare)
> Auto-immune haemolytic anaemia (rare)
> Disseminated intravascular coagulation
> Wilson's disease (hepatolenticular degeneration)
> Haemolytic uraemic syndrome
> Infections
> Periarteritis and disseminated lupus
> Drugs
> Solvent sniffing

This list is by no means complete, but it does include the more important conditions.

The most common cause of anaemia on the first day of life is *haemolytic disease,* and this is almost certainly the diagnosis if in addition there is jaundice. The possibility of prenatal blood loss must be remembered. *As treatment may be urgently needed, it is vital that an exact diagnosis should be established immediately, with the help of the Blood Transfusion Laboratory or other laboratory service.*

Vitamin E deficiency may be associated with haemolysis in preterm babies [4].

Haemolysis may occur in necrotizing enterocolitis.

*Acholuric jaundice.* A family history of acholuric jaundice or unexplained anaemia should alert one to the diagnosis. The spleen is almost always enlarged. There is a rare hereditary non-spherocytic haemolytic anaemia.

*Sickle-cell anaemia.* The sickle-cell trait is found in 9 per cent of American Negroes, in parts of India and in 45 per cent of some African tribes. It is a chronic debilitating disease with symptoms of anaemia, thromboses in various organs or limbs and consequent pain and fever. There may be haemolytic or aplastic crises, often precipitated by infections. No coloured child should be treated for iron deficiency anaemia without sickle-cell anaemia being considered. If there is no response to iron in 4 weeks, full laboratory investigation for sickling and other conditions should be carried out.

*Thalassaemia* occurs in the Mediterranean area, parts of India, Bangladesh and Sri Lanka. In mild forms there is a mild persistent anaemia; in severe forms there is progressive severe anaemia with gross splenomegaly unless repeated transfusions are given. A characteristic facies develops owing to the thickening of the bones of the face and skull.

*Glucose-6-phosphate dehydrogenase deficiency* occurs in some millions of persons including Greeks, Cypriots, Turks, Chinese, Indians, Saudi Arabians, Filipinos and Jews from Iran and Iraq. It leads to haemolysis particularly when certain drugs are administered, notably antimalarial drugs, BAL, diphenhydramine, naphthalene, nitrofurantoin, phenacetin, salicylates, sulphonamides and vitamin K. Haemolysis may also occur if broad beans are eaten, and *favism* is due to deficiency of this enzyme. There may be haemolysis with some infections, such as infective hepatitis or glandular fever. *Pyruvate kinase deficiency* is a rare enzyme deficiency associated with haemolysis.

*Auto-immune haemolytic anaemia.* This occurs in association with a variety of unrelated conditions, including virus infections (herpes, infective hepatitis), pyelonephritis, disseminated lupus erythematosus, periarteritis nodosa and dermatomyositis.

*Drugs* may cause haemolysis, apart from glucose-6-phosphate dehydrogenase deficiency. They include antibiotics, antimalarials, cytotoxic drugs, dapsone in breast milk, non-steroidal anti-inflammatory drugs, quinine and vitamin K.

*The haemolytic uraemic syndrome* is a mysterious condition in which the child develops haemolytic anaemia, fever, abdominal pain, arthralgia, jaundice and signs of renal failure, often with thrombocytopenic purpura [2]. There is commonly a mild gastroenteritis or upper respiratory tract infection, followed in 2 to 5 days by acute symptoms—vomiting, abdominal pain, oliguria or anuria, oedema, convulsions and intestinal haemorrhages. There may be hepatosplenomegaly. In the urine there are red cells, casts and albumin. Outbreaks have occurred in certain areas, and a virus cause has been suspected. The diagnosis depends on the demonstration of haemolysis, thrombocytopenia and renal failure, with characteristic burr cells (odd-shaped cells) in the blood smear. The condition is more common in the first 4 years, especially the first year. The mortality is high (40 per cent). Recovery follows in others after 4 to 8 weeks. The condition may be the same as *thrombotic thrombocytopenic purpura*. *Disseminated intravascular coagulation* is manifested by haemorrhage state, haemolytic anaemia and thrombosis, commonly in association with severe systemic disease.

Haemolysis may occur in *mycoplasma* infection.

**Nutritional anaemia**

- Prolonged breast feeding
  Poor diet; mental handicap; fad diets
  Anaemia of prematurity
  Rickets
  Scurvy
  Steatorrhoea

By far the commonest cause of anaemia in a child after about 9 months of age is *nutritional anaemia*. This may be due to a poor diet with inadequate protein and iron content, and an excess of milk and carbohydrate. It occurs in tropical countries as a result of prolonged breast feeding and commonly results from 'fad' diets such as vegetarian or macrobiotic diets. One must not be deterred by the claim that the child is receiving a good mixed diet; such a history is frequent, but there is no doubt that the child has not been receiving an appropriate diet. Mentally handicapped children (including those with cerebral palsy) are liable to develop anaemia because of the difficulty which they experience in chewing and therefore in taking solid foods. They have to be maintained on thickened feeds, and nutritional anaemia or avitaminoses may develop.

*The anaemia of prematurity* is not strictly a nutritional anaemia, but it is convenient to include it here. If small preterm infants are not given additional iron they are likely to become anaemic, especially after the age of 6 months.

*Nutritional rickets* is itself associated with hypochromic anaemia. The diagnosis can be made in severe cases by the finding of the markedly thickened epiphysis of the radius and ulna at the wrist, but the diagnosis must be confirmed by X-ray of the wrist, along with estimation of the plasma calcium, phosphorus and alkaline phosphatase.

*Scurvy* is now rarely seen, but is more likely to occur in mentally handicapped children who are unable to chew and cannot take an ordinary mixed diet. The diagnosis is suggested by spongy bleeding gums, anaemia and severe pain in a leg due to subperiosteal haemorrhages.

The anaemia of *steatorrhoea* is due to malabsorption, and so must be included under the heading of nutritional anaemia.

## Defective red cell production

> Infections
> Drugs
> Lead-poisoning
> Hypoplastic and aplastic anaemia
> Megaloblastic anaemia
> Thyroid deficiency
> Miscellaneous
> > Malignant disease
> > Leukaemia
> > Liver disease
> > Bone disease
> > Uraemia
> > Lipoid storage disease (rare)
> > Letterer–Siwe disease (rare)

*Infections.* When a 3- or 4-week-old baby gradually becomes anaemic, the cause may be a low-grade infection. The umbilicus must be examined for infection, and a blood culture should be performed if there is doubt. In older infants and children, a low-grade infection, such as pyelonephritis, may cause a persistent mild anaemia.

*Drugs.* Numerous drugs are capable of causing anaemia. They include antibiotics, anticonvulsants, antihistamines, antithyroid drugs, chlorothiazide, mepacrine, non-steroidal anti-inflammatory drugs, pyrimethamine, quinidine, quinine, salicylates and tranquillizers. Over 400 drugs or chemicals are known to cause blood dyscrasias. It follows that, when a child presents with anaemia, one should ask in detail about all drugs taken in the previous few months.

Various poisons, such as cleaning agents, paints, paint removers, lacquers and hydrocarbons may cause anaemia, often hypoplastic in type.

*Lead poisoning* in some areas, especially in low social classes, is an important cause of anaemia, especially where there is pica. It is commonly acquired by eating paint which is flaking off window-sills or lead-impregnated plaster or from dust and other objects. Manifestations include abdominal pain, encephalopathy, headache, vomiting, anorexia, incoordination, weight loss and peripheral neuritis. Stippling of the red cells is unreliable. An X-ray may show increased density at the end of long bones, but the diagnosis is established by blood lead estimation.

*Hypoplastic and aplastic anaemia* may remain unexplained after the fullest investigation, but it may be due to drugs and poisons, including lead, infections or exposure to irradiation, or inborn errors of vitamin $B_{12}$ metabolism.

One form of hypoplastic anaemia (*Fanconi's syndrome*) is associated with skeletal deformities (notably an absent radius), skin pigmentation, hypogenitalism, dwarfism, microcephaly and webbed neck. In some cases there is an arrest in the maturation of the red cell for no discoverable reason, leading commonly to severe anaemia between the age of 2 and 18 months. Many cases of 'hypoplastic' or 'aplastic' anaemia prove eventually to be due to leukaemia.

*Megaloblastic anaemia* may be due to steatorrhoea, pernicious anaemia, liver disease, drugs (anticonvulsants, nitrofurantoin), leukaemia or tapeworms. It may be caused by chronic infection in a malnourished child.

*Hypothyroidism* may be associated with anaemia which responds to treatment with thyroxine.

A variety of other conditions cause anaemia, of which the most common is *malignant disease*, including leukaemia. Certain *bone diseases*, especially osteopetrosis, are associated with anaemia. *Renal failure* is usually accompanied by anaemia.

## Conclusion

Anaemia in the newborn period is an acute emergency, requiring immediate hospital investigation and treatment.

Many children are treated with iron for a non-existent anaemia—

and many other children, especially coloured ones, have an anaemia which is not diagnosed, and so do not receive treatment.

Iron deficiency is the commonest cause of anaemia after the newborn period, but the diagnosis should only be made with the help of a blood count. If there is not a good rise of haemoglobin after treating a child with ferrous sulphate for a month, and if one can be sure that he really took the iron, the child should be properly investigated by a hospital laboratory.

## References

1 Aballi PJ. Vitamin K at birth will not prevent late hemorrhagic disease. *Pediatrics* 1985; **75**: 373.
2 British Paediatric Association. Communicable Disease Surveillance Centre. *Br Med J* 1986; **1**: 115.
3 Lane PA, Hathaway WE. Vitamin K in infancy. *J Pediatr* 1985; **106**: 351.
4 Lo SS, Frank D, Hitzig WH. Vitamin E and hemolytic anemia in premature infants. *Arch Dis Child* 1973; **48**: 360.
5 O'Brien RT, Pearson HA. Physiological anemias of the newborn infant. *J Pediatr* 1971; **79**: 132.
6 Rausen AR, Seki M, Strauss L. Twin transfusion syndrome. *J Pediatr* 1965; **66**: 613.
7 v. Kries R, Maase B, Becker A, Göbell U. Latent Vitamin K deficiency in healthy infants. *Lancet* 1985; **2**: 1421.

# Purpura

As the causes of purpura differ in the newborn baby from those in older children, the subject will be discussed in relation to the child's age.

## The newborn

Petechial haemorrhages over the face and forehead are normal, and retinal haemorrhages can be found in about 20 per cent of all newborn babies, except those born by Caesarian section, and in 50 per cent of those born by vacuum extraction [1].

Neonatal purpura may be due to the following conditions:
> Maternal infections—rubella, cytomegalovirus, herpes, toxo-
> plasmosis, AIDS
> Maternal auto-immune disease—thrombocytopenia, systemic
> lupus [4]
> Drugs taken by the mother—anticoagulants, anticonvulsants,
> chloroquine, quinine, salicylates, thiazide diuretics
> Drugs of addiction
> Congenital leukaemia
> ABO incompatibility
> Septicaemia
> Renal vein thrombosis
> Fanconi syndrome (absent radius)
> Galactosaemia
> Cold injury [3]
> Disseminated intravascular coagulation—especially if the
> infant had a low birth weight, hypoxia, acidosis, hypo-
> thermia, infection, incompatible transfusion, abruptio
> placentae [2]
> Cavernous haemangioma

## Purpura after the newborn period

The common causes of purpura after the newborn period are as
follows:
> Trauma (e.g. child abuse)
> Henoch–Schönlein or anaphylactoid purpura
> Idiopathic thrombocytopenic purpura
> Leukaemia
> Petechiae after a convulsion
> The effect of drugs

Less common causes are:
> Aplastic anaemia
> Haemolytic uraemic syndrome
> Uraemia
> Meningococcal septicaemia and other severe infections
> Common infectious diseases
> Haemophilia and allied diseases
> Histiocytosis X

Scurvy
Hereditary telangiectasia (rare)
Purpura with eczema (Wiskott–Aldrich syndrome—rare)
Disseminated lupus erythematosus (rare)
Ehlers–Danlos syndrome (rare)

*Henoch–Schönlein purpura* is more common in boys than girls. It occurs particularly around the age of 5 or 6 years. Preceding haemolytic streptococcal infection is not usually a factor. There are commonly petechiae on the extensor surface of the limbs and around the buttocks, frequently associated with urticaria and effusion into joints and with abdominal pain and often bleeding from the bowel. The face is usually spared except in infants, but there may be some periorbital oedema. Nephritis with haematuria complicates the condition in about 40 per cent of cases. *Special investigations give entirely negative results*—an important diagnostic feature. The platelet count, bleeding and clotting time and capillary fragility tests are normal. Provided that the diagnosis is correct, there is probably no indication for hospital treatment, as no specific treatment is available, but it would be unwise to keep at home an early case complicated by nephritis, because complications of nephritis (such as hypertensive encephalopathy) have to be treated in hospital. It would be a disaster to diagnose Henoch–Schönlein purpura when the child in fact had meningococcal septicaemia. *Berger's disease* may be the same as Henoch–Schönlein purpura without a rash [5].

*Thrombocytopenic purpura* is by far the commonest type of purpura in children after the Henoch–Schönlein type. The child having been previously well is found to have bruises in various parts of the body without history of injury. It is more common between the age of 3 and 7 than at other ages. The limbs are always involved, and there is commonly bleeding from the bowel, vagina or urinary tract. The course may be acute, lasting for 3 or 4 weeks, but it may last for many months. It is important to note that the spleen is not usually palpable; an enlarged spleen would strongly suggest some other diagnosis, such as leukaemia. The capillary fragility test is positive; the blood pressure cuff is inflated to a point halfway between the systolic and diastolic pressures, and the pressure is maintained for 8 min. In a ring 1·5 cm in diameter 2·5 cm below the crease of the elbow the number of petechiae are counted half a minute after removal of the cuff. The test is positive if more than twenty are found. The diagnosis is confirmed

in the laboratory by the prolonged bleeding time, thrombocytopenia
and a normal blood film. It has to be distinguished above all from
leukaemia by the blood film and bone marrow examination. A child
with suspected thrombocytopenic purpura should be referred to a
specialist for laboratory investigation, because other conditions may
be confused with it and only eliminated by laboratory means. For
instance, purpura may be due to meningococcal septicaemia, and a
mistaken diagnosis would be likely to lead to the child's death.

Purpura may be due to *drugs*. Those causing thrombocytopenia
include acetazolamide, antibiotics, anticonvulsants, antihistamines,
antithyroid drugs, atropine, chlorothiazide, corticosteroids, cytotoxic
drugs, digoxin, iodides, non-steroidal anti-inflammatory drugs,
penicillamine, quinine, salicylates, tartrazine and tranquillizers.
Numerous *poisons* affect the blood; they include paints, lacquers,
paint removers and cleaning agents.

Purpura may be due to *hypoplastic or aplastic anaemia, Wiskott–
Aldrich syndrome* of eczema, purpura and recurrent infections,
*disseminated lupus erythematosus* and the *haemolytic uraemic syndrome*
(p. 57).

The possibility of *uraemia* should be remembered in an ill child with
unexplained purpura at any age, including infancy. The blood
pressure will be raised, and this part of the examination should not be
forgotten.

Petechiae or more obvious purpura occur in meningococcal or
*haemophilus influenzae* septicaemia, and sometimes in rubella,
chickenpox, measles, diphtheria, whooping cough, salmonella infections, toxoplasmosis and subacute bacterial endocarditis. Purpura
may follow 1 to 10 days after the onset of the rubella rash, and may
follow mumps vaccine.

A few petechiae may result from *whooping cough* or follow a *major
convulsion*.

Bruising may be a feature of *haemophilia, Christmas disease*, and
other bleeding disorders. A full laboratory investigation is essential.
In *von Willebrand's disease* there are epistaxes and bleeding from the
gums and gastrointestinal tract. The bleeding time is prolonged, but
the clotting time and platelet count are normal. The diagnosis is made
by capillary microscopy and other means.

Purpura occurs in *hereditary telangiectasia*, in which telangiectases can be seen on the face, on the fingers and in the nasal or buccal mucosa, and in the *Ehlers–Danlos syndrome* in which there are over-extensible joints and a hyperelastic skin.

Thrombocytopenic purpura is one of the less common manifestations of *cold injury* [3]. Infants present with a misleading ruddy complexion, lethargy, oedema, anorexia, and sometimes melaena, haematemesis, haematuria and convulsions (especially on over-rapid rewarming, due to hypoglycaemia).

### References

1 Baum JD, Bulpitt CJ. Retinal and conjunctival haemorrhage in the newborn. *Arch Dis Child* 1970; **45**: 344.
2 Chesterman CN. Disseminated intravascular coagulation and related disorders. *Medicine UK* 1980; **No. 28**: 1428.
3 Cohen I, Amir J, Gedaliah A, *et al*. Thrombocytopenia of neonatal cold injury. *J Pediatr* 1984; **104**: 620.
4 De Swiet M. Maternal autoimmune disease and the fetus. *Arch Dis Child* 1985; **60**: 794.
5 Meadow SR, Scot DG. Berger disease: Henoch–Schönlein syndrome without the rash. *J Pediatr* 1985; **106**: 27.

# Poor Appetite

When a newborn baby goes off his food, the most likely cause is an infection, in the urinary tract, the ear or the meninges. Cold injury or developing kernicterus are other causes—the latter only if there has been hyperbilirubinaemia.

I have discussed the problem of a poor appetite in detail elsewhere [1]. By far the commonest cause of a poor appetite, other than that due to an acute infection, is *food forcing*. This consists of feeding the child with a spoon, often by force, persuading him to eat more, offering him bribes if he will finish his dinner, threatening punishment if he does not eat, smacking him for not eating, allowing him to choose exactly what he would like to eat, allowing him to eat snacks at any time he likes between meals, and using various methods of distraction, so that when his attention is distracted some food can be put in by spoon.

Food forcing is itself due to a variety of causes, the chief of which are probably the following:

Excessive anxiety about the child's nutrition and weight

Dawdling with food—the child giving the impression that he has no appetite

Failure to realize that because of his small build (which is usually a familial feature, or related to his low birth weight) he has a smaller than average food requirement

The mother may confuse the average weight with the normal weight—thinking that if the child is below the average weight, he must have something wrong with him. She does not realize that all children are different and that a child may be kilograms below the average weight and yet be normal. Many mothers are concerned because the child's appetite is less in the second six months of his life than in the first six months. Mothers should be told how the weight gain falls off as the child grows older—averaging 7 oz per week (198 g) in the first three months, 5·3 oz per week (150 g) from four to six months, 3½ oz per week (99 g) from seven to nine months, and 2½ oz per week (71 g) from ten to twelve months.

When babies are beginning to feed themselves, from 9 to about 18 months, they characteristically dawdle with their food, playing with it, patting it with the back of the spoon, and giving the impression that they are not hungry. The mother then becomes worried and tries to make them eat.

Well children vary in their appetite. There are little eaters and big eaters. In general the active wiry child eats less than the fat placid one. Efforts to make little eaters eat more always lead to the opposite of the effect desired.

The mother's anxiety about her child's appetite is bound up with many other factors. The problem is more common in an only child or in a child born many years after the previous one. It is more common when the parents are elderly and cannot have another child.

When food forcing occurs, food refusal results for two main reasons. The child resists because of his normal negativism which is a feature from 9 months to 3 years. In addition he becomes conditioned against food because whenever food is presented to him it is associated with unpleasantness, forcing methods and often punishment, so that he develops a real dislike for food.

A breast-fed infant may have a poor appetite as a result of the *chloride deficiency syndrome* (p. 7).

When a child is older, *depression* may manifest itself by a poor appetite.

*Anorexia nervosa*, though predominantly seen in adolescence and early adult life, may occur in children, boys or girls. Jacobs & Isaacs [2] described 20 cases, with severe loss of weight and, as in adolescents, a morbid fear of putting on weight. There is the usual distorted body image, and often obsessional behaviour, vomiting, abdominal pain and depression.

*Certain drugs* may reduce the appetite—apart from amphetamine and the appetite suppressants. They include aminophylline, amitriptyline, antihistamines, antimetabolites, carbamazepine, chlordiazepoxide, digoxin, ephedrine, ethionamide, ethosuximide, indomethacin, methotrexate, methylphenidate, metronidazole, nitrofurantoin, penicillamine, phenytoin, sodium valproate, sulphasalazine and vitamin A or D excess.

If, in addition to a poor appetite, the child does not appear well, one must look for organic causes, such as chronic urinary tract infection, coeliac disease or other cause of 'failure to thrive' (p. 1).

### References

1 Illingworth RS. *The normal child.* 9th edn. London: Churchill Livingstone, 1987.
2 Jacobs BW, Isaacs S. Prepubertal anorexia nervosa: a retrospective controlled study. *J Child Psychol Psychiat* 1986; **27**: 237.

# Pica (dirt eating)

Pica, or dirt eating, occurs particularly in the first 4 or 5 years. It is more prevalent in the lower social classes than in the upper ones. It is often associated with emotional deprivation, neglect or child abuse [1]. It is more common in mentally handicapped children than in those of normal intelligence, partly because mentally handicapped children

continue to take objects to the mouth long after the normal child has
ceased to do so.

It has been thought by some that pica was associated with iron
deficiency anaemia, but the association is often coincidental—iron
deficiency anaemia and pica both being related to the low social class
and to malnutrition. There is commonly a family history of pica, so
that the child may have merely followed the example of others.

The danger of pica is the risk of infection, ingestion of worms and
lead poisoning. In all cases the haemoglobin and blood lead should be
determined.

### Reference

1  Singhi S, Singhi P, Adwani GB. Role of psychosocial stress in the cause of
   pica. *Clin Pediatr (Phila)* 1981; **20**: 783.

# Nausea

Apart from the nausea which usually precedes vomiting, nausea is not
a common symptom of childhood. The usual causes are:

        Psychogenic, including attention-seeking and distaste for
            school. Unpleasant sights or smells

Morning nausea
Dislike for certain foods
Fatty foods
Vasomotor disturbance—posture, anaemia
Infective hepatitis
Urinary tract infection
Cerebral tumour
Drugs

Nausea in the morning when *getting ready for school* may or may not
signify the child's preference for staying at home. It is not always easy
to be sure, because some children and adults do feel nausea in the
morning—and have little breakfast. One needs to ask whether the
morning nausea is as frequent in the weekends and holidays as it is in

term time. Nausea may represent an attention-seeking device—when a mother expresses anxiety over the child's various symptoms.

Nausea on *changing posture* occurs in some older children. It is a vasomotor disturbance and is more common when there is anaemia.

*Subclinical infective hepatitis* may cause nausea and lassitude. Liver function tests will help if the urine examination for bile does not reveal the diagnosis.

*Urinary tract infection* may show itself by vague unwellness and nausea.

It is a mistake to assume that the vomiting due to a *cerebral tumour* is not accompanied by nausea.

Numerous *drugs* may cause nausea. They include antibiotics, anticonvulsants, clonidine, nitrofurantoin, penicillamine, salicylates, tranquillizers and many others.

To establish the diagnosis a full physical examination is necessary, including culture of the urine in order to eliminate a urinary tract infection.

# Vomiting

It is probable that all children vomit, at least sometimes; but some vomit more readily than others. Almost all normal babies bring some milk up after feeds. Either it wells up into their mouth, or else vomited material shoots out with a belch of wind. The difficulty lies in deciding whether vomiting can be disregarded as being within the range of normality, or whether it is necessary to investigate to determine whether disease is present.

The causes of vomiting are legion, and it would not be profitable to attempt to give a complete list. Hence the discussion to follow is inevitably and intentionally incomplete; but I have tried to include the most important causes. For convenience I have related the discussion to three age periods—the newborn infant, the infant after the newborn period, and the child after infancy. There will be some overlapping between these three groupings.

**The newborn infant**

The following causes of vomiting may be important:

      Normal possetting
      Sucking and swallowing difficulties (p.182)
      Infections. Meningitis. Septicaemia
      Intracranial—oedema, haemorrhage, kernicterus, hypoxia
      Obstruction—oesophagus, duodenum, small intestine
        Vascular ring, meconium plug or ileus
        Bezoars
      Chalasia
      Perforation of stomach or pharynx
      Renal insufficiency, urethral obstruction
      Metabolic disorders (rare)—phenylketonuria, galactosaemia, carbohydrate intolerance, organic acidurias, adrenocortical hyperplasia
      Drugs

It is common for the normal newborn baby to bring some milk up after feeds. When the vomiting is frequent one has to consider the possibility of organic disease. When only small amounts come up after feeds and the child is well, taking the feeds normally and gaining weight (after the first 2 or 3 days), disease is unlikely. It has been suggested, on what evidence I am not sure, that much vomiting in the newborn period is due to irritation of the stomach by amniotic contents, meconium or blood swallowed during delivery. Since all babies *in utero* constantly swallow amniotic fluid, it seems unlikely that amniotic fluid would cause vomiting after birth. It is at least true to say that some newborn babies vomit fairly frequently in the first few days after birth, sometimes causing anxiety, and then settle down without further trouble and without treatment.

The features which would make one seriously consider organic disease are as follows:

1  Hydramnios.

2  Persistent vomiting, as distinct from occasional vomiting.

3  The presence of bile in the vomit (green vomitus). This would suggest obstruction below the ampulla of Vater, but green vomitus may occur when there is a serious infection or birth injury. *Green vomitus should be regarded as being due to intestinal obstruction until proved otherwise.* Green vomitus should be distinguished from yellow

colostrum or from vomitus containing meconium. It is not always possible to find an organic cause of vomiting of green material in the newborn period; in a series of forty-five cases, no organic cause was found in thirty-one, and recovery in the remainder was complete [13].

4  Drowsiness, failure to suck well, failure to demand feeds.

5  Abdominal distension. This suggests obstruction in the lower part of the intestinal tract. There is commonly no distension in the presence of high intestinal obstruction.

6  Failure to gain weight or loss of weight.

7  Dehydration.

8  Fever. This may be due to dehydration or infection.

9  Failure to pass meconium in the first 24 hrs. This suggests meconium ileus, Hirschsprung's disease or intestinal obstruction. The passage of a stool in the first 24 hrs does not, however, exclude obstruction.

10  Visible peristalsis from right to left, suggesting obstruction in the jejunum, ileum or colon.

11  The presence of a palpable mass—meconium ileus, enlarged kidneys, reduplication of the intestine or a palpable bladder.

12  The presence of a bulging fontanelle, suggesting cerebral oedema or an intracranial haemorrhage.

These and other conditions will now be discussed in more detail.

### Obstruction in the alimentary tract

*Hirschsprung's disease* is perhaps the commonest cause of intestinal obstruction in the newborn.

*Atresia of the oesophagus* is suggested when the infant's mother had hydramnios. In such a case it is the practice to pass a catheter down the infant's oesophagus immediately after birth, in order to make sure that there is no atresia, and until that has been done a feed must not be given. If there is atresia, the catheter commonly meets an obstruction 4 in (10 cm) from the lips. The lower end of the catheter may coil itself in the blind upper pouch of the oesophagus, and one may be misled unless an X-ray photograph is taken. Atresia is suspected when the infant's mouth is overflowing with mucus and saliva. It will be suspected when a baby chokes and vomits on being given his first feed, or vomits nothing but mucus between feeds. The diagnosis of atresia is usually confirmed by a straight X-ray.

According to Ducharme, Bertrand & Debie [5] *perforation of the pharynx* in the newborn causes symptoms identical with those of the oesophageal atresia. It may be impossible to pass a nasogastric tube in either condition, and radiological studies are confusing. A *vascular ring* will be considered if there is stridor, usually inspiratory and expiratory, commonly with vomiting. *Chalasia of the oesophagus*, or lax cardio-oesophageal sphincter, is an unusual cause of vomiting in the newborn period.

*Duodenal stenosis* would be suspected when a baby vomits repeatedly without abdominal distension. Bile will be present in the vomitus only when the obstruction is below the ampulla. Duodenal stenosis or atresia may be a feature in Down's syndrome.

A *meconium plug* consists of greyish brown inspissated material which precedes the passage of normal meconium. The plug may sometimes be expelled after digital examination of the rectum.

*Meconium ileus* may be suspected when meconium is not passed in the first 24 hrs. Multiple masses may sometimes be felt in the distended abdomen. As it is usually a manifestation of cystic fibrosis, there may be a history of that condition in a sibling. It is more likely to occur in low-birth-weight infants. Signs are mainly abdominal distension, abdominal mass, vomiting, diarrhoea and sometimes signs of gastric perforation.

*Intestinal atresia* may be associated with other congenital abnormalities of the alimentary tract, such as oesophageal atresia or imperforate anus. The symptoms and signs are persistent vomiting with bile in the vomitus, abdominal distension, often visible peristalsis and constipation. Vomiting tends to occur later and to be less profuse when the obstruction is in the lower part of the alimentary tract, but distension is more marked. Obstruction may be caused by malrotation or volvulus.

Vomiting, blood in the stool and abdominal distension may follow perforation of the colon after a replacement transfusion (p. 124). Obstruction a few days after birth may result from *inspissated milk (lactobezoar)*, usually resulting from milk being insufficiently diluted [18] or from the use of gaviscon. Other bezoars are trichobezoars (hair balls), phytobezoars (vegetable matter), polystyrene, vaseline [6] and antacid bezoars (aluminium hydroxide [17]. Human milk bezoars have occurred in preterm infants [24].

*Ganglion-blocking drugs* given in pregnancy to the mother for hypertension may be followed by ileus in the newborn baby for the first week or two.

A second serious cause of vomiting in the newborn period is an *infection*. This may be septicaemia, resulting from an infected umbilicus, urinary tract infection, meningitis, necrotizing enterocolitis or gastro-enteritis. *Meningitis in the young baby is commonly manifested by drowsiness, loss of appetite, vomiting and sometimes fits. There may or may not be a bulging fontanelle. There is commonly no neck stiffness or other sign of meningism. The unexplained drowsiness and illness without other discoverable cause demands a lumbar puncture in order to exclude pyogenic meningitis. The diagnosis of this condition is a matter of great urgency. Delay in instituting treatment is likely to be fatal or to lead to serious permanent sequelae, such as mental handicap.*

In a serious infection the vomited material may be green, as it is when there is intestinal obstruction.

Vomiting may be an important symptom of *cerebral oedema or of an intracranial haemorrhage, such as a subdural haematoma.* The signs are often bulging of the fontanelle and wide separation of the sutures. The child may have an abnormal high-pitched cry and be unduly drowsy or irritable—with an exaggerated startle reflex and even twitching, frank convulsions or cyanotic attacks. The Moro reflex may be exaggerated or absent. There may be retinal haemorrhages—though it must be remembered that small haemorrhages may be found in normal newborn babies. Vomited material may be green. Depression of the respiratory centre as a result of increased intracranial pressure may cause atelectasis, so that respiratory symptoms may outweigh the cerebral ones. Failure to diagnose a *subdural effusion* causes serious brain damage and progressive hydrocephalus.

*Kernicterus* is now rare in Britain because it can usually be prevented by replacement transfusion when the serum bilirubin reaches a dangerous level, but sometimes it occurs in a fulminating septicaemia, causing a rapid rise of serum bilirubin, with possibly unavoidable brain damage. It is said to be relatively common in Chinese children, and Yeung [23] described 152 cases; 53 per cent had non-haemolytic conditions, including cephalhaematoma, and 44 children had glucose-6-phosphate dehydrogenase deficiency. Thirty had ABO incompatibility. Symptoms usually commence about the fifth to ninth day, and consist of vomiting, loss of appetite, arching of the back, spasticity, rolling of the eyes and sometimes convulsions. There may be a peculiar pronation of the wrist.

Renal causes of vomiting include *hydronephrosis* from *urethral obstruction*. A useful pointer to the diagnosis would be a distended bladder with a poor urinary stream—or failure to pass urine.

*Metabolic causes* of vomiting include many inborn errors of metabolism, such as galactosaemia, lactose or fructose intolerance, adrenocortical hyperplasia, organic acidurias and urea cycle disorders. Vomiting due to these causes may occur in the newborn period, but is usually later. The diagnosis of *phenylketonuria* has to be suspected when a sibling has the disease; phenylpyruvic acid does not usually appear in the urine in the first days, and the diagnosis should be made within a few days of birth by estimation of the serum phenylalanine and tyrosine.

### Infancy after the newborn period

The following causes should be considered:

Non-organic
  Normal possetting. Food coming up with wind
  Incorrect feeds
  Overfeeding (preterm babies only)
  Careless handling after feeds
  Rumination
  Giving solids before the baby can chew. Food forcing
  Delay in giving solids
  Crying causing vomiting
  Travel sickness
  Migraine
  Allergy (p. 13)
  Achalasia. Oesophageal reflux
  Bezoars
Organic
  Infection—otitis media, gastroenteritis, whooping cough, winter vomiting disease, etc.
  Intracranial
  Obstruction
  Peptic ulcer

Coeliac disease
Appendicitis
Metabolic diseases. Diabetes
Rare—uraemia, phenylketonuria, galactosaemia, carbo-
hydrate intolerance, ketotic hypoglycaemia, adreno-
cortical hyperplasia, Reye's syndrome, Riley's
syndrome (p. 46)
Drugs and poisons

Probably all normal infants bring some milk up after feeds, but some
bring up more than others, or bring it up more frequently. The
difficulty in such cases lies in deciding whether the vomiting is within
normal limits or not, and so whether it is desirable to investigate for
organic disease.

The first feature which guides one is the weight gain. If there is a
story of vomiting over a prolonged period, and the child's weight in
relation to his birth weight is average or above average, one is less
likely to miss organic disease than if he is underweight. The child may
be an average weight because he was previously overweight before
the vomiting began. One is frequently asked to see an infant who is
said to have vomited the whole of every feed every day for some
weeks, and who is above the average weight for his age. One then
knows that the mother, in her anxiety or desire to impress, is exag-
gerating. It would not be safe to assume that organic disease in such a
case could be absolutely excluded, for he might have a hiatus hernia.
Organic disease is more likely if the child is underweight.

Another feature of importance would be the presence of blood in
the vomitus, for that would suggest *oesophageal reflux* (p. 153).
*Achalasia* is rare [1]: it may cause vomiting, dysphagia and retrosternal
pain.

By far the commonest non-organic cause of vomiting is *excessive
wind*. In a breast-fed baby this is due to the baby sucking too long on
the breast, or sucking on an empty breast so that he swallows air.
Sometimes a breast fed baby swallows air as a result of gulping milk
rapidly. He does this not because he is 'greedy', but because the milk
is flowing out of the breast rapidly—usually at the first feed in the
morning, when the breast is distended. The young baby commonly
does not bring his lips tightly around the nipple and sucks in air at the
angle of the mouth. In a bottle-fed baby the almost invariable cause of

excessive wind is the presence of too small a hole in the teat. A bottle feed should not take more than 10 or 15 min. I am repeatedly told by mothers of 'windy' babies that the feeds take 45 to 60 min. All that time the baby is swallowing air. A baby may swallow an excess of air if he is allowed to suck when the teat has flattened as a result of a vacuum having been created in the bottle. If the bottle is not tilted so that the teat is not kept full of milk, the baby will suck milk and air; for this reason he is likely to suffer from wind if he is left to suck on a bottle which has been propped up on a pillow. Two babies were referred to me on account of excessive wind because the mother in each case had filled the bottle up with sago pudding and expected the baby to be able to suck it through the teat.

Theoretically the baby may be sick as a result of wrong food. In fact this is rare in my experience, though one must always ask a mother not just how much milk the baby is being given, but how much milk powder and water is being given at each feed. I have seen some impressive mistakes. It is a regrettable fact that many doctors and nurses, when faced with a baby who cries, vomits, or has other symptoms, still advise mothers to change from one dried food to another in order to find one which 'suits' the baby. The differences between the dried milks are so trivial that *it is never necessary to change from one dried milk to another,* except in the case of the rare metabolic diseases such as hypercalcaemia or carbohydrate intolerance. Yet I have seen hundreds of babies who had been tried on one dried milk after another in an effort to find one which 'suits' the baby—when his symptoms were due to something different, such as congenital pyloric stenosis. An occasional baby, however, is allergic to cow's milk: in that case a soya milk preparation may be tried—but he may become allergic to that too. The symptoms, which may follow only after a few hours, may include vomiting, diarrhoea, constipation, wheezing, or muscle and joint pains [15].

Some would say that *overfeeding* is an important cause of vomiting.

*Careless handling* of the baby after a feed may cause milk to be brought up. This applies particularly to the preterm baby in which the cardio-oesophageal sphincter is lax. If his nappy is changed after a feed, and the buttocks and therefore lower part of the body are elevated, milk may be brought up.

*Rumination* is an unusual non-organic cause of vomiting [2]. The baby, usually between 6 weeks and a year, but sometimes older, seems to try to get the milk up, pushes his abdomen in and out, arches his back, and eventually brings it up, with apparent satisfaction. He may appear almost to gargle with it, the milk disappearing and reappearing in his throat. There may be associated sucking movements in the lips and cheeks. His action stops when he is watched or when he is actively interested in something. It is commonly ascribed to emotional deprivation, but it is wise to eliminate a hiatus hernia by radiological examination, for these conditions are associated with rumination, making it easier for the baby to regurgitate [8].

A baby is likely to vomit if given *solids before he can chew*. Most babies begin to chew at 6 or 7 months; they can be given thickened feeds before then, but not solids. A retarded child is later than the normal child in beginning to chew, and so is liable to vomit from this cause. If a child is not given solids at a time when he has recently become able to chew, he is likely to refuse solids and to vomit them. This probably depends on the sensitive or critical period [10].

Some infants may develop a strong *dislike for certain foods,* and vomit them if the mother insists on giving them. Some mothers force their infants to take foods which are thought to be good for them, or try to compel them to take more than they need, with the result that they vomit.

Some infants have an unfortunate way of vomiting if they are *left to cry* for any length of time. This may be due to the baby air-swallowing when crying, or to his putting his thumb or finger into the back of the throat.

*Travel sickness* may begin in young infants 5 or 6 months of age.

*Migraine* begins as vomiting. It may first appear in infancy (p.101). Cyclical vomiting is usually an early manifestation of migraine but other conditions cause recurrent vomiting, and one has several times seen serious errors in diagnosis of cyclical vomiting. Conditions which cause confusion include recurrent volvulus, urinary tract infection urea cycle disorders, ketotic hypoglycaemia and lactose intolerance. Familial dysautonomia (p. 46) ia a rare cause of confusion.

An *organic cause* for vomiting would be suspected if the child suddenly began to vomit after being previously well; if he were ill or febrile in addition to vomiting; if there were other symptoms; if he had an inadequate weight gain or lost weight; or if there were blood in the vomitus. It would be dangerous to diagnose migraine or 'periodic syndrome' if the child were unwell between the attacks.

When a previously well infant becomes ill and vomits, the possible causes are numerous. The most likely is an *infection*. These include otitis media, gastroenteritis, urinary tract infection, whooping cough, 'winter vomiting' and meningitis. Otitis media is suspected when an infant has a cold or has just recovered from one. Gastroenteritis may cause some difficulty in the diagnosis for a few hours, in that vomiting may precede diarrhoea. A history of diarrhoea in another member of the family makes the diagnosis easier. For necrotizing enterocolitis, see p. 92.

*Whooping cough* is an important cause of vomiting (p. 151), and it may be the presenting symptom; but on direct questioning one finds that the vomiting is the result of coughing.

The term *'winter vomiting'* disease is not a good one, for it occurs in summer and winter. This is a virus infection, due commonly to the orbivirus, rotavirus or calcivirus. It has been well described in a report by the College of Practitioners [4], in which 1300 cases were recorded by 106 family doctors. Three children with this condition were found to have a CSF pleocytosis, suggesting a neurotropic virus [7]. Normally the only symptom is vomiting, nearly always in the night. Diarrhoea, if it occurs at all, is most unusual. The child is afebrile and is well until he suddenly vomits without previous nausea and without warning. The vomiting may recur.

*Congenital pyloric stenosis* occurs in one in 150 boys and one in 775 girls. There is a genetic factor. The onset of vomiting is nearly always between 3 and 6 weeks of age, though rarely it can begin in the newborn period. If vomiting begins after the age of 10 weeks, it is exceedingly unlikely to be due to pyloric stenosis: in about 1 per cent vomiting is delayed until the third month. The essential feature is projectile vomiting immediately after or during a feed. There is one big vomit and almost the whole feed comes up. If the baby is merely bringing small quantities up at intervals between one feed and the next, e.g. an hour or two after a feed, pyloric stenosis can be almost excluded. Rarely a child may have one big vomit immediately after or during a feed, and bring small quantities up for an hour or two, like a normal baby frequently does; but this is an unusual picture. There is no bile in the vomitus, but there is occasionally some blood. Jaundice is a rare feature. The vomiting begins with one feed and may then occur in every subsequent feed or not until the next day. It rapidly becomes more frequent, so that in 2 or 3 days the baby is vomiting at almost every feed. As a result of vomiting the baby becomes constipated and dehydrated. Peristaltic waves may be seen crossing from left to right in the upper abdomen. The expert will feel a pyloric tumour which comes and goes and is commonly the size of a pea, slightly to the right of the umbilicus and usually a little above. It is often larger if symptoms have been present for a longer than usual period. He feels the baby during a feed. If the stomach is distended when he is about to begin, he will wash the stomach out first, because it is often impossible to feel a tumour when the stomach is distended.

Owing to the infrequency with which pyloric stenosis is seen in general practice, the family doctor should not rely on his ability to feel the tumour. He should suspect the diagnosis and ask the paediatrician to express an opinion on examination. The diagnosis is established by feeling the tumour. X-ray examination or ultrasound investigation is nearly always unnecessary. There is no place for a therapeutic test of atropine methyl nitrate, for the correct treatment is surgical. The majority of babies with congenital pyloric stenosis seen in hospital have been tried on one dried food after another to find one which suits the baby.

*Pylorospasm* in my opinion is probably a non-existent condition in infants, though some will disagree. I can certainly say that I have never recognized a case, or seen a case thought by somebody else to be pylorospasm and which did not appear to me to be incorrectly diagnosed. I have seen no evidence that such a condition exists. I usually find that babies thought to have this condition are suffering from excessive wind, congenital pyloric stenosis or are merely normal 'possetters'.

*Gastro-oesophageal reflux* with or without hiatus hernia is an important cause of vomiting [21]. The vomiting is commonly effortless, but may be projectile. Theoretically it should be more prominent when the child is lying down rather than sitting upright, but this is unreliable. When asked to see a persistent vomiter, one always asks whether there is blood in the vomitus, for that immediately suggests oesophagitis from reflux. The vomiting may lead to a failure to thrive.

In about 12 per cent of cases there are pulmonary complications consisting of cough and patchy consolidation. Rarely in the young infant the regurgitation may lead to apnoeic episodes [1].

Gastro-oesophageal reflux is sometimes a feature of children who are mentally subnormal or have cerebral palsy [20] or have cystic fibrosis [18]. The association of reflux with torticollis or opisthotonos is described on p. 229.

The possibility of a *tracheo-oesophageal fistula* should be considered if there is persistent unexplained vomiting, especially if there has been another anomaly of the alimentary tract, such as an imperforate anus: it was found in 3 per cent of 760 preterm infants [9]. The diagnosis, if not made by X-ray, may be made by the passage of a stomach tube, with the proximal end of the tube under water: when the tube is slowly withdrawn up the oesophagus, bubbles reveal a fistula.

*Peptic ulcers* can occur at any age. Johnson, L'Heureux & Thompson [10] described sixteen under the age of 11 weeks; nine of them presented with recurrent vomiting and seven with bleeding or perforation.

*Coeliac disease* (p. 10) may present as vomiting when gluten-containing foods are introduced.

*Appendicitis* can occur at any age (p. 110). In infancy it commonly presents as an abdominal mass, peritonitis and diarrhoea.

*Metabolic diseases* which may present with vomiting include diabetes mellitus, Reye's syndrome and a variety of rare diseases.

*Ketotic hypoglycaemia* may present as vomiting and fits. It is more common in low-birth-weight infants.

*Reye's syndrome* affects infants and young children [12]. Five to six days after the onset of respiratory infection, especially influenza A or B, or chickenpox, there is vomiting, followed in some cases in a few hours by irritability, delirium, convulsions, hypoglycaemia and coma. There is hepatic dysfunction, with elevated serum transaminases [13]. The cause is unknown; there has been an apparent association with administration of salicylates. For a full review see the symposium edited by Yamashita *et al.* [22] and for a review of the differential diagnosis see Robinson [16], who includes liver failure, haemorrhagic shock encephalopathy, toxic shock encephalopathy, and other rare metabolic diseases.

*Drugs and poisons.* Innumerable drugs may cause vomiting. Poisoning should always be considered when a previously well child begins to vomit without discoverable cause. It must be remembered that the possibility of poisoning may be stoutly denied by a parent, and in that case it may be a form of *non-accidental injury*.

## Vomiting after infancy

*Non-organic causes*

Vomiting because of psychological factors is common in children. These causes may be grouped as follows:

1 Excitement. Some children may vomit as the result of excitement, such as the prospect of going to a party.

2 Fear or anxiety. Anxiety about going to school, or about leaving home, may cause vomiting in school-age children in the morning before departure for school.

3 Suggestion and imitation. Vomiting may be suggested by anxious parents on a car journey. Vomiting may result from the child seeing another child vomit.

4 Attention-seeking device. Vomiting may occur as an attention-seeking device if the child sees that sickness causes consternation and anxiety.

5 Insertion of finger into the throat. Some small children make themselves sick, probably accidentally, by insertion of a finger into the throat—sometimes when the throat is sore as a result of tonsillitis.

6 Migraine. Though it may be argued that migraine is an example of organic disease, emotional factors may precipitate attacks. Migraine, also termed in children the periodic syndrome, is described elsewhere (p. 101).

7 Travel sickness.

8 In older children—self-induced vomiting in association with anorexia nervosa (p. 67).

*Organic* causes are suggested if the vomiting is of sudden onset, or if the child between attacks of vomiting is not well and is lacking in energy—though these symptoms may be psychological in origin. They are certainly suggested if there is loss of weight. The periodic syndrome can be confused with other conditions such as recurrent volvulus, herniation of the stomach through the diaphragm, ketotic hypoglycaemia, or recurrent urinary tract infection; and even if a child is known to suffer from migraine, he may also develop a different condition such as acute appendicitis, which also causes abdominal pain and vomiting.

Organic causes include the following:

> Infection, especially tonsillitis or otitis media
> Meningitis
> Winter vomiting disease
> Appendicitis, mesenteric lymphadenitis
> Intestinal obstruction
> Torsion of the testis (p. 330)
> Poisons and drugs

As in the younger child, the commonest organic cause of vomiting is *an infection*—such as otitis media, tonsillitis, pyelonephritis, whooping cough, gastro-enteritis or the winter vomiting disease. Meningitis is another possible cause, but in the case of the older child signs of meningism are usually but not invariably present.

Unexplained vomiting may be due to *drugs or poisons*. Innumerable medicines cause vomiting. They include aminophylline, anthelmintics, antibiotics, antidepressants, anticonvulsant drugs, antihistamines, cytotoxic drugs, morphia, pethidine, salicylates, tranquillizers and other drugs. Digitalis intoxication may cause vomiting, diarrhoea, confusion and blurring or yellow vision [3].

Vomiting may be a symptom of *lead poisoning*.

## References

1 Berquist WE, Byrne WJ, Ament ME, Fonkalsrud EW, Euler AR. Achalasia: diagnosis, management and clinical course in 16 children. *Pediatrics* 1983; **71**: 798.

2 *British Medical Journal*. Six month old persistent vomiters. Leading article. 1979; **2**: 459.

3 *British Medical Journal*. Digitalis intoxication: a new approach to an old problem. 1983; **1**: 1533.

4 College of Practitioners. Epidemic winter vomiting. Symposium by the epidemic observation unit of the college of general practitioners. *Research News Letter No. 8* (no date).

5 Ducharme JC, Bertrand R, Debie J. Perforation of the pharynx in the newborn. A condition mimicking esophageal atresia. *Can Med Ass J* 1971; **104**: 785.

6 Goh DW, Buick R. Inestinal obstruction due to ingested vaseline. *Arch Dis Child* 1987; **62**: 1167

7 Haworth JC, Tyrell DAJ, Whitehead JEM. Winter vomiting disease with meningeal involvement. *Lancet* 1956; **2:** 1152.
8 Herbst JJ. Gastro-esophageal reflux. *J Pediatr* 1981; **98:** 859.
9 Hrabovsky EE, Mullett M. Gastrooesophageal reflux and the premature infant. *J Pediatr Surg* 1986; **21:** 583.
10 Illingworth RS, Lister J. The critical or sensitive period, with special reference to certain feeding problems in infants and children. *J Pediatr* 1964; **65:** 839.
11 Johnson D, L'Heureux P, Thompson P. Peptic ulcer disease in early infancy: clinical presentations and roentgenographic features. *Acta Paediatr Scand* 1980; **69:** 753.
12 *Lancet.* Reye's syndrome. Leading article. 1982; **1:** 941.
13 Liechtenstein PK, Heubi JE, Daughterty CC. Grade I Reye's syndrome. *N Engl J Med* 1983; **309:** 133. Leading article 179.
14 Lilien LD, Srinivasan G, Pyati SP, Yeh TF, Ildes RS. Green vomiting in the first 72 hours in normal infants. *Am J Dis Child* 1986; **140:** 662.
15 McCarty EP, Frick OL. Food sensitivity: keys to diagnosis. *J Pediatr* 1983; **102:** 645.
16 Robinson RO. Differential diagnosis of Reye's syndrome. *Develop Med Child Neurol* 1987; **29:** 110.
17 Rosenberg HK. Antacid bezoars in a premature infant. *Clin Pediatr (Phila)* 1982; **21:** 503.
18 Schreiner RL, Brady MS, Franken EA, *et al.* Increased incidence of lacto-bezoars in low birth weight infants. *Am J Dis Child* 1979; **133:** 936.
19 Scott RB, O'Loughlin EV, Gall DG. Gastro-esophageal reflux in patients with cystic fibrosis. *J Pediatr* 1985; **106:** 223.
20 Sondheimer JM, Morris BA. Gastro-esophageal reflux among severely retarded children. *J Pediatr* 1979; **94:** 710.
21 Weissbluth M. Gastro-esophageal reflux. *Clin Pediatr (Phila)* 1981; **20:** 7.
22 Yamashita F, *et al.* Reye's syndrome. *Acta Paediatr Japonica* 1986; **28:** 650–764.
23 Yeung CY. Kernicterus in term infants. *Australian Paediatr J* 1985; **21:** 273.
24 Yoss BS. Human milk bezoars. *J Pediatr* 1984; **105:** 819.

# Haematemesis

Before accepting the diagnosis of haematemesis, one must be sure that what was thought to be altered blood was not chocolate. When a child brings blood up from the stomach, the following are the conditions to consider first:

In a newborn infant
Swallowed blood during delivery

Swallowed blood from the mother's nipple
Haemorrhagic disease of the newborn
Drugs taken in pregnancy—anticoagulants, diuretics, sali-
    cylates (rare cause)
Drugs taken by the infant
Cold injury (p. 65)
Infancy after the newborn period
    Gastro-oesophageal reflux
    Chalasia of the oesophagus
    Blood diseases
    Congenital pyloric stenosis
After infancy
    Gastro-oesophageal reflux
    Severe retching for any reason
    Nose bleeds
    Acute tonsillitis, adenovirus
    Oesophageal varices
    Peptic ulcer (especially when on corticosteroids)
    Intestinal obstruction (altered blood)
    Blood diseases
    Uraemia
    Poisons (corrosive substances, ferrous sulphate overdose)
    Drugs
*Rare causes*
    Enterogenous cyst
    Disseminated intravascular coagulation
    Tyrosinosis (p. 126)
    Gaucher's disease (p. 126)
    Hypernatraemia
    Zollinger–Ellison syndrome
    Curling's ulcer (burns)
    Polycystic disease of the liver and kidney
    Foreign body in oesophagus
    CNS injury

When a newborn in his first 3 or 4 days vomits blood, one needs to
know whether it is the baby's or the mother's blood. He may have
swallowed the mother's blood during delivery, or blood from the
mother's cracked nipple. The two are readily distinguished by the

chemical test described on p. 55: if it is the baby's blood, the most likely cause is haemorrhagic disease of the newborn, commonly due to *hypoprothrombinaemia*. In this case he requires treatment, and a careful watch must be kept to ensure that the blood loss is not such that a transfusion is necessary.

The gut mucosa may be damaged by aspirin or *indomethacin* given as prostaglandin inhibitor in the management of a patent ductus [3]. Indomethacin may also prolong the bleeding time and act on the platelets.

After the newborn period, blood-streaked vomiting is commonly caused by a *hiatus hernia*. It is a rare finding in *pyloric stenosis*.

At any age haematemesis may be a feature of *blood diseases*.

*Severe retching* may lead to streaking of vomitus with blood.

Other causes of blood in the vomitus of a child are *blood swallowed after a nose bleed or from acute tonsillitis*—presumably as a result of rupture of a blood vessel in the acutely inflamed nose or throat.

Haematemesis has been caused by an adenovirus infection [2].

*Oesophageal varices* only occur in association with *cirrhosis of the liver, portal hypertension or hypersplenism* or may be the late result of an operation for biliary atresia.

In *portal hypertension* there may be a history of omphalitis, hepatitis, exchange transfusion by an umbilical vein catheter, or umbilical sepsis. It may be the result of cirrhosis of the liver or an abnormal vascular arrangement.

*Aspirin* may cause bleeding from the stomach. This may be due to particles of aspirin tablets eroding the gastric mucosa; it may also be due to hypoprothrombinaemia or thrombocytopenia. Haematemesis may result from an overdose of aminophylline. The possibility of *poisoning* by a corrosive substance or other material (such as ferrous sulphate), or boric acid poisoning, must be remembered. It could be due to the deliberate administration of a toxic dose of iron or other medicine (Munchausen syndrome). Blood may have been added to the vomitus by the mother.

*Peptic ulceration* may occur in children, though it is a rare cause of haematemesis. The possibility should be remembered when a child receiving corticosteroids, or non-steroid anti-inflammatory drugs, complains of abdominal pain.

*The Zollinger–Ellison syndrome* is more common in boys; it consists of peptic ulceration with a non-beta-cell islet tumour of the pancreas or liver [1]. The symptoms include abdominal pain, vomiting, haematemesis, diarrhoea and melaena.

Altered blood in the vomitus is a feature of *intestinal obstruction*.

### References

1 Buchta RM, Kaplan JM. Zollinger–Ellison syndrome in a nine-year-old child: a case report and review of this entity in childhood. *Pediatrics* 1971; **47**: 594.
2 Bye AM, Rice SJ, Koh T, Brown R, Price E. Haematemesis as a presentation of adenovirus Type 7 infection. *Australian Paediatr J* 1983; **19**: 184.
3 Rennie JM, Doyle J, Cooke RW. Early administration of indomethacin to preterm infants. *Arch Dis Child* 1986; **61**: 233.

# Constipation

The causes of constipation include the following: those without disease are the commonest.

Non-disease

Breast-fed babies—normal infrequent stools (not true constipation). Rarely—excess of fatty foods, cream, etc. taken by lactating woman

Bottle-fed—insufficient sugar or fluid in the feed. Undiluted cow's milk. Allergy to cow's milk

Toilet training errors

Unexplained normal variations

Drugs—chronic use of laxatives, etc.

Disease

Obstruction: imperforate anus, meconium plug, Hirschsprung's disease, anorectal stenosis, ectopic anus

Severe vomiting

Polyuria (see p. 324)

Severe hypotonia. Congenital absence of abdominal muscles (prune-belly syndrome)

Hypothyroidism
Lead-poisoning
Coeliac disease or cystic fibrosis

**Non-disease**

Normal fully breast-fed infants may have very infrequent stools, maybe one every 5 days or so. The stools are loose—the same as those of breast-fed babies who have frequent stools—maybe several a day. Rarely, if a mother mistakenly takes a gross excess of protein and fat, a breast-fed baby's stools may be firmer and pultaceous.

Occasional bottle-fed babies, with no evidence of disease, pass hard stools. This may occur if the baby is given insufficient fluid, especially in a hot climate, or is perspiring excessively, because of over-clothing. If a baby in the first 4 months or so is given undiluted cow's milk, constipation may result. If he finds it painful to pass a stool because it is hard or because there is an anal fissure, he may withhold stools and become even more constipated. It is said that *allergy to cow's milk* may present as chronic constipation [1].

Constipation after about 9 months of age may be due to *unwise toilet training*—compelling the child to sit on the potty against his will. The baby becomes conditioned against using the potty and troublesome constipation results. But not all constipation can be explained by errors of toilet training—though it is customary for child psychologists to blame a mother for it. There are differences in intestinal fluid absorption and rates of peristalsis. It may be found that gut hormones—such as the vasoactive intestinal polypeptides—may play a part. Dietary or genetic factors may be relevant. I am uncertain whether deficiency of fibre in the diet is a cause of constipation.

Various *drugs* may cause constipation. They include amitriptyline, chlordiazepoxide, imipramine and vincristine. Constipation may follow the chronic use of laxatives.

*Constipation with disease*

An *imperforate anus* will not long pass unnoticed, but *anorectal stenosis* may escape detection for a long time until someone performs a rectal examination. Sometimes a history of the child passing stools shaped like expelled toothpaste may point to the diagnosis. Constipation may result from an anterior ectopic anus [5].

Ninety per cent of infants pass meconium in the first 24 hrs. Delay in passing meconium (e.g. until after 36 hrs) strongly suggests *Hirschsprung's disease* (p. 14) but it could be due to a meconium plug which can be released by insertion of a finger into the rectum [4]. Hirschsprung's disease may affect only a terminal ultra-short segment [2]. Cases of Hirschsprung's disease with late onset of symptoms have been described [3]. Constipation may be caused by other forms of intestinal obstruction.

Vomiting for any cause, such as congenital pyloric stenosis, leads to constipation. Constipation may be due to polyuria, such as in renal acidosis, hypercalcaemia or nephrogenic diabetes insipidus. If a child is being investigated for 'failure to thrive' the history of gross constipation, with palpable faecal masses in the abdomen, strongly suggests one of the metabolic causes of polyuria.

Rare causes include hypotonia, the prune-belly syndrome, thyroid deficiency, diabetes or lead-poisoning.

Anything which causes vomiting, such as *excessive possetting* or *pyloric stenosis*, will cause constipation.

*Coeliac disease* and *cystic fibrosis* may present as constipation.

## References

1 Chin KC, Tarlow MJ, Alfree AJ. Allergy to cow's milk presenting as chronic constipation. *Br Med J* 1983; **2**: 1593.
2 Clayden GS, Lawson JON. Investigation and management of long-standing chronic constipation in childhood. *Arch Dis Child* 1976; **51**: 918.
3 Doig CM. Childhood constipation and late presentation of Hirschsprung's disease. *J Roy Soc Med* 1984; **77** (supl. 3): 3.
4 Ellis D, Chatworthy HW. The meconium plug revisited. *J Pediatr Surg* 1966; **1**: 54.
5 Leape LL, Ramenofsky ML. Anterior ectopic anus, a common cause of constipation in children. *J Pediatr Surg* 1978; **13**: 627.

# Encopresis and Faecal Incontinence

There is disagreement as to the definition of faecal incontinence and encopresis. Some regard the term encopresis as signifying faecal incontinence without a structural cause such as spina bifida. It commonly presents as diarrhoea alone, diarrhoea with soiling, or soiling alone. One has often seen children treated with drugs for 'diarrhoea' when the cause of the 'diarrhoea' was gross constipation.

Soiling, faecal incontinence or encopresis is usually associated with constipation, and is especially common in mentally handicapped children [1, 2]. It occurs in otherwise normal children most commonly at the age of 6 to 8 years; it is more common in boys. On rectal examination it is found that the rectum is loaded with a huge mass of faeces. The 'diarrhoea' is due to liquid material leaking round the edge of the faecal mass. There may be associated urinary incontinence especially if the soiling is not due to constipation. In about a third there is a history of early bowel-training difficulties. About half the affected children have never controlled the bowel, and have acquired the encopresis, usually after an emotional disturbance such as the birth of a sibling, starting school, or separation from the mother. The constipation is occasionally due to ultra-short segment Hirschsprung's disease, causing failure of the anus to relax. Soiling without constipation is a more troublesome behaviour problem due to emotional disturbance and insecurity. It is commonly associated with urinary incontinence.

Faecal incontinence may be due to a gross neurological abnormality such as *meningomyelocele, lipoma* involving the spinal cord, *diastematomyelia, spina bifida* or *absent sacral segments* (p. 312).

## References

1 Bentley JFR. Faecal soiling and achalasia. *Arch Dis Child* 1978; **53:** 185.
2 Levine MM. Children with encopresis: a descriptive analysis. *Pediatrics* 1975; **56:** 412.

# Diarrhoea

Many infants and children are said by their mothers to have diarrhoea when in fact their stools are normal.

Fully breast-fed babies always have loose stools, unless they have Hirschsprung's disease. Their stools are explosive, contain curd (in the early weeks), and may be bright green in colour. They may be frequent, as many as 24 stools in the 24 hrs. Fully breast-fed babies virtually never suffer from gastroenteritis.

The so-called *starvation stools* may be confused with diarrhoea. These are loose green frequent small stools, containing little faecal matter. They are due to gross deficiency of food intake. It is a disaster if foods are restricted on the grounds that the child has gastroenteritis or is being overfed. I doubt whether *overfeeding* causes diarrhoea. Many infants are said to be suffering from overfeeding when the correct diagnosis is underfeeding.

Many older children are referred to the paediatrician on account of chronic diarrhoea and on examination it is found that weight is average. If the mother is asked to bring sample stools on a subsequent occasion, it is found that they are normal. It is important to see stools if there are reasons for doubting the mother's story.

It is vital to remember that *diarrhoea is never due to teething*.

> *Causes*
> Excess of sugar in infant's feeds
> Phototherapy
> Toddler's diarrhoea ('irritable colon')
> Psychogenic
> Child abuse
> Infections
> Toxic shock syndrome
> Haemolytic uraemic syndrome
> Surgical or semisurgical conditions
>> Hirschsprung's disease
>> Appendicitis, intussusception, peritonitis, biliary atresia, chylous ascites
>> Malrotation

Short gut syndrome
Ulcerative colitis, regional ileitis, polyposis
Tumours—lymphoma, carcinoid, neural tumours
Radiation diarrhoea
Malabsorption—fat, carbohydrate, protein
Intestinal lymphangiectasia
Abetalipoproteinaemia
Allergy—cow's milk, soya, etc.
Immune deficiency. Auto-immune diseases
Endocrine diseases—thyrotoxicosis, hypoparathyroidism
Zollinger–Ellison syndrome (p. 85)
Pancreatic insufficiency, adrenocortical hyperplasia or insufficiency
Miscellaneous rare diseases—congenital chloride diarrhoea, acrodermatitis enteropathica (p. 362), Wiskott–Aldrich syndrome (p. 64)
Drugs

For an extensive review of the subject of diarrhoea, see Milla [15].

*Excess of sugar* in the feeds of a bottle-fed baby is a common cause of diarrhoea.

*Phototherapy* for neonatal jaundice is sometimes followed by diarrhoea, possibly as a result of temporary intestinal lactase deficiency [1].

*Toddler's diarrhoea*—termed by some the 'irritable colon syndrome' or 'chronic non-specific diarrhoea of early childhood'—is common in well thriving toddlers aged 9 months to 3 years [6, 22]. It occurs in well, thriving children with normal weight gain. Dietary alteration and medicines have little effect—but it has been suggested [4] that some respond to an increase of fat in the diet. I have not seen confirmation of that by others. There is no evidence of malabsorption or of infection. Dodge and his colleagues [7, 8] showed that affected children have raised prostaglandins, especially $PGF_2\alpha$, and that the diarrhoea was reduced by prostaglandin inhibitors, indomethacin and aspirin.

*Psychogenic diarrhoea* occurs in older children—often in relation to anxieties or distaste for school.

Diarrhoea can be due to *child abuse*. I have seen cases in which the diarrhoea was due to the deliberate administration of purgatives in the absence of constipation.

The commonest cause of acute diarrhoea is infection, usually due to the contamination of food, but also due to respiratory tract organisms; pathogenic *E. coli*; viruses (notably the rotavirus); AIDS; legionnaires' disease; malaria; giardia; urinary tract infection; septicaemia; cryptosporidiosis [17]—sometimes in association with *Shigella* organisms, *Yersinia* (sometimes with abdominal pain, vomiting, fever, mesenteric adenitis, arthritis or erythema nodosum [20]), or *Campylobacter* [13]. Prolonged diarrhoea may be a feature of AIDS in children.

The *toxic shock syndrome* [2, 19] includes fever, diarrhoea, shock, melaena, renal and hepatic dysfunction, acidosis, disseminated intravascular coagulation and encephalopathy, myalgia, drowsiness, a red throat or conjunctiva, and later desquamation of hands and feet.

*Necrotizing enterocolitis* affects particularly low-birth-weight babies fed on cow's milk, especially when given hyperosmolar feeds, or when there was hypoxia, respiratory distress syndrome, apnoeic attacks or an exchange transfusion [21]. The features are bile-stained vomiting, abdominal distension, diarrhoea, often with blood in the stool, and sometimes perforation or terminal jaundice.

*Pseudomembranous enterocolitis* [18] is precipitated by antimicrobial *drugs*, in particular lincomycin, clindamycin and ampicillin, but sometimes by penicillin, cotrimoxazole, cephalosporins, chloramphenicol, gold or metronidazole: the organism commonly found is *Clostridium difficile*.

Other important infective causes of diarrhoea include dysentery and salmonella, and, in developing countries, giardiasis, bilharzia, trichuriasis, amoebiasis and malaria. Giardiasis is associated with steatorrhoea, diarrhoea, abdominal distension or abdominal pain [3]. For the *haemolytic uraemic syndrome*, see p. 57. There is sometimes a family history of *coeliac disease* (p. 10). *Granulomatous disease* is similar.

*Hirschsprung's disease* may present in the newborn baby with diarrhoea, thus confusing the diagnosis.

*Acute appendicitis*, which can occur at any age, including infancy, may be associated with diarrhoea, especially when there is peritonitis, or when the appendix is pelvic, retrocaecal or retroileal (p. 110), and intussusception may be accompanied by diarrhoea (p. 113).

*Ulcerative colitis* may begin in early infancy as intermittent attacks of diarrhoea, in the first place without blood or mucus in the stool. Later blood and mucus appear, sometimes with weight loss, defective physical growth, fever, clubbing of the fingers, arthritis, anaemia, thrombocytosis, stomatitis and enlargement of the liver. *Granulomatous colitis* is similar. The so-called *short gut* or short bowel syndrome [23] follows massive resection of the small intestine. It causes chronic diarrhoea and malabsorption.

For diarrhoea with blood in the stool, see the next section.

The catecholamine-secreting *neural tumours,* especially the ganglioneuroma, may cause chronic diarrhoea, possibly through vasoactive intestinal polypeptides [14].

For *malabsorption syndromes* see p. 9. Gastroenteritis or prolonged starvation may cause secondary lactase deficiency and so chronic diarrhoea.

Carbohydrate intolerance may be simulated by intolerance to lactulose in baby milk [10]. Symptoms ascribed to allergy to cow's milk may be related to lactose intolerance [9].

For allergy to cow's milk protein, see p. 13. Diarrhoea could be due to allergy to other substances, such as egg, fish or rice [15]. Allergy to soya [5] may cause diarrhoea, vomiting and weight loss.

*Congenital chloride diarrhoea* [11] is an autosomal recessive condition. There is often a history of hydramnios and a family history of the same complaint. There is persistent diarrhoea, failure to thrive, abdominal distension, hypochloraemia, hyponatraemia and high faecal chlorides.

For acrodermatitis enteropathica see p. 362.

Numerous *drugs* cause diarrhoea apart from those causing pseudomembranous colitis. Penicillin and ampicillin by mouth commonly cause diarrhoea. Other drugs include acetazolamide, antibiotics (e.g. rifampicin), boric acid poisoning, cimetidine, cytotoxic drugs, digoxin, ergotamine, fenfluramine, griseofulvin, ipecacuanha, iron, metronidazole, nalidixic acid, non-steroidal anti-inflammatory drugs, salicylates, thyroxin overdose, tranquillizers and viprynium.

*Unknown causes*

In either acute or chronic diarrhoea, the cause cannot always be determined [12]; further research will reduce the number of unexplained cases. In his review of severe protracted diarrhoea Milla [15] found that in 30 per cent of cases the cause was not known. It may have an auto-immune basis [16].

## References

1 Bakken AF. Temporary intestinal lactase deficiency in light treated jaundiced infants. *Acta Paediatr Scand* 1977; **66**: 91.

2 Buch DAL, Levin M, Wilkins B, *et al.* Toxic shock syndrome. *Arch Dis Child* 1985; **60**: 563.

3 Burke JA. Giardiasis in childhood. *Am J Dis Child* 1975; **129**: 1304.

4 Cohen SA, Hendricks KM, Mathis RK, Laramee S, Walter WA. Non-specific diarrhoea. *Pediatrics* 1979; **64**: 402.

5 Committee on nutrition. Soy-protein formulas: recommendation for use in infant feeding. *Pediatrics* 1983; **72**: 359.

6 Davidson M, Wasserman R. The irritable colon of childhood (Chronic nonspecific diarrhoea). *J Pediatr* 1966; **69**: 1027.

7 Dodge JA. Essential fatty acids, prostaglandins and the gastrointestinal tract. *Acta Paediatr Japonica* 1985; **27**: 153.

8 Dodge JA, Hamdi IA, Burns GM, Yamashiro Y. Toddler diarrhoea and prostaglandins. *Arch Dis Child* 1981; **56**: 705.

9 Harrison M, Kilby A, Walker-Smith JA, France NE, Wood CBS. Cow's milk intolerance; a possible association with gastroenteritis, lactose intolerance and IgA deficiency. *Br Med J* 1976; **1**: 1501.

10 Hendrickse R, Woolridge M, Russell A. Lactulose in baby milks causing diarrhoea, simulating lactose intolerance. *Br Med J* 1977; **1**: 1194.

11 Holmberg C, Perheentupa J, Launiala K, Hallman N. Congenital chloride diarrhoea. *Arch Dis Child* 1977; **52**: 255.

12 Larcher VF, Shepherd R, Francis DEM, Harries JT. Protracted diarrhoea in infancy. *Arch Dis Child* 1977; **52**: 597.

13 Levin M, Hjelm M, Kay JD, *et al.* Haemorrhage shock and encephalopathy: a new syndrome with a high mortality in young children. *Lancet* 1983; **2**: 64.

14 Long RD, Bryant MG, Mitchell SJ, *et al.* Clinicopathological study of pancreatic and ganglioneuroblastoma tumours secreting vasoactive intestinal polypeptide (vipomas). *Br Med J* 1981; **1**: 1767.

15 Milla PJ. Severe protracted diarrhoea in infancy. *Acta Paediatr Japonica* 1985; **27**: 178.

16 Mirakian R, Richardson A, Milla PJ. Protracted diarrhoea of infancy; evidence in support of an autoimmune variant. *Br Med J* 1986; **2**: 1132.

17 Pearl M, Kaufman DL, Helmick CG, *et al.* Cryptosporidiosis in tourists returning from Caribbean Islands. *N Engl J Med* 1985; **312**: 648.

18 Pittman FE. Antibiotic associated colitis, an update. *Adverse Drug Reaction Bulletin* 1979; **No. 75**: 268.

19 Public Health Laboratory Service Committee Disease Surveillance Centre. Toxic shock. *Br Med J* 1985; **1**: 1578.

20 Rodgers B, Karn G. Yersinia enterocolitis. *J Pediatr Surg* 1975; **10**: 497.

21 Santulli TV, Schnullinger JN, Heird WC, *et al.* Acute necrotizing entero-colitis in infancy. *Pediatrics* 1975; **55**: 376.

22 Savilahti E, Simell O. Chronic non-specific diarrhoea. *Arch Dis Child* 1985; **60**: 452.

23 Young WF, Swain VAJ, Pringle EM. Long term prognosis after major resection of small bowel in early infancy. *Arch Dis Child* 1969; **44**: 465.

# Blood in the Stool

When a newborn baby passes blood in the stool or vomits blood one determines whether it is the mother's blood or his own (p. 54). The bleeding may be due to vitamin K deficiency, especially if the baby is fully breast-fed; it may occur as late as a month or two after birth (p. 55).

If the stool is lined with blood, the source is commonly low in the alimentary tract. When there is red blood in a baby's stool, the source may be fairly high, while red blood in the stool of an older child would suggest a low source. These observations, however, are not entirely reliable.

Blood may have been added to a child's stool by the mother (p. 95).

The commonest causes of blood in the stool are constipation (trauma by hard stools) or dysentery.

The following is a classification based largely on anatomial distribution: there is overlap between the various groupings.

Bleeding from the nose or throat

Bleeding from the oesophagus. Hiatus hernia. Chalasia. Varices. Foreign body

Bleeding from the stomach. Gastritis. Peptic ulcer. Congenital pyloric stenosis

Bleeding from the intestine. Duplication. Volvulus. Meckel's diverticulum. Intussusception

Angioma. Telangiectasia. Polyp

Gardner's syndrome. Perforation

Mesenteric thrombosis

Necrotizing enterocolitis, dysentery, salmonella, campylobacter

In the tropics—amoebiasis, ancylostoma, malaria, bilharzia, trichuriasis

Ulcerative colitis, regional ileitis, granulomatous disease

Non-specific ulceration of the ileum [5]

Bleeding from fissure *in ano*, piles, prolapse

Bleeding from constipation—hard stools

Bleeding from trauma—thermometer, foreign body, child abuse

Cold injury (p. 65)
Allergy
Blood diseases. Wiscott–Aldrich syndrome (p. 64)
   Disseminated intravascular coagulation
   Haemolytic uraemic syndrome (p. 57)
Toxic shock syndrome
Tyrosinosis (p. 126)
Drugs
Cause not discovered

A rare cause, which, however, one has seen several times, is bleeding as a result of *acute rhinitis* or *tonsillitis.*

When one is asked to see an apparently well infant with long-lasting persistent vomiting (possetting), one asks whether there is blood in the vomitus. That would suggest hiatus hernia.

Bleeding from *congenital pyloric stenosis* is rare. Probably the most likely cause of a bleeding gastric ulcer is a drug (see below).

*Duplication of the intestine* or duplication cysts can cause considerable blood loss and abdominal distension.

A *haemangioma* of the intestine [2] or *intestinal telangiectasia* may be difficult to diagnose. Facial telangiectasia may provide the clue, as may the finding of blue naevi [3] or Turner's syndrome. Other rare vascular anomalies may be responsible [6].

When the bleeding is from *Meckel's diverticulum,* the blood is usually dark [4]. There is an association between Meckel's diverticulum and Turner's syndrome.

A survey of fifty cases of *rectal polyposis* [7] showed that all had rectal bleeding and seven had abdominal pain. Most of the children were aged 2 to 6 years. *Gardner's syndrome* [1] consists of intestinal polyposis, multiple osteomata and epidermoid tumours.

For *allergy to cow's milk or soya,* see p. 13.

For the *toxic shock syndrome,* see p. 92.

*Drugs* are an important cause of bleeding. Aspirin and non-steroidal anti-inflammatory drugs are the chief offenders (p. 85). Other drugs include acetazolamide, chlortetracycline, cytotoxic drugs and thiazide diuretics. Bleeding has resulted from severe *hypernatraemia* due to accidental or deliberate addition of salt to an infant's feeds.

*No known cause.* It is often impossible to determine the cause of blood in the stool despite full investigation.

## References

1 Jones EL, Cornell WP. Gardner's syndrome: review of the literature. *Arch Surg* 1966; **92:** 287.
2 Nader PR, Margolin F. Hemangioma causing gastrointestinal bleeding. *Am J Dis Child* 1966; **111:** 215.
3 Rook A, Wilkinson DS, Ebling FJG. *Textbook of dermatology*. Oxford: Blackwell Scientific Publications, 1979.
4 Rutherford RB. Meckel's diverticulum; a review of 148 paediatric patients with special reference to the pattern of bleeding and to mesodiverticular bands. *Surgery* 1966; **59:** 618.
5 Sunaryo FP, Boyle JT, Ziegler MM, Heyman S. Primary non-specific ileal ulceration as a cause of massive rectal bleeding. *Pediatrics* 1981; **68:** 247.
6 Taube M. Vascular abnormalities in the bowel. *Hospital Update* 1983; **9:** 261.
7 Toccalino G, Guastavino E, De Pinni F, O'Donnell JC, Williams M. Juvenile polyps of the rectum and colon. *Acta Paediatr Scand* 1973; **62:** 337.

# The Colour of the Stools

The following are the principal colour changes in stools:
  Black
      Meconium
      Bilberries
      Altered blood
      Iron, bismuth, lead
      Possibly liquorice
      Charcoal
      Eating earth or coal
  Abnormally pale
      Obstructive jaundice, including infective hepatitis
      Steatorrhoea
      Aluminium hydroxide
      The periodic syndrome. Stools are often pale in the attacks
  Green
      Breast feeding. It is normal for the stools of fully breast-fed or
        bottle-fed babies to be bright green in colour at times.
        They may be green when passed, or become green on
        standing

Diarrhoea
Red
  Blood
  Viprynium (for threadworms)
  Dioralyte
  Red gelatin desserts
  *Serratia marcescens*
Pink
  Diazepam syrup
  Phenolphthalein in teething powders; the stool is sur-
    rounded by a salmon-pink collar which changes to
    mauve when hot water is poured on to it
The non-pathogenic organism *Serratia marcescens* may produce an
alarming red colour in the baby's nappy.


# Pain—General Comments


When we attempt to assess the significance and severity of pain or
what we think is pain, we face the difficulty of assessing someone
else's pain. In fact we can only assess it by inference.

The infant shows that he has pain by crying. There are many causes
of crying other than pain, and many an infant is thought to have pain
when he has no such thing. The fact that he draws his legs up and cries
does not mean that he has pain, for babies usually 'draw up their legs'
when they cry for any reason. I have had numerous babies referred to
me on account of 'acute indigestion' and 'terrible wind', which was
supposed to be the reason for the cries in the night, when the crying
was due entirely to the usual causes of sleep problems—mainly bad
habit formation and parental anxiety. Infants may rub their ears when
they have earache, or roll or hold their head when they have a
headache, but infants rub the ear and roll or hold the head when they
have no pain. It may be difficult to decide whether the infant has pain
or not. Severe pain causes a child to emit high-pitched screams. The
cry of pain is different from that of fatigue, boredom, loneliness or
other causes. The pain is not severe if the crying stops as soon as he is
picked up.

When the child is old enough to express his feelings in words, it is easier to decide whether he really feels pain. Even so, one has to assess the severity of his pain not by what he says, or even entirely on what the mother says about the pain, but by associated signs. For instance, a pain is not likely to be severe if it does not stop him playing, if it does not stop him eating, if it does not keep him awake, or if there is no change in his colour. A severe pain usually makes the child cry, though some children are more stoical than others. A severe abdominal pain is likely to make him double up. *It is always profitable to ask the mother whether she would know that he had the pain if he did not tell her. If she would not know, the pain is not severe.*

We have to assess the child's pain not only by the presence or absence of associated signs, but by our assessment of the mother's personality. The question of whether or not the child is taken to the doctor on account of his pain depends on the parental threshold for anxiety. Some loving mothers will take him to the doctor if he has the most trivial and short-lasting pain; others take him to the doctor only when the pain is severe and frequent. Some mothers aggravate a child's pain by displaying anxiety about it, by rubbing his abdomen, petting him and giving him pleasant warm drinks, so that he complains all the more as an attention-seeking device. In order to assess his pain, one has to assess the family pattern of behaviour as a whole and to determine whether other members of the family have similar pains. This is not merely because migraine or peptic ulcer commonly has a hereditary basis; it is because a child may imitate his parents, consciously or unconsciously, or fear that he has the same symptoms. If his father frequently complains about his gastric symptoms, or has had to go to hospital on their account, or if the mother is seen to have incapacitating attacks of migraine, it would not be surprising if the child also experienced pains, not necessarily due directly to peptic ulcer or migraine. When talking to a child about pain, it is important to ask whether any of his friends have a similar pain. The answer is frequently in the affirmative.

A child may experience pain (particularly in the head or abdomen) as a result of worries and anxieties about school. He may be in difficulty with a particular subject such as arithmetic, or he may be worried by a teacher's loud voice or threats of punishment. He may be worried because of bullying or because of teasing about his clothes, appearance or obesity. He may experience the pain when he is getting ready to go to school. He is not necessarily malingering; he is not pretending; he may really experience the pain, though it is entirely psychological in origin.

Pain may be suggested by an anxious mother. A few minutes after I had talked to a mother about her boy's abdominal pain, telling her that I had found no disease to explain it, she was overheard saying to the boy, 'Of course you have pain in your tummy, darling, haven't you?' He had.

Diagnostic errors may result from referred pain. Familiar examples are the following:

| Site of pain | Source of pain |
|---|---|
| Abdomen | Chest, testis, spine |
| Shoulder | Pulled elbow (p. 277), ruptured spleen, pleura, pancreas, diaphragm, gall bladder |
| Ear, face | Molar tooth |
| Wrist, shoulder | Elbow (e.g. pulled elbow) |
| Knee | Hip |

When a child (or adult) suffers two fractures to a limb, as in a road traffic accident, pain may be localized to the site of one fracture, so that the other fracture may be missed.

# Headache

Headache is a common symptom in childhood. Oster & Nielsen [9] found that 20·6 per cent of 2178 school children experienced headaches.

The commonest cause of headache before puberty is migraine [1] or an acute infection. Other common causes of headache are a stuffy room, lack of fresh air, climatic conditions (e.g. thunder), hunger, and emotional factors.

*Psychological causes of headache*

Emotional factors include worry about school work, an unkind teacher or bullying. The 'headache of convenience' may bring about a happy release from the arithmetic class. A headache may be an attention-seeking device.

## Migraine

For reviews see Bille [2], Collins [5], Selby & Lance [12] and Barlow [1]. Bille's review was based on a study of 9000 Swedish school children.

Symptoms of migraine commonly begin in early childhood. Vomiting attacks which recur and which later turn out to be due to migraine may begin as early as 6 months of age. Selby & Lance [12] found that 30 per cent of their 500 cases of migraine began before the age of 10. One in five also had travel sickness. Limb pains ('growing pains') are often an associated feature.

Migraine may manifest itself in childhood by any combination of the following symptoms—headache, vomiting, abdominal pain or fever, often associated with the passage of pale stools [3]. This group of symptoms is commonly termed the 'periodic syndrome'. It used to be called 'cyclical vomiting'.

There may be premonitory visual, auditory, sensory or mental symptoms, aphasia, blurring of vision, paraesthesia, or photophobia—sometimes occurring without a headache. The commonest visual aura consists of fortification figures or scintillating scotomata. It is said that a convulsion can occur in the premonitory phase.

The headache, commonly throbbing, is unilateral or bilateral. Selby & Lance [12] found that 38 per cent of their 500 cases had hemicrania, 21 per cent always had the headache on the same side and 38 per cent had pain all over the head. The attacks may last an hour or two or 2 to 3 days. They commonly last a few hours and are relieved by sleep. It is important to note that between attacks the child is entirely well and free from headache.

There are several variants of migraine. In *basilar artery migraine* there may be transient visual disturbance, vertigo, ataxia, dysarthria, ptosis, paraesthesia, tinnitus or vomiting, sometimes without a headache. It is more common in girls and usually begins before the fourth year. The attacks clear completely [7]. *Cluster headaches* consist of short-lasting attacks of eye pain or headache, sometimes with lacrymation and nasal discharge, with flushing or Horner's syndrome [13], occurring especially at night. They last up to half an hour, and often occur in clusters of several attacks a day, for a few weeks at a time. *Ophthalmoplegic migraine* consists of an attack of migraine followed, especially when the headache subsides, by ophthalmoplegia. It has been seen as early as 5 months of age [14]. In *hemiplegic migraine* there is headache localized to the eyes, followed by third nerve palsy on the same side. There may be ptosis, paralysis of pupillary constrictor fibres, nausea and vomiting. It occurs especially in infancy or early childhood. Sometimes the hemiplegia occurs first on one side and then on the other. It has been suggested that 'benign paroxysmal vertigo' (p. 204) is a migraine equivalent.

In 90 per cent of cases of migraine there is a family history of the complaint—an important diagnostic feature. I would suspect the diagnosis if there were not a family history of it.

The attacks are precipitated by many different factors—emotional disturbance, fatigue, menstruation, hunger, exposure to the sun, bright lights, loud noise, long car journeys, infections or head trauma. Certain foodstuffs are common precipitating factors. They include monoamine-containing foods, especially cheese (containing tyramine), and chocolate (containing phenylethylamine), monosodium glutamate (Chinese restaurant or Kwok disease) [4, 10] and other food additives. In Kwok disease there may be numbness of the face and neck, vertigo, headache, vomiting and abdominal pain. The role of food allergy or hypersensitivity, apart from the above, is disputed, but there is some evidence of it [6].

The initial symptoms of migraine are associated with vasoconstriction of the intracranial arteries, leading to visual and other symptoms, followed by dilatation of the vessels with the development of the headache.

*Organic causes of headache*

There are many organic causes of headache, and the differential diagnosis may be difficult—largely because there are no pathognomonic signs of migraine. The recurrent attacks of migraine may give a false sense of certainty of diagnosis. A child may have several attacks of migraine, followed by an attack with similar symptoms, but due to pyogenic meningitis.

The nature of the headache is of some value in diagnosis. An occipital headache is more likely than a frontal one to be due to an organic lesion, though a supratentorial tumour commonly causes a frontal headache. The headache of increased intracranial pressure is liable to be affected by change of posture, or by coughing or sneezing; it is worse on rising in the morning, or on stooping or straining. It is often a dull throbbing or bursting pain, while a headache of nervous origin is more likely to consist of a feeling of pressure. The headache of migraine may be of a throbbing nature.

In order to make the diagnosis of migraine and distinguish it from other conditions, one must determine whether, as in the case of epilepsy, the child is entirely well between attacks. If a child, thought to have migraine, is unwell between the attacks, is tired, has a poor appetite, has lost weight or has become clumsy in movement, serious intracranial disease is the likely diagnosis. Nevertheless, in the case of an older child, in which the headaches are thought to be psychological in origin ('tension headache') and not migraine, the child might not be entirely free from symptoms between attacks; there might, for instance, be a mild headache with acute exacerbations: but the story of increasing symptoms, especially of lassitude and certainly weight loss or neurological symptoms, would suggest organic disease (see epilepsy p. 390). Symptoms suggestive of a cerebral tumour [8] would be a headache of recent onset, a changing character of headache, increasing frequency or severity of headache, onset especially on awakening, a headache which repeatedly awakens the child, the occurrence of vomiting, behaviour change or deteriorating school performance.

Organic causes of headache include the following:

Infection. Earache. Toothache

Hypertension, kidney disease, phaeochromocytoma (p. 46)

Intracranial causes—tumour, abscess, meningitis, encephalitis, benign intracranial hypertension, vascular abnormalities

Head injury

Glaucoma (rare)

Eye strain (very rare)

Chronic antrum infection (rare cause)

Basilar impression syndrome

Drugs. Lead poisoning

The routine clinical examination of children complaining of headache readily excludes hypertension as the cause; but one has seen serious errors made because the examination had not included blood pressure determination and ophthalmoscopy.

One is concerned about the possibility of an *intracranial aneurism* when a child has neurological symptoms and signs such as aphasia, paraesthesiae or hemiplegia in association with apparent migraine attacks. Scanning procedures make the diagnosis easier than it was in the past.

Unless there is laceration of the brain, *head injuries* are infrequently followed by sequelae in the way of headaches. Emotional factors prior to the head injury are relevant. Nevertheless, when headaches follow a head injury, one must eliminate subdural effusion and other conditions by a scan and other methods.

*Benign intracranial hypertension,* with a sudden onset of a sixth nerve palsy and papilloedema, may follow a respiratory infection, otitis media or head injury. It may be caused by *drugs*—ampicillin, corticosteroids, nalidixic acid, nitrofurantoin or tetracyclines.

*Eye strain* is a most unlikely cause of headache, unless the symptom of eye strain, with severe myopia, is obvious. Glaucoma is a rare cause in children.

A *chronic antrum infection* is a most unlikely cause of recurrent headaches, especially in the first 7 or 8 years. One would find a history of a persistent purulent nasal discharge or postnasal discharge between colds.

Headache may be referred pain from the face or teeth.

The *basilar impression syndrome* causes persistent occipital headache. There is a short neck, cranial nerve palsy, nystagmus, ataxia or spasticity. It is due to a congenital abnormality of the upper cervical spine and base of the skull. It may be associated with the Klippel–Feil syndrome.

*Drugs* may cause headaches. They include acetazolamide, alcohol, anticonvulsants, antihistamines, ephedrine, ethambutol, fenfluramine, griseofulvin, isoniazid, methylphenidate, nalidixic acid, niclosamide, nitrofurantoin, non-steroidal anti-inflammatory drugs, sulphasalazine, theophylline, thiobendazole, trimethoprim, tranquillizers (e.g. benzodiazepines, sulphasalazine, tricyclics), and vincristine. Prolonged use of ephedrine nose drops may cause hypertension [11].

Lead-poisoning may cause headaches.

## References

1 Barlow CF. *Headaches and migraine in childhood.* Clinics in Developmental Medicine No. 91. Oxford: Blackwell Scientific Publications.

2 Bille B. Migraine in school children. *Acta Paediatr Uppsala* 1962; **51:** Suppl. 136.

3 Brown JK. Migraine and migraine equivalents. *Dev Med Child Neurol* 1977; **19:** 683.

4 Cochran JW, Cochran AH. Monosodium glutamania. The Chinese restaurant syndrome revisited. *JAMA* 1984; **252:** 899.

5 Collins KJ. Headache. *Austral Paediatr J* 1985; **21:** 245.

6 Egger J, Carter M, Wilson J, Turner MW, Soothill JF. Is migraine food allergy? *Lancet* 1983; **2:** 865.

7 Golden GS, Lapkun ML. Basilar artery migraine. *Am J Dis Child* 1978; **132:** 278.

8 O'Donohoe NV. Headache and tumours in children. *Br Med J* 1982; **2:** 4.

9 Oster J, Nielsen A. Growing pains. *Acta Paediatr Scand* 1972; **61:** 329.

10 Rief-Lehrer L. Monosodium glutamate intolerance in children. *N Eng J Med* 1975; **293:** 1204.

11 Saken R, Kates GL, Miller K. Drug induced hypertension in infancy. *J Pediatr* 1979; **95:** 1077.

12 Selby G, Lance JW. Observation on 500 cases of migraine and allied vascular headaches. *J Neurol Neurosurg Psychiat* 1960; **23:** 23.

13 Shinnar S, D'Souza BJ. The diagnosis and management of headaches in children. *Pediatr Clin N Am* 1982; **29:** 82.

14 Woody RC, Blaw ME. Ophthalmoplegic migraine in infancy. *Clin Pediatr (Phila)* 1986; **25:** 83.

# Abdominal Pain

## Acute abdominal pain

*General comments*

Joseph Brennemann, famous Chicago paediatrician, wrote 'After 40 years of extensive experience I still approach the acutely painful abdomen of a child with much apprehension and a greater feeling of uncertainty than any other domain of childhood.'

## The history

A detailed history is an essential step in the diagnosis. In the first place one needs to know how long the child has had the pain, asking in particular whether he ever had it before the date mentioned, and whether he was well before that date.

One next needs to know whether the pain is continuous or intermittent. If it is intermittent, one needs to know how frequent the attacks are, how long they last, and whether they are becoming more or less frequent. One often finds that the pain is infrequent—for example once in 3 or 4 months, and that when it occurs it only lasts for a minute or two. This is important, because one has to try to assess the significance of the complaint. In the case of an acute abdominal pain, it is usually true to say that a pain which comes and goes is unlikely to be due to appendicitis, the pain of which is more often continuous.

One needs to know where the pain is. Most of the non-organic recurrent abdominal pains of childhood are localized vaguely in the umbilical region. Apley [2] remarked that the further the pain is localized away from the umbilicus, the more likely is an underlying organic disorder. When a child complains of pain in one part of the body one day and a different part on another, and there is no constant localization, organic disease is less likely than when the pain is always localized to one area. An obvious exception to this is the pain of acute appendicitis, which may begin in the umbilical region and settle in the right iliac fossa.

The severity of the pain has to be assessed. Zachary [44] suggested that one should ask the child 'whether it is different from ordinary tummy-ache'. Apley found that a quarter of the children with recurrent abdominal pain without organic disease suffered from severe pain. He wrote that the truly severe pain, causing the child to thresh and writhe in agony, is hardly ever organic in origin. Whether the pain is continuous or intermittent, one must determine whether the pain is getting better or worse. One pays more attention to a pain which is becoming worse.

The nature of the pain may be helpful in diagnosis. A stabbing pain, feeling as if needles are being pushed in, may be pleural or peritoneal in origin. A pain which regularly comes and goes, lasting for a minute or two, with corresponding free intervals, suggests an alimentary origin.

The mode of onset may be important. A pain of instantaneous onset lasting a few minutes only and followed by sleep may be due to epilepsy. The duration of the pain is important. *An attack of abdominal pain lasting more than 3 hrs should be regarded as an abdominal emergency until proved otherwise.*

It may be useful to ask what brings the pain on, what relieves it and what makes it worse. A pleural pain (and sometimes a peritoneal pain) is worse on breathing or coughing.

It is vital to enquire about associated symptoms. An associated headache may point to migraine, though headache may be a symptom of fever. Associated diarrhoea suggests an alimentary origin. Associated urinary symptoms suggest a lesion of the urinary tract. In the case of acute abdominal pain, associated vomiting should indicate the need for great caution in the diagnosis, for it may well point to a condition for which surgical treatment will be needed. When the pain is due to an acute surgical condition, it usually precedes other symptoms, such as vomiting.

Finally one must assess the family as a whole. One must know whether other members of the family have abdominal pains. One must assess the personality of the parents, noting whether they are tense, anxious, worried or placid characters, for this will help one to establish the diagnosis.

## The examination

When a child presents with abdominal pain, the whole child must be examined, if for no other reason but the fact that many extra-abdominal conditions cause pain in the abdomen.

Many a small child steadfastly refuses to lie down when asked to do so, and determined efforts to get him to lie down will inevitably lead to tears, so that it becomes impossible to examine the abdomen adequately. It is reasonably satisfactory to examine the child's abdomen when he is standing or kneeling. Sometimes it is impossible to get the child to relax, and in that case, if accurate examination is vital, he should be given a sedative. Even if the child is crying, increased vigour of crying may help to localize the site of pain and tenderness.

Medical students commonly make the mistake of keeping the eyes on the abdomen when palpating it. I commonly tell them that omphaloscopy does not help in establishing the diagnosis. It is essential to watch the child's face in order to detect signs of abdominal tenderness. Another common mistake is to examine the abdomen when the head is elevated on two or more pillows. Unless the head is flat on the bed, or only slightly elevated on a low pillow (which is often preferable), it may be impossible to detect splenic enlargement.

Tenderness over the descending colon is not of importance. There may be only deep tenderness when an inflamed appendix is retrocaecal. Rectal examination is advised for any child with acute abdominal pain. One notes particularly whether there is more tenderness or heat on one side than on the other. Inspection of the scrotum and hernial orifices must not be omitted, e.g. for strangulated hernia or torsion of the testes.

Auscultation of the abdomen may contribute to the diagnosis of ileus, the absence of peristaltic sounds being the important feature of that condition.

## The diagnosis

The following are the main conditions which should be considered:

Infantile colic

Dietary indiscretion

Pain from vomiting, coughing or diarrhoea

Pain referred from the chest—lobar pneumonia, pleurisy, pleurodynia

Pain referred from the spine (rare)—discitis, (p. 284)

Diaphragmatic hernia

Alimentary tract—appendicitis, intussusception, obstruction, strangulated hernia, volvulus, Hirschsprung's disease
  Rare—Crohn's disease, Meckel's diverticulum

Food allergy

Mesenteric lymphadenitis, mesenteric cyst

Peritonitis

Pancreas—cystic fibrosis, diabetic acidosis, hypoglycaemia
  Rare—acute pancreatitis, pancreatic pseudocyst, Zollinger–Ellison syndrome (p. 85)

Liver—infective hepatitis

Gall bladder (rare)

Kidney—acute nephritis, calculus, Wilms' tumour, urinary tract infection

Phaeochromocytoma
Testis—torsion
Ovary (rare): twisted pedicle, ruptured cyst
Blood diseases—sickle-cell crises, haemophilia
   Anaphylactoid purpura
Hereditary angio-oedema
Infections—infectious mononucleosis, rheumatic fever
   Tropics—malaria, roundworm, strongyloides, bilharzia, trichuriasis
Collagen diseases (rare)
Porphyria (rare before puberty)
Drugs
   Lead poisoning
Trauma

A useful review is that of Hatch [15].

## Infantile colic

The term 'colic' is a term often wrongly applied to any infant who cries more than usual: it is not a diagnosis. Often it is due to excessive wind. If the baby is breast-fed it is due to sucking too long on the breast or sucking on an empty breast, and if he is bottle-fed it is almost always due to the feed taking too long because the hole in the teat is too small.

*Evening colic,* also called *three month colic* because it usually ceases by 3 months of age [18], affects well thriving babies, breast- or bottle-fed, largely confined to the evenings at about 18.00 hours, and therefore with a characteristic circadian rhythm. Occasionally it occurs at other parts of the day, and is then more likely to be confused with other causes of crying (p. 296). There may be an apparent recurrence of colic at about 6 months of age. The pain may be mild, merely causing the child to be restless in the evenings, or severe, with rhythmical screaming attacks, lasting a few minutes at a time, alternating with equally long quiet periods in which he almost goes to sleep, before another attack starts.

The rhythmical timing of the attacks, with the loud borborygmi, and the relief obtained by the passage of flatus *per rectum,* indicates an intestinal origin. I think that it may prove to be related to intestinal prostaglandins, vaso-active intestinal polypeptides or gut hormones (e.g. motilin, enteroglucagon, neurotensin, opioids), with their action on gut motility and secretions. The attacks are not due to gastric flatulence, but may well be due to intestinal spasm and wind becoming blocked in a loop of bowel.

Colicky pain in infants may sometimes be due to allergy to cow's milk protein, soya or other substances [18, 30]. It is possible that pain suffered by breast-fed infants may be due to substances such as cow's milk taken by the mother [20].

Attacks of infantile colic have surprisingly been confused with infantile spasms (p. 241). They could more justifiably be confused with colicky pain due to *intussusception*.

Abdominal pain may be due to *vomiting, coughing* or *diarrhoea*. It is common for infants or children (or adults) to experience pain in association with diarrhoea; the pain may precede diarrhoea. I saw an adult with acute abdominal pain and marked abdominal rigidity for 2 hrs before acute diarrhoea developed (due to Shiga dysentery): the pain had been promptly relieved by a saline infusion before the diagnosis was clear. Pain may be an early feature of *Hirschsprung's disease* in an attack of enterocolitis.

*Lobar pneumonia and pleurisy.* Referred pain from pleurisy with or without pneumonia is a common source of confusion in a child with acute abdominal pain. The finding of reduced air entry at one base, possibly with a slight alteration in the character of the breath sounds, or the so-called indux crepitations, should indicate lobar pneumonia. An X-ray of the chest confirms the diagnosis. *Epidemic pleurodynia* (Bornholm disease) may give rise to severe abdominal pain.

Abdominal pain may be a complaint when a child has *tonsillitis* or other respiratory tract infection, including measles. Sometimes it may be due to mesenteric lymphadenitis (see below).

### Appendicitis

The symptoms and signs of appendicitis are so well known that I do not propose to describe them here. Instead I shall draw attention to the common sources of error in diagnosis. Jackson of Newcastle [19] described many of these sources of confusion. They are as follows:

1   The appendix is not always in the 'typical' position. Of Jackson's 313 cases in childhood, the appendix was in the typical site in 32 per cent, retrocaecal in 27 per cent, pelvic in 23 per cent, and elsewhere (retro-ileal, subhepatic, splenic, or left iliac fossa) in 11 per cent. When the appendix is retrocaecal there may be no abdominal tenderness.

**2** It is only in 30 per cent of cases that the pain begins in the periumbilical region and then settles in the right iliac fossa. In 20 per cent the pain is confined to the central area, in 25 per cent it is confined to the right iliac fossa, whereas in the remaining 25 per cent it is situated elsewhere in the abdomen.

**3** Though the pain of appendicitis is usually continuous from the onset, it is occasionally intermittent. It was intermittent throughout in 12 per cent of Jackson's cases, and in a further 22 per cent it was intermittent first and continuous later.

**4** The pain may be mild or even absent. In four of Jackson's 313 cases there was no complaint of pain at all. Mildness of the pain may lead to delay in diagnosis.

**5** There is not always vomiting.

**6** There may be urinary symptoms and signs, particularly in children in whom the appendix is in the pelvis. About 12 per cent experience some dysuria. There may be an excess of white blood cells in the urine.

**7** Instead of the usual constipation there may be diarrhoea. About 10 per cent experience this symptom, which may cause serious confusion in the diagnosis. Diarrhoea is especially liable to occur in the infant or very young child, or when the appendix is pelvic, retrocaecal or retro-ileal. Hatch [15] suggested that in gastro-enteritis vomiting commonly precedes the onset of diarrhoea, while in acute appendicitis the vomiting is likely to follow the development of abdominal pain.

**8** Though the temperature is not usually high, above 5 per cent have a temperature of over 39°C.

**9** Appendicitis is rare under the age of 3 (though it can occur in early infancy), and when it does occur the diagnosis may be missed. In that age group acute appendicitis is likely to present as an abdominal mass due to perforation, general peritonitis, diarrhoea or dysuria, with fever and vomiting.

Auldist [3] reviewed 203 cases of appendicitis under the age of 5 years. He found anorexia in 99 per cent, vomiting in 94 per cent, pain in 93 per cent, fever in 68 per cent, respiratory symptoms in 31 per cent, and diarrhoea and constipation each in 26 per cent. In 38 per cent there was a palpable mass in the right iliac fossa. Shaul [37], writing about the diagnosis of acute appendicitis in the newborn, stated that, while the usual symptoms were irritability, vomiting and abdominal distension, often with excess of white cells in the urine, an important feature in some infants was oedema of the abdominal wall, often localized to the right flank, sometimes with erythema.

**10** Previous attacks of abdominal pain. In about one in every ten cases of acute appendicitis, there is a history of previous attacks of pain. Recurrent attacks of abdominal pain favour the diagnosis of a non-organic cause, though a child may have had a history of recurrent abdominal pain followed on this occasion by a different pain with fever due to appendicitis.

**11** Appendicitis may coexist with other conditions, notably acute tonsillitis, but also with pneumonia, urinary tract infection or even gastro-enteritis.

For *anaphylactoid purpura* see p. 63.

*Acute peritonitis* should be considered when a child is acutely ill with abdominal pain and fever, and generalized rigidity is found on abdominal examination. The commonest cause of peritonitis is a perforated appendix, but the peritonitis may be due to the pneumococcus or other pyogenic organism. Holgersen & Stanley-Brown [17], analysing 100 cases of acute appendicitis with perforation, found that vomiting, fever and abdominal pain were the main symptoms, but in 40 per cent there was an unlocalized abdominal pain, and in 5 per cent there was no pain at all. In one child the pain was confined to the testis. Four had had previous abdominal pain. The white cell count was not helpful in infancy, eight infants having a white cell count of less than 10,000. In twenty-eight there was albuminuria, in nine haematuria, and in sixteen acetonuria. There was a significant increase of white cells in the urine of twenty-four children.

*Mesenteric lymphadenitis.* This is difficult to distinguish from acute appendicitis. It is said that a shifting of the point of maximum tenderness on turning the patient on his side is in favour of mesenteric adenitis. It is not a reliable sign. The temperature tends to be higher in mesenteric adenitis than in appendicitis, but it is not always so. There may be tonsillitis in either case. There is usually more true rigidity over the right iliac fossa in a child with acute appendicitis. When there is doubt, and this is frequent, one will establish the diagnosis by laparotomy. *Mesenteric adenitis* may be due to *Yersinia, adenovirus, Coxsackie* or *Influenza B infection* [32].

## Intussusception

The common age at which intussusception occurs is 5 to 9 months. It is unusual after the first 2 years. In about half of all cases there is an associated infection by the *adenovirus* or *rotavirus* [25]. After the age of about 2 years, it may be associated with *Meckel's diverticulum, intestinal polypi, Henoch–Schönlein purpura* or *cystic fibrosis*. It is said to be more common in babies who are above the average weight and who are artificially fed. Intussusception should be strongly suspected when an infant becomes suddenly ill with abdominal pain, vomiting and pallor. The most common initial symptom is pain, and vomiting usually follows shortly after. The onset may be so sudden that the mother may be able to state the exact time at which the pain started. The pain is commonly rhythmical in character, coming and going. The child characteristically becomes pale in each spasm. He rapidly becomes ill and goes off his food, becoming pale and collapsed. In some cases there may be no pain at all, the only sign being sudden collapse with pallor and shock. These sudden attacks of pallor have led to the incorrect diagnosis of fits. Ein & Minor [13] found that there was no pain in fifty-six (13 per cent) of 422 cases of intussusception seen in Toronto. When there is no pain, early signs [33] may be apathy and listlessness, perhaps following an attack of vomiting. The colic commonly lasts for 2 or 3 min, recurring every 15 to 20 min. After three or four attacks the child is likely to be pale and drowsy. Intussusception should be suspected if attacks of colic persist for over 2 hrs. The passage of blood in the stool is not usually an early symptom. A history of previous attacks of abdominal pain is a point in favour of the diagnosis.

On examination in an early case there may be a palpable mass in the right upper quadrant of the abdomen; later there may be a tumour to the left of the midline. The mass is best felt during a spasm of pain. It is most often felt in the right hypochondrium but may be felt anywhere along the line of the colon. When in doubt and the child is crying, one palpates the abdomen after a sedative has been given. Even when one cannot feel a mass, there may be guarding over the upper part of the right rectus muscle. On rectal examination the rectum is empty; there may be blood on the finger stall.

In one series the full picture of abdominal pain, vomiting, rectal bleeding and a palpable mass was found in only 17 per cent [39].

Snares in diagnosis include the fact that some children pass a stool in the first 24 hrs after the onset of symptoms, so that intestinal obstruction is not suspected; there may be diarrhoea at the onset; there may be no blood in the stool, at least in the early stages; in about half of the cases, there is no vomiting for 6 to 12 hrs; there is often an elevation of temperature, and there is often a history of preceding upper respiratory tract infection; there may be a polymorphonuclear leucocytosis; and, most difficult of all, there may be no pain, the child presenting with unexplained shock and pallor of sudden onset.

Chronic intussusception may present with a history of days or weeks of abdominal pain, vomiting, constipation and the presence of blood and mucus in the stools. The diagnosis of ulcerative colitis or salmonella infection could easily be made in error [33].

The clinical diagnosis is confirmed by a scan or straight X-ray of the abdomen, followed, if necessary, by a barium enema.

### Other causes

Amongst other causes of intestinal obstruction, *intermittent volvulus* may result from a non-fixed but normally rotated intestine [21].

*Meckel's diverticulitis* may cause pain in the right iliac fossa. A previous history of blood in the stool, or in the presence of blood in the stool in the present attack, would suggest the diagnosis.

*Crohn's disease* (regional ileitis) is an important though rare cause of abdominal pain, often leading to unnecessary appendicectomy (p. 11).

Children with *cystic fibrosis* may experience attacks of abdominal pain, sometimes as a result of faecal impaction or gall bladder disease. Abdominal pain is an important symptom of *diabetic acidosis* or *hypoglycaemia*.

*Acute pancreatitis* is usually due to mumps [10] but may be due to biliary disease, or cystic fibrosis [40]. Three or four days after the swelling of the parotid gland in mumps there is vomiting, periumbilical pain, shock and then diarrhoea. There may be fever, bulky stools and polyuria.

Pancreatitis may be due to other virus infections, injury, cystic fibrosis, choledochal cyst, gallstones, hypercalcaemia, hyperlipoproteinaemia, malnutrition and drugs [5]. Symptoms are midabdominal pain (sometimes radiating to the back), abdominal tenderness, vomiting, fever and jaundice [22]. There is a hereditary (autosomal dominant) pancreatitis in childhood [16].

A *pancreatic pseudocyst* may develop about a month after injury in a cycle accident. The symptoms are abdominal pain, vomiting, fever and an abdominal mass, suggesting a diagnosis of appendicitis and perforation. The serum amylase is usually but not always raised [22]. The pancreatic pseudocyst may be the result of non-accidental injury [8].

Various *drugs* cause pancreatitis, particularly prednisolone [27]. Other drugs which may cause pancreatitis include diphenoxylate, chlorothiazide, frusemide, sulphasalazine, rifampicin, immunosuppressants, non-steroidal anti-inflammatory drugs, isoniazid, paracetamol, salicylates, sulphonamides, sodium valproate and tetracycline.

*Infective hepatitis.* Some children at the onset of infective hepatitis experience pain in the right upper quadrant of the abdomen. The diagnosis should be established by icterus and the presence of bilirubin in the urine.

*Cholecystitis* is rare in children [1]. It is accompanied by pain in the right upper quadrant of the abdomen, vomiting, fever and abdominal distension. It is difficult to distinguish from intestinal obstruction or a high retrocaecal appendicitis.

*Gallstones,* though rare, especially in the absence of acholuric jaundice, do occur in childhood, usually, but not always, with a family history of gall bladder trouble. They may complicate cystic fibrosis, or sickle cell disease. Gallstones may also occur in malformations of the biliary tract, small bowel dysfunction, Wilson's disease and metachromatic leucodystrophy [43]. Chang and colleagues [6] described fifteen children with congenital bile duct dilatation, probably choledochal cysts, presenting as abdominal pain, jaundice or fever, or a combination of those symptoms. Roslyn *et al.* [35] reported that jaundice developed in nine of twenty-one children receiving long-term parenteral nutrition.

*Hydrops of the gall bladder* [36] may present as an acute illness, with distension of the gall bladder without gallstones, with vomiting and abdominal pain: it can be confused with appendix abscess, intussusception or volvulus.

A child at the onset of *acute nephritis* may experience pain in the abdomen, leading to a diagnosis of appendicits. The diagnosis should be established by examination of the urine for albumin, red cells, granular and cellular casts.

*Renal colic* is an unusual cause of abdominal pain in children. It may result from sulphonamide crystalluria or from prolonged recumbency.

Abdominal pain only rarely results from *urinary tract infection*.

Pain from *torsion of the testis* may be referred to the abdomen.

An *ovarian cyst*, rupture of a *follicular cyst* or *twisted ovarian pedicle* may cause lower abdominal pain with shock and vomiting. Ein, Darte & Stephens [12] described seventy-five children presenting with abdominal pain, vomiting, nausea and abdominal swelling, due to ovarian tumour.

For *anaphylactoid purpura*, a common cause of acute abdominal pain, see p. 63. Rarely the pain may precede the development of purpura.

*Infections* are an important cause of abdominal pain, and include any which cause diarrhoea. *Acute rheumatic fever* may present with severe pain in the right iliac fossa.

*Sickle-cell anaemia crises* in coloured children may cause severe abdominal pain. The diagnosis is made by the haematologist. The pain may be accompanied by rigidity of the abdominal wall, pains in the legs, arthritis, flank pain or convulsions. Jaundice usually follows in 2 or 3 days.

*Glandular fever and acute infectious lymphocytosis* may be associated with abdominal pain.

Pain may be precipitated in *porphyria* by sulphonamides or barbiturates. There may be a history of vomiting and colicky abdominal pain, sometimes with photosensitivity, exposure to sunlight causing a vesicular or bullous eruption. There may be hypertrichosis, limb pains and tenderness of muscles, and red-coloured urine when sulphonamides or barbiturates are given.

*Drugs* which may cause abdominal pain include antibiotics, anticonvulsants, chloroquine, corticosteroids, cytotoxic drugs, dichlorophen, ergotamine, iodides, iron, metronidazole, non-steroidal anti-inflammatory drugs, piperazine, tranquillizers and viprynium.

*Lead poisoning* is a possible cause of abdominal pain.

*Conclusion*

The diagnosis of the cause of acute abdominal pain in a child may be a matter of the greatest difficulty. It is certainly a matter of the utmost importance, and many tragedies are caused by over-confidence, which so often involves delay in the diagnosis of some condition which could readily have been cured by prompt surgical treatment. It follows that there should be no hesitation in calling in expert advice when one is faced with the problem of a child with acute abdominal pain.

## Recurrent abdominal pain

Levine & Rappaport [27], discussing the difficulty in diagnosing the cause of recurrent abdominal pain, wrote 'It often is a test of stamina, or diagnostic self-confidence, of fiscal restraint and of vigilance for rare conditions. The clinician is apt to be haunted by the lingering question "Am I missing something?"' They then listed some seventy-five possible causes, rightly expressing doubt about the validity of the usual emphasis on psychological factors.

When faced with a child suffering from recurrent abdominal pain, the following conditions should be considered [7].

Psychological factors. Sexual abuse
Periodic syndrome
Hydronephrosis, urinary tract infection
Peptic ulcer
Abdominal epilepsy
Abdominal allergy
Sickle-cell anaemia
Lactose intolerance
Constipation
Worm infestation
Lead-poisoning
Torsion of testis
Malrotation
Rare—periodic peritonitis
    chronic relapsing pancreatitis
    hereditary angio-oedema
    regional ileitis

*Psychological factors* are of importance. In his monograph on *The child with abdominal pains* Apley [2] described a study of 1000 schoolchildren in Bristol. The incidence of abdominal pains was 12·2 per cent in girls and 9·5 per cent in boys. In 92 per cent of children referred for recurrent abdominal pain, no organic cause could be found after full investigation. In half of the affected children there was another member of the family who suffered from pains. Two out of three had associated vomiting, one out of two had pallor in the attacks, and one out of five had headaches. One out of four went to sleep after the attack. Various comparisons were made between affected children and controls. The incidence of appendicectomy was seventeen times greater than in controls and headaches were three times more frequent. The incidence of convulsions, however, was three times greater in controls than in the children with abdominal pains. There was a much greater incidence of headaches, nervous breakdowns and other nervous symptoms in the family of affected children than in the family controls. With regard to intelligence, there was no difference between the affected children and controls. The pain was umbilical in two-thirds; it consisted usually of a dull ache, and in a quarter it was severe. It occurred in the day or night, and occasionally in holidays. The duration and frequency varied considerably from child to child. Of thirty children followed up 8 to 12 years later, nine were symptom-free and three had migraine.

The possibility of *sexual abuse*, commonly with resulting depression, has to be remembered.

The *periodic syndrome* or migraine (p. 101) is a common cause of recurrent abdominal pain, commonly with fever, vomiting or pale stools.

In a study of 6000 Buckinghamshire schoolchildren, it was found that, up to the age of 10 years, 4 per cent had recurrent abdominal pain, at the age of 12 to 13 years 15 per cent had it and from 14 to 15 years 25 per cent had it [38]. In a study of 117 children with recurrent abdominal pain in Israel, organic disease was found in 10 per cent [42]. But I suspect that, as in the case of evening colic and toddlers' diarrhoea, a physiological basis will be found in time (e.g. related to prostaglandins or gut hormones) [10, 24, 31].

Complaints of pain may be an attention-seeking device. If the mother expresses anxiety about the child's complaints, rubs his abdomen, gives him sweets, medicine or a warm drink and makes him lie down, the pain is likely to recur.

A child may complain of pain in imitation of one of his parents, who is constantly complaining of his pains. He may feel worried about his parent's symptom and express his anxiety by feeling the same pain as that of his parent. Pains may be due to worry and anxiety—worries about bullying at school, fear of a teacher or dislike of being teased.

*Hydronephrosis* can cause troublesome abdominal pain. The pain is by no means always localized to the loins. It is frequently impossible to palpate the kidney and the urine may be normal on examination. Even if there is a pyonephrosis, the flow of urine from the affected kidney may be blocked, so that the urine examined is normal. One can never entirely eliminate hydronephrosis as a cause of abdominal pain without a pyelogram or ultrasound examination. Abdominal pains in children are common, and one wants to avoid pyelography where possible for four important reasons: it is unpleasant for the child; it involves irradiation; the child has to be deprived of fluid before the procedure and the hyperosmolar injection may cause dehydration; and there is a small risk of dangerous iodine sensitivity. One has to use one's judgment, therefore, in deciding whether an intravenous pyelogram is needed. The further danger of a retrograde pyelogram is the introduction of infection by instrumentation. Even if one finds a double renal element as a result of pyelography, one cannot be sure whether the pain is related to the renal anomaly or not. For urinary tract infection, see p. 320.

There are widely differing views as to the frequency of *peptic ulceration* in children. Some regard it as common while some think it is rare. Many adults with proved peptic ulcer date the onset of abdominal symptoms to childhood. The symptoms in a child are more vague and indefinite than they are in an adult [26]. An analysis of fifty cases [40] showed that twenty had no pain at all; only twenty-eight had epigastric pain; five with a perforated duodenal ulcer (and one other) had pain in the right lower quadrant, suggesting appendicitis; twenty-nine had gastrointestinal bleeding, suggesting Meckel's diverticulum. Pain is often nocturnal. Diagnosis is likely to be established by fibre-optic endoscopy.

Drugs which in particular may be responsible are aspirin and non-steroidal anti-inflammatory drugs.

One has seen several examples of recurrent volvulus which had been wrongly thought to have been the periodic syndrome (migraine) or pains of psychological origin [23].

*Abdominal epilepsy* is a possible cause of recurrent abdominal pain [11]. In order to make the diagnosis one must obtain a history that the attacks are of sudden onset, last a few minutes only and are followed by sleep. An electro-encephalogram may confirm the diagnosis, but the EEG is frequently normal in epilepsy of grand mal type. The therapeutic test of phenytoin in full dosage is perhaps a more reliable method of establishing the diagnosis.

Though some would say that *allergy* is a common cause of abdominal pain, I have seen few children for whom I found this diagnosis satisfactory [7]. Nevertheless, one should ask whether any particular food causes the child's pain. One may then try to prevent the pain by elimination diets. So-called *milk allergy* may prove to be *lactose or sucrose intolerance* [4, 29]. Liebman [29] found lactose intolerance in eleven of thirty-eight children with recurrent abdominal pain.

*Constipation* is commonly blamed for abdominal pain in children. Unless there is impaction of faeces causing intestinal obstruction, I am doubtful whether constipation ever causes abdominal pain in children. Children with gross constipation, often with soiling, rarely suffer from abdominal pain as a result, but a child may have pain on passing a hard stool. If they do not have pain, it seems unlikely that children with a much less degree of constipation would have pain either. Davidson [9] ascribed many recurrent abdominal pains to hypertonus of the colon with excessive drying of the stool and therefore constipation. Attacks of intestinal obstruction, abdominal pain and faecal impaction in older children, termed meconium ileus equivalent, are said to be fairly common [14].

*Worm infestation* with ascaris may cause pain. It is probably rare in Britain. Unless *threadworms* block the appendix. I find it difficult to believe that they would cause pain. I cannot imaging the mechanism whereby minute threads, averaging a few millimetres in length and lying loosely in the intestine would cause abdominal pain.

Reimann [33] described three *genetic causes of recurrent abdominal pain*: periodic peritonitis, occurring especially in Jews, Armenians, Turks and Arabs, sometimes with pleurisy; hereditary angioneurotic oedema (p. 49); and chronic relapsing pancreatitis.

*Unknown causes.* Usually there is no discoverable cause of recurrent abdominal pain in otherwise well children.

## References

1 Andrassy RJ, Treadwell TA, Ratner IA, Buckley CJ. Gall bladder disease in children and adolescents. *Am J Surgery* 1976; **132:** 19.
2 Apley J. *The child with abdominal pains.* Oxford: Blackwell Scientific Publications, 1975.
3 Auldist AW. Appendicitis in patients under five years of age. *Austr Paed J* 1967; **3:** 144.
4 Barr RG, Levine MD, Watkins JB. Recurrent abdominal pain of childhood due to lactose intolerance. *N Engl J Med* 1979; **30:** 1449.
5 Buntain WL, Wood JB, Woolley MM. Pancreatitis in childhood. *J Pediatr Surg* 1978; **13:** 143.
6 Chang GM, Wang T, Chen C, Hung W. Congenital bile duct dilatation in children. *J Pediatr Surg* 1986; **21:** 112.
7 Crook WG. Recurrent abdominal pain. *Am J Dis Child* 1980; **134:** 326.
8 Dahman B, Stephens CA. Pseudocyst of the pancreas after blunt abdominal trauma in children. *J Pediatr Surg* 1981; **16:** 17.
9 Davidson M. Recurrent abdominal pain. *Am J Dis Child* 1971; **121:** 179.
10 Dodge JA. *Topics in pediatric gastroenterology.* London: Pitman Medical, 1976.
11 Douglas EF, White PT. Abdominal epilepsy—a reappraisal. *J Pediatr* 1971; **78:** 59.
12 Ein SH, Darte JMM, Stephens CA. Cystic and solid ovarian tumors in children. *J Pediatr Surg* 1970; **5:** 148.
13 Ein SH, Minor A. The painless intussusception. *J Pediatr Surg* 1976; **11:** 563.
14 Hanly JG, Fitzgerald MX. Méconium ileus equivalent in older patients with cystic fibrosis. *Br Med J* 1983; **1:** 1411.
15 Hatch EI. The acute abdomen in children. *Pediatr Clin N Am* 1985; **32:** 1151.
16 Hilmer RS, Nayanar VV, Bohane TJ. Hereditary pancreatitis presenting in childhood. *Austr Paediatr J* 1985; **21:** 201.
17 Holgerson LO, Stanley-Brown EG. Acute appendicitis with perforation. *Am J Dis Child* 1971; **122:** 288.
18 Illingworth RS. Infantile colic revisited. *Arch Dis Child* 1985; **60:** 981.
19 Jackson RH. Parents, family doctors and acute appendicitis in childhood. *Br Med J* 1963; **2:** 277.
20 Jacobsson I, Lindberg T. Cow's milk proteins cause infantile colic in breast fed infants: a double blind crossover study. *Pediatrics* 1983; **71:** 268.
21 Janik JS, Ein SH. Normal intestinal rotation with non fixation: a cause of chronic abdominal pain. *J Pediatr Surg* 1979; **14:** 670.
22 Jordan SC, Ament ME. Pancreatitis in children and adolescents. *J Pediatr* 1977; **91:** 211.

23 Kullendorf CM, Mikaelsson C, Ivancen K. Malrotation in children with symptoms of gastrointestinal allergy and psychosomatic abdominal pain. *Acta Paediatr Scand* 1985; **74**: 296.

24 *Lancet*. (Leading article re prostaglandins) Primary dysmenorrhoea. 1980; **1**: 800.

25 *Lancet*. Acute intussusception in childhood. Leading article. 1985; **2**: 250.

26 *Lancet*. Duodenal ulcer in childhood. Leading article. 1987; **2**: 891.

27 Lendrum R. Drugs and the pancreas. *Adverse Drug Reaction Bulletin* 1981; **No. 90**: 328.

28 Levine MD, Rappaport LA. Recurrent abdominal pain in school children: the loneliness of the long-distance physician. *Pediatr Clin N Am* 1984; **31**: 969.

29 Liebman WM. Recurrent abdominal pain in children. Lactose and sucrose intolerance. *Pediatrics* 1979; **64**: 43.

30 Lothe L, Lindberg T, Jacobsson I. Cow's milk formula and infantile colic. *Pediatrics* 1982; **70**: 7.

31 Lucas A, Mitchell MD. Prostaglandins in human milk. *Arch Dis Child* 1980; **55**: 950.

32 Prince RL. Evidence for an aetiological role for adenovirus type 7 in the mesenteric adenitis syndrome. *Med J Austr* 1979; **2**: 56.

33 Rachmel A, Rosenbach Y, Amir J, *et al*. Apathy as an early manifestation of intussusception. *Am J Dis Child* 1983; **137**: 701.

34 Reimann HA. Three periodic diseases as causes of recurrent abdominal pain in childhood. *Arch Dis Child* 1976; **51**: 244.

35 Roslyn JJ, Berquist WE, Pitt HA, *et al*. Increased risk of gallstones in children receiving total parenteral nutrition. *Pediatrics* 1983; **71**: 784.

36 Rumley TO, Rodgers BM. Hydrops of the gallbladder in children. *J Pediatr Surg* 1983; **18**: 138.

37 Shaul WL. Clues to the early diagnosis of neonatal appendicitis. *J Pediatr* 1981; **98**: 473.

38 Shepherd M, Oppenheim B, Mitchell S. *Child behaviour and mental health..* London: Univ. of London Press, 1971.

39 Sparnon AL, Little KET, Morris LL. Intussusception in childhood: a review of 139 cases. *Austr NZ Surg* 1984; **54**: 353.

40 Tam PKH, Saing H, Irving IM, Lister J. Acute pancreatitis in childhood. *J Pediatr Surg* 1985; **20**: 58.

41 Tam PKH, Saing H, Lau JTK. Diagnosis of peptic ulcer in children: the past and present. *J Pediatr Surg* 1986; **21**: 15.

42 Versano I, Zeidel A, Matoth Y. Recurrent abdominal pain in children. *Paediatrician* 1977; **6**: 90.

43 *Year Book of Pediatrics*. Gallstones. Editorial. 1984; 165.

44 Zachary RB. Diagnosis of the acute abdomen in childhood. *Br Med J* 1965; **1**: 635.

# Abdominal Distension

*Non-disease*

Abdominal distension is not necessarily due to disease. Infants swallow large quantities of air during a feed. Excessive wind experienced by a breast-fed baby is likely to be due to his sucking too long on the breast or sucking on an empty breast. By far the commonest cause of a formula-fed baby having excessive wind is too small a hole in the teat, so that the sucking is prolonged. Babies swallow air when crying for a prolonged period, with resulting abdominal distension.

Many toddlers are thought to have a big abdomen when they are normal. If there is lordosis the abdomen may appear to be unduly large. One occasionally sees marked distension as a result of severe constipation (without Hirschsprung's disease). A fat child may have a large abdomen.

For reasons which are not clear, a child suffering severe emotional deprivation (non-accidental injury) may have an unusually large abdomen (p. 8).

*Neonatal abdominal distension*

The most important organic causes of abdominal distension in the very young infant are as follows [5]:

  Phototherapy
  Intestinal obstruction, meconium ileus or plug, lactobezoar
  Perforation of alimentary, biliary or urinary tract
  Congenital heart disease
  Tracheo-oesophageal fistula, forcing air into the stomach
  Hirschsprung's disease
  Tumours and cysts, especially renal tumours, intestinal
      duplication
  Infection—septicaemia, peritonitis, necrotizing enterocolitis,
      pneumonia
  Congenital nephrotic syndrome (rare)

Urethral obstruction: distended bladder
Low potassium
Drugs—chloramphenicol

After *phototherapy* a baby may have abdominal distension and loose stools.

*Rupture of the stomach* of the newborn baby leads to abdominal distension, respiratory distress, vomiting and melaena, commonly on about the third day [3]. On auscultation no bowel sounds can be heard. Oedema of the abdominal wall suggests peritonitis. Even in newborn infants, *appendicitis* may occur, usually with perforation. The symptoms are vomiting, abdominal distension and shock. *Perforation of the colon* of a newborn baby suggests Hirschsprung's disease or meconium peritonitis. Colonic perforation may follow an exchange transfusion [4]. Four to 15 hrs after the transfusion the child becomes poorly, develops abdominal distension and vomits, and there is usually blood in the stool. On auscultation no bowel sounds are heard.

*Perforation of the rectum* by a rectal thermometer is a well-known hazard [7].

*Intestinal duplication or duplication cysts* may cause considerable swelling of the abdomen. The cysts are often mobile and may reach a considerable size. There may be abdominal pain and rectal bleeding. A ladder pattern of visible peristalsis indicates obstruction.

Byrne *et al.* [1] described eleven children with '*pseudo obstruction*'. There were episodes of abdominal pain and distension, vomiting and constipation or diarrhoea. There was abnormal oesophageal motility and delayed gastric emptying. The prognosis was poor.

*Infections* may cause abdominal distension. When a newborn baby develops septicaemia, in addition to distension of the abdomen there is often vomiting, diarrhoea, jaundice, lethargy, respiratory distress and apnoeic attacks. It may be due to Gram-negative bacteria or group B streptococci. For necrotizing enterocolitis see p. 92.

When there is *urethral obstruction* (due to urethral valves, etc.) there may be gross enlargement of the bladder. The diagnosis, suspected on account of the fact that the swelling involves the lower abdomen more than the upper part, is confirmed by observation of the stream of urine and by running an opaque substance into the bladder and inverting the baby, so that the material will run into the patulous ureters. There may be perforation of the urinary tract when obstruction is severe, with ascites. *Neonatal ascites* should be regarded as due to obstructive uropathy until proved otherwise.

*Ascites* can be due to congenital heart disease, nephrosis, congenital cirrhosis, congenital cytomegalovirus infection or peritonitis due to meconium or syphilis. The ascites can also be chylous, as a result of malformation of the lymphatic system, rupture of a mesenteric cyst, neoplasm, trauma or obstruction of the lymphatic system: often the cause cannot be determined.

*Chloramphenicol* in an overdose in the newborn period causes abdominal distension, cyanosis, shock and other manifestations of the 'grey syndrome'.

### Abdominal distension subsequent to the newborn period

The causes after the newborn period include the following:

Aerophagy

Intestine—obstruction, ileus, perforation, duplication, cysts, Hirschsprung's disease

Omentum and mesentery—cysts, mesenteric thrombosis

Ascites—diseases involving the heart (congestive failure)

Pericardium (constrictive pericarditis)

Kidney (acute nephritis, nephrotic syndrome)

Liver (cirrhosis, portal hypertension)

Pancreas (chronic pancreatitis)

Inferior vena cava—thrombosis, other obstruction

Lymphatic obstruction: congenital, chylous ascites, trauma, tuberculosis, Hodgkin's disease

Hypoproteinaemia: beriberi

Liver—cyst, tumour, storage diseases, tyrosinosis, sub-capsular haematoma

Gall bladder—choledochal cyst, perforation of bile ducts, cholecystitis (p. 115)

Kidney—tumour, hydronephrosis, polycystic disease, renal vein thrombosis

Adrenal—neuroblastoma, haemorrhage

Spleen—leukaemia, haematoma

Pancreatic cyst (p. 115)

Sclerosing peritonitis from a ventriculoperitoneal shunt [6]

Ovary—cyst

Vagina—hydrocolpos
Uterus—pregnancy
Sacrococcygeal teratoma, dermoid, anterior meningocele
Hypokalaemia
Carbohydrate or fat malabsorption
Allergy to cow's milk

*Aerophagy* sometimes occurs in older children [2].

*Tyrosinosis* presents in early infancy with failure to thrive, fever, diarrhoea, vomiting, hepatomegaly and abdominal distension. There may be melaena, haematemesis, haematuria and jaundice, with glycosuria and generalized aminoaciduria.

*Gaucher's disease* occurs in two forms—acute infantile, with moderate hepatosplenomegaly and bulbar palsy, ending fatally by the age of 2 to 6 years, and the chronic form, with early abdominal enlargement, splenomegaly rather than hepatomegaly and bone pain.

*Drugs* which may cause abdominal distension include diphenoxylate and indomethacin.

## References

1 Byrne WJ, Cipel L, Euler AR, Halpin TC, Ament ME. Chronic idiopathic intestinal pseudo-obstruction syndrome in children. *J Pediatr* 1977; **90:** 585.
2 Gauderer MWL, Halpin TC, Izant R. Pathological childhood aerophagia: a recognizable clinical entity. *J Pediatr Surg* 1981; **16:** 301.
3 Gwinn JL, Lee FA. Rupture of the stomach in the newborn infant. *Am J Dis Child* 1970; **119:** 257.
4 Hardy JD, Savage TR, Shirodaria C. Intestinal perforation following exchange transfusion. *Am J Dis Child* 1972; **124:** 136.
5 Koop CE. Abdominal mass in the newborn infant. *N Engl J Med* 1973; **289:** 569.
6 La Ferla G, McColl KE, Crean GP. Cerebrospinal fluid induced sclerosing peritonitis: a new entity? *Br J Surg* 1986; **73:** 7.
7 Wolfson JJ. Rectal perforation in infants by thermometer. *Am J Dis Child* 1966; **111:** 197.

# Jaundice

## Jaundice in infancy

The following statements can be made with little fear of contradiction:

**1** The diagnosis of the cause of prolonged jaundice in a young infant is commonly one of great difficulty.

**2** Jaundice on the first day of life must be considered to be due to haemolytic disease until proved otherwise.

**3** Physiological jaundice is not seen in the first 24 hrs. With rare exceptions, jaundice after the first week in a full-term baby is not physiological and must be investigated; but breast milk jaundice may last for several weeks.

**4** In physiological jaundice, including breast milk jaundice, the urine and stools are a normal colour. There is no bilirubin in the urine and the stools contain normal bile pigments.

**3** Pale-coloured stools with a dark urine containing bilirubin signify an obstructive element. The commonest cause is neonatal hepatitis.

**6** In the newborn period, infection is an important cause of jaundice (e.g. septicaemia), particularly when the jaundice begins after the fourth day. The bilirubin is partly direct and partly indirect, so that the stools may be pale.

**7** It is essential that every effort be made to establish the correct diagnosis because some of the conditions demand urgent treatment.

### The diagnosis

Jaundice must be distinguished from the yellow colour of the skin caused by *carotenaemia*. This is due to the lipochrome carotene, predominantly present in carrots, but also in other yellow vegetables, including yellow corn, and in greens, in which the yellow is obscured by chlorophyll [11]. Chronic yellow staining of the hands and feet has been caused by tangerines and satsumas [5]. Yellow staining of the skin is usually due to an excess of carrots in the diet of a lactating mother, or an excess of puréed carrots in the baby's diet. Carotenaemia is also associated with *hypothyroidism, diabetes mellitus* and the *nephrotic syndrome*.

A similar condition is *lycopenaemia*, in which the skin is an orange-yellow colour, usually due to a large amount of tomatoes in the diet. Lycopene is an isomer of beta-carotene, and is the colouring matter in tomatoes (and tomato juice), beetroots and rosehips. Both pigments are present in commercial infant foods.

The skin is stained yellow by *mepacrine*.

The baby's skin may be yellow as a result of meconium staining in *postmaturity* and the *placental dysfunction syndrome*.

At the risk of some oversimplification, one can state that there are four main groups of causes of jaundice in the infant and young child. More than one of these causes may be operative at the same time. They are as follows:

**1** *Deficiency of the enzyme glucuronyl transferase.* Bilirubin is fat-soluble, and, before it can be excreted by the liver into bile or excreted in the urine, it must be converted into a water-soluble form by conjugation with glucuronic acid. In the absence of glucuronyl transferase this indirectly reacting pigment ('unconjugated') accumulates in the plasma and may damage the nervous system.

The following are the conditions in which deficiency of the enzyme glucuronyl transferase plays a part:

> Jaundice following severe hypoxia
> Hypothyroidism
> Breast milk jaundice
> Drugs given to the mother or newborn
> Rare causes
> > Maternal diabetes
> > Congenital pyloric stenosis
> > Crigler–Najjar syndrome
> > Gilbert's syndrome
> > Galactosaemia
> > Adrenocortical hyperplasia
> > Fructose intolerance
> > Hirschsprung's disease

*Physiological jaundice* is due to a combination of immaturity of the liver with consequent transferase deficiency, and the breakdown of red cells immediately after birth. The jaundice of prematurity, whose basis is the same, is more severe than that of the mature baby, because of greater immaturity of the enzyme system. Severe hypoxia during delivery or cold injury after delivery tends to increase the jaundice.

Physiological jaundice is not seen in the first 24 hrs. In a full-term baby it begins at the end of the second day and lasts for 2 or 3 days. It rarely lasts into the second week. If jaundice lasts into the second week in a full-term baby, the cause should be sought elsewhere.

The jaundice of a preterm baby begins later, is more severe and lasts longer. One would not expect physiological jaundice in a premature baby in the first 48 hrs. Physiological jaundice reaches its maximum about the fifth or sixth day (depending on the degree of immaturity), and in the smallest ones may last up to the 18th day. When food is withheld for 48 to 72 hrs after birth, the jaundice is increased. It is reduced by early feeding. Physiological jaundice is sometimes prolonged in hypothyroidism because of deficiency of the transferase enzyme.

*Breast milk jaundice*, for unknown reasons, has become common. The mean serum bilirubin is significantly higher in breast-fed infants than in those on formula feeds [1]. There is no correlation between the level of serum bilirubin and the degree of weight loss. The breast milk jaundice may occur as early as the third or fourth day. The jaundice clears as soon as breast feeding is discontinued and returns when it is restarted. It appears to be harmless, and has not caused kernicterus; there is no need to take the baby off the breast, and the jaundice disappears after a time without treatment. The theroy that it was due to an abnormal steroid in breast milk has been discarded—and the later theory, that it was related to lipoprotein lipase, found no support with Greek workers [6]. It may, in some way as yet unknown, be due to delayed maturation or inhibition of glucuronyl transferase [12]; but it is of interest that it may occur in only one of a family, and is therefore difficult to explain on a maternal metabolic basis. It is said [7] that the earlier the baby is put to the breast, and the more frequent the feeds, the lower is the serum bilirubin.

Drugs taken by the mother during pregnancy may be a factor in neonatal jaundice. They include corticosteroids, diazepam, novobiocin, phenothiazines, salicylates, sulphonamides and excess dosage of vitamin K. Oxytocin, given to start labour, increases the fetal bilirubin, probably by interfering with the glucuronyl transferase. Buchan [4] suggested that the oxytocin raised the infant's serum bilirubin by increasing the breakdown of red cells. Wood *et al.* [16], on the other hand, suggested that the apparent increase in the incidence of neonatal jaundice was more related to factors in breast milk or to epidural anaesthesia.

The *Crigler–Najjar syndrome* is a rare recessive condition in which there is a deficiency of transferase. Extrapyramidal rigidity develops in a few weeks and persists. The picture is similar to that of kernicterus. There is no evidence of haemolysis or of obstruction. The bilirubin is unconjugated.

*Gilbert's disease* is a much less serious congenital disease due to deficiency of the same enzyme. Mild jaundice with lassitude persists throughout life. It is non-haemolytic, and more common in males. It is inherited as an autosomal dominant. The bilirubin is unconjugated.

Occasionally infants with *congenital pyloric stenosis* have jaundice with raised serum bilirubin of indirect type. The explanation of this is unknown, but Bleicher *et al.* [3] suggested that it was due to inhibition of glucuronyl transferase by hypergastrinaemia.

The jaundice of *galactosaemia* may be due to delayed development of transferase or a toxic damage to the liver cells. When milk is given, the child goes off his food, vomits, loses weight, becomes jaundiced, and his liver and spleen enlarge.

Jaundice is sometimes an early feature of *adrenocortical hyperplasia* and of *fructose intolerance.*

It will be noted that in none of the above conditions is there bile in the urine, and in all of them the stools are of normal colour. In none of them is there haemolysis. The serum bilirubin is of the indirect or unconjugated variety.

**2** *Increased bilirubin production—mainly due to haemolysis.* The main conditions are as follows:

> Congenital haemolytic disease (rhesus or ABO incompatibility; more rarely Kell, Kidd or Duffy group)
> Hereditary spherocytosis or acholuric jaundice. Thalassaemia. Sickle-cell anaemia
> Drugs—vitamin K, neomycin, camphor, sulphonamides
> Infections—septicaemia, syphilis, Weil's disease
> Absorption of blood from a large cephalhaematoma or other haemorrhage

Glucose-6-phosphate dehydrogenase deficiency (p. 57)

Rarely pyruvate kinase deficiency

Jaundice on the first day must be regarded as *haemolytic disease* due to blood group incompatibility until proved otherwise. It is essential that a child with jaundice on the first day should be referred immediately to hospital for investigation and treatment, which may well consist of a replacement transfusion. Failure to do so without delay may lead to the death of the child or to kernicterus which is either lethal or crippling for life.

Though haemolytic disease due to rhesus incompatibility does not occur in the first pregnancy unless there has been a previous incompatible transfusion, that due to ABO incompatibility may occur in the first pregnancy, and it cannot be anticipated by tests during pregnancy. In this case the mother is usually group O and the baby group A, but the baby may be group B. Rarely the mother is group A and the infant group B, or vice versa. The Coombs test in the infant with ABO incompatibility is commonly negative.

The diagnosis of *congenital spherocytosis or acholuric jaundice* is readily established by the family history of that complaint, together with examination of the child's blood for spherocytes, reticulocytosis and abnormal red cell fragility.

*Vitamin K* in an overdose increases the level of jaundice by three possible mechanisms—haemolysis, a toxic action on the liver or by competing for conjugating enzymes. It should be remembered that if the mother is given large doses of vitamin K during delivery it is likely to affect the baby.

If nappies have been stored in *camphor balls,* the baby may absorb the camphor and develop haemolytic anaemia. Neomycin may cause some degree of haemolysis.

*Infections* cause jaundice partly by haemolysis and partly by a toxic action on the liver which may interfere with the transferase system [13]. The serum bilirubin is mostly unconjugated (indirect) but partly conjugated (direct). Jaundice appearing rapidly after the fourth day in a full-term infant should always be considered as infective in origin until proved otherwise; it may cause kernicterus. The relevant infections include septicaemia and syphilis. Sometimes the jaundice is the only manifestation of a urinary tract or other bacterial infection. The diagnosis of septicaemia would be strongly suggested by a moist umbilicus and would be confirmed by blood culture. An important cause is group B streptococcal infection from the mother's vagina. Jaundice may result from *legionnaires' disease* (p. 151) and *Kawasaki disease* (p. 39).

If a *cephalhaematoma* is a large one, the absorption of blood may lead to a rise in the serum bilirubin. A *subaponeurotic haemorrhage* is more likely to cause a significant rise in the serum bilirubin.

**3** *Interference with protein binding.* Sulphonamides or flucloxacillin may increase the jaundice of a newborn baby by competing with bilirubin for protein binding and displacing bilirubin into the tissues [8]. These drugs should therefore be avoided.

**4** *Obstructive jaundice.* The following are the main causes in the newborn infant:

> Neonatal hepatitis due to maternal rubella, coxsackie virus, adenovirus, herpes, listeriosis, toxoplasmosis, cytomegalovirus, syphilis
> Biliary atresia
> Inspissated bile, cystic fibrosis
> Urinary tract infection
> Rare
> > Choledochal cyst
> > Gallstones
> > Dubin–Johnson syndrome
> > $Alpha_1$ antitrypsin deficiency
> > Tyrosinosis
> > Galactosaemia
> > Fructose intolerance (p. 12)
> > Glycogen storage disease type IV
> > Gaucher's disease
> > Mucopolysaccharidosis
> > Porphyria
> > Drugs

*Neonatal hepatitis* is a somewhat mysterious condition of uncertain aetiology. It has occurred in two or three children of the same family. In some, the rubella virus has been isolated. It may be the end result of several conditions such as serum hepatitis in the mother. The relationship of neonatal hepatitis to biliary atresia is uncertain. Jaundice due to neonatal hepatitis may be present at birth or appear during the first week or two. It is of varying duration and may last for several months before clearing.

There are no certain means of distinguishing neonatal hepatitis from *biliary atresia*. An American paper on neonatal jaundice described seventy-three liver function tests recommended for this age period. Even a liver biopsy may not provide a definite answer. It is important to determine whether there is an obstructive lesion of the biliary tract which can be corrected with surgery: only a small number of cases can be corrected, but one must give the child the benefit of the doubt. This can be determined by limited laparotomy with a cholangiogram after injecting dye into the gall bladder and biopsy of a specimen of liver. If nothing is or can be done for an infant with biliary atresia, he continues to have severe jaundice with biliary cirrhosis and dies in a few months, or rarely a few years.

Hepatitis due to *toxoplasmosis or cytomegalovirus* is rare, but that due to maternal rubella is relatively common. The diagnosis is made by serological methods.

*Alpha-1-antitrypsin deficiency* may cause hyperbilirubinaemia following physiological jaundice; or the jaundice may not develop for 3 to 4 months. It usually lasts 2 or 3 months, after which the child is well, but enlargement of the liver remains, cirrhosis developing later in childhood [10].

Jaundice may be the only obvious symptom of *urinary tract infection*. The bilirubin is partly direct and partly indirect [14]. The jaundice develops commonly between the 8th and 56th day, mostly in boys, and is usually associated with an *E. coli* infection.

Obstructive jaundice may occasionally develop in infants suffering from haemolytic anaemia due to *blood group incompatibility*. This has been ascribed to inspissated bile blocking the bile duct. It is rare, but there have been instances in which the jaundice has cleared after the duct has been washed through at laparotomy.

A *choledochal cyst* is a rare cause of obstructive jaundice. The chief signs are jaundice and a palpable mass [9].

The *Dubin–Johnson syndrome* is a rare type of chronic jaundice with bile in the urine, due to inability of the hepatic cells to excrete conjugated bilirubin. The bilirubin is partly direct and partly indirect. It is an autosomal dominant condition, and is probably the same as the Rotor syndrome.

In *tyrosinosis* the phenistix test is positive. In galactosaemia the clinitest is positive, but the clinistix is negative.

## Jaundice after infancy

### Obstruction

By far the commonest cause of jaundice after infancy is *infective hepatitis*. There will be bile in the urine and the stools will be clay-coloured. It could also be due to serum hepatitis, if the child has had a transfusion, or has been given injections with a contaminated needle.

Toxic hepatitis can be caused by scores of *drugs*. These include acetazolamide, amphetamine, anabolic steroids, antibiotics, anticonvulsants, chloroquine, clonidine, cytotoxic drugs, dioctyl sulphosuccinate, gold, griseofulvin, halothane, iron, ketoconazole, non-steroidal anti-inflammatory drugs, paracetamol, pyrimethamine, quinine, salicylates, thiouracil and tranquillizers.

It can also be caused by a wide variety of poisons, such as phosphorus, iron, arsenic, bismuth or fungi. Obstructive jaundice has been traced to a chlorinated hydrocarbon in breast milk [2].

In the tropics, *malaria* and *bilharzia* cause jaundice. Ingestion of certain poisons or moulds (alpha toxins) may be relevant.

Jaundice could be caused by *solvent sniffing*.

*Cirrhosis of the liver* in its late stages causes jaundice as in adults. Valman, France & Wallis [15] described four children with prolonged obstructive jaundice and cystic fibrosis—possibly because of increased density of bile. Rare causes to consider include Wilson's disease (p. 231), tyrosinosis and Niemann–Pick disease.

*Weil's disease* (leptospirosis) is a rare cause of jaundice. It is characterized by jaundice, fever, leucocytosis, albuminuria and haemorrhages. It is diagnosed by agglutination tests, isolation of the spirochaete in the blood or inoculation of a guinea-pig.

Jaundice occasionally occurs in association with acute pancreatitis (p. 114).

*Infectious mononucleosis* is on rare occasions complicated by jaundice.

## Haemolysis

In jaundice due to haemolysis the urine does not contain bile and the stools are of normal colour. The causes include congenital spherocytosis (acholuric jaundice), sickle-cell anaemia and thalassaemia, and acquired (auto-immune) haemolytic anaemia.

**References**

1 Adams JA, Hey DJ, Hall RT. Incidence of hyperbilirubinemia in breast-vs-formula fed infants. *Clin Pediatr (Phila)* 1985; **24:** 69.
2 Bagnell PC, Ellenberger HA. Obstructive jaundice due to a chlorinated hydrocarbon in breast milk. *Can Med Ass J* 1977; **117:** 1047.
3 Bleicher MA, Reiner MA, Rapaport SA, Track NS. Extraordinary hyperbilirubinaemia in a neonate with hypertrophic pyloric stenosis. *J Pediatr Surg* 1979; **14:** 527.
4 Buchan PC. Pathogenesis of neonatal hyperbilirubinaemia after induction of labour with oxytocin. *Br Med J* 1979; **2:** 1255.
5 *Communicable Disease Report 1983* 23 December, p. 3.
6 Constantopoulos A, Messaratakis J, Matsaniotis N. Breast milk jaundice: the role of lipoprotein lipase and the free fatty acids. *Europ J Pediatr* 1980; **134:** 35.
7 De Carvalho M, Klaus MH, Merkatz RB. Frequency of breast feeding and serum bilirubin concentration. *Am J Dis Child* 1982; **136:** 737.
8 Hanefeld F, Ballowitz L. Flucloxacillin and bilirubin binding. *Lancet* 1976; **1:** 433.
9 Harris VJ, Kahler J. Choledochal cyst: delayed diagnosis in a jaundiced infant. *Pediatrics* 1978; **62:** 235.
10 *Lancet.* Childhood liver disease with alpha₁-antitrypsin deficiency. Leading article. 1977; **1:** 82.
11 Lascari AD. Carotenemia. *Clin Pediatr (Phila)* 1980; **20:** 25.
12 Poland RL. Breast milk jaundice. *J Pediatr* 1981; **99:** 86.
13 Rooney JC, Hill DJ, Danks DM. Jaundice associated with bacterial infection in the newborn. *Am J Dis Child* 1971; **122:** 39.
14 Seeler RA, Hahn K. Jaundice in urinary tract infection in infancy. *Am J Dis Child* 1969; **118:** 553.
15 Valman HP, France NE, Wallis PG. Prolonged neonatal jaundice in cystic fibrosis. *Arch Dis Child* 1971; **46:** 805.
16 Wood B, Culley P, Roginski C, Powell J, Waterhouse J. Factors affecting neonatal jaundice. *Arch Dis Child* 1979; **54:** 111.

# Persistent Cyanosis

*Peripheral cyanosis* is a normal feature of newborn infants. The limbs are cyanosed, while the face and trunk are a normal pink. The cyanosis lasts a few days only. Cyanosis of hands and feet are a feature of the chilblain type of circulation in child or adult.

Causes of *persistent generalized cyanosis* in an infant include the· following:

Congenital heart disease

Severe chest disease. Respiratory distress syndrome, cor pulmonale

Cerebral oedema or haemorrhage

Methaemoglobinaemia (rare)

   (i) Congenital

   (ii) Absorption of aniline from laundry marks on clothes

   (iii) Other poisons—acetanilide, dinitrophenol, nitrites, phenazopyridine, potassium perchlorate

   (iv) Phenytoin taken by breast-feeding mother

Sulphaemoglobinaemia (rare)

*Congenital heart disease* is the most common cause of persistent cyanosis in an infant. In the newborn period, the usual causes are complete transposition of the great vessels or cor triloculare. Other causes are truncus arteriosus or tricuspid atresia. In the first two of these there may be no cardiac murmur. After the newborn period the usual lesion is Fallot's tetralogy. It can also be due to a right-to-left shunt when there is a patent ductus arteriosus with coarctation of the aorta proximal to the ductus. Other causes are a hypoplastic left heart, the Eisenmenger complex, patent ductus with pulmonary hypertension, isolated pulmonary stenosis or atresia, tricuspid atresia and a persistent truncus. The diagnosis is established by the usual investigations—X-ray of the chest for heart shape and size, ECG, cardiac catheterization and angiocardiography.

*Severe chest disease* is an unlikely cause of persistent cyanosis in a baby, except in an acute illness such as the respiratory distress syndrome or atelectasis.

A baby may rapidly develop respiratory distress, bronchitis, cyanosis and intercostal retraction after the accidental *inhalation of talcum powder* [2].

Persistent generalized cyanosis in association with dyspnoea is likely to be due to *atelectasis*, or possibly *pneumothorax, mediastinal or lobar emphysema* or a large *diaphragmatic hernia*. Atelectasis may itself be due to a *cerebral haemorrhage*. One must not forget to palpate the anterior fontanelle and the sutures for evidence of increased intracranial pressure.

*Methaemoglobinaemia* may be congenital, or it may result from the absorption of aniline from laundry marks which have been applied *after* the nappies or clothes have been boiled. If they are applied before boiling, absorption does not occur. Methaemoglobinaemia has occurred in rural areas as a result of the presence of *nitrates* in well water used for making up the feeds [1]. They have been used as fertilizers in the fields, and have percolated into the water. A variety of other rather unlikely poisons may cause the condition. When a lactating mother takes phenytoin, the baby may be cyanosed as a result.

Babies may develop cyanosis and methaemoglobinaemia as a result of eating spinach, especially if they are also given the water in which it was boiled. It is due to the nitrates in the spinach. It has resulted from taking carrot juice [3].

Cyanosis may result from polycythaemia or nitrofurantoin.

*Sulphaemoglobinaemia* is a rare congenital metabolic disorder. Cyanosis, abdominal distension and collapse may be part of the *'grey syndrome'* due to chloramphenicol overdosage in the newborn.

In the older age group the likely causes of persistent cyanosis are *congenital heart disease, pulmonary hypertension, pulmonary fibrosis* or *cystic fibrosis*.

## References

1 *British Medical Journal*. Annotation. Spinach, a risk to babies. 1966; **1**: 250.
2 *British Medical Journal*. Accidental inhalation of talcum powder. 1969; **4**: 5.
3 Keating JP, Lell ME, Strauss AW, Zarkowski H, Smith GE. Infantile methaemoglobinaemia caused by carrot juice. *N Engl J Med* 1973; **288**: 824.

# Respiratory Problems in the Newborn

## Apnoeic attacks

Everyone who looks after newborn babies is conversant with cyanotic attacks ('apnoeic attacks'). A baby, usually in his first few days, but sometimes a little later, is found to be ashen grey in colour and not breathing. The condition is far more common in the preterm baby than in the full-term one, and the smaller the preterm baby the more common are the apnoeic attacks. These attacks are particularly common during feeds because of milk entering the trachea.

The causes of apnoeic attacks may be grouped as follows:

Depression of the respiratory centre
   Preterm delivery
   Hypoxia
   Cerebral oedema or haemorrhage
   Analgesic or anaesthetic drugs in labour
   Respiratory distress syndrome
   Meningitis or septicaemia
Obstruction of the airway by meconium, vomitus, milk, mucus, medicine
   Nasal obstruction. Choanal atresia
   Laryngeal obstruction
Convulsions
Pertussis
Primary alveolar hypoventilation (rare)
Obstructive sleep apnoea: excessive snoring

In a study in Sheffield, we found that congenital heart disase was a rare cause of apnoeic attacks in the newborn.

*Depression or immaturity of the respiratory centre* is an important cause of cyanotic attacks, probably mainly by hypoxia [11, 12]. Attacks are sometimes precipitated by a sudden stimulus, such as a suction catheter. In small preterm babies phasic respiration, including Cheyne–Stokes breathing, is a normal finding; some cyanotic attacks are due to failure to restart breathing after the normal brief apnoeic stage. After the newborn period cyanotic attacks may be a feature of congenital heart disease, especially Fallot's tetralogy [23]. When a 1- or 2-week-old baby who has been previously well develops apnoeic attacks, pyogenic meningitis must be remembered as a possible cause.

*Obstruction of the airway* is a major cause of apnoeic attacks. Nasal obstruction may cause apnoeic attacks because the newborn baby does not usually open his mouth to breathe when the nose is blocked. *Choanal atresia* is rare but of the utmost importance, in that the correct treatment is easy to apply and lifesaving [9]. It is due to a web or membrane behind the palate. If it is complete, the child gasps for breath or has apnoeic attacks, but his distress is immediately relieved by crying or by the insertion of an oral airway pending elective surgery.

Many apnoeic attacks are convulsions (see p. 234).

*Pertussis* is an important cause of apnoeic attacks, even in the newborn period. In a New Zealand study of eighty-five infants admitted because of pertussis, thirteen had apnoeic attacks. They usually occurred spontaneously, but might follow a coughing spasm [6]. In a Scandinavian study of fifty-seven infants admitted for pertussis, three had such severe apnoeic attacks that artificial ventilation was needed for up to a week [5].

*Primary alveolar hypoventilation* (Ondine's curse) consists of abnormally shallow breathing, often with apnoeic attacks, and chronic respiratory acidosis, probably due to failure of the central mechanism of respiration [25].

Australian workers [2] found that some children who snore heavily have periods of apnoea which, if frequent, they term the 'obstructive sleep apnoea syndrome'. They described twenty children who showed morning irritability, excessive sleepiness during the day, lethargy and failure to thrive. They ascribed the symptoms to the triad of severe asphyxia, sleep deprivation and cardiovascular impairment.

### Dyspnoea and tachypnoea

The following conditions should be considered (not in order of frequency):

    Cerebral hypoxia or haemorrhage
    Respiratory distress syndrome
    Group B streptococcal infection

Massive aspiration of amniotic fluid or meconium
    Aspiration of talcum powder [4]
Intrauterine pneumonia
Choanal atresia (p. 139). Pierre Robin syndrome (p. 183)
Transient tachypnoea of the newborn
    Maternal fluid overload
    AIDS
    Rib fractures in delivery
Drugs taken during labour. Narcotic withdrawal
Wilson–Mikity syndrome
Atelectasis, mediastinal or lobar emphysema, pneumothorax, air cyst, chylothorax, pulmonary lymphangiectasia, pulmonary haemorrhage. Amnionitis. Histiocytosis X
Thoracic dysplasia. Bronchopulmonary dysplasia
Tracheo-oesophageal fistula
Diaphragmatic hernia or paralysis
Cystic fibrosis. Pancreatic pseudocyst (rare)
Heart failure. Total anomalous venous drainage
    Pulmonary atresia
    Endocardial fibroelastosis
Anaemia. Loss of blood: bleeding into liver or adrenal
Foregut duplication (rare)

For a comprehensive discussion, the reader is referred to the books by Schaffer & Avery [20] and Williams & Phelan [26].

It is often difficult to determine whether respiratory symptoms are primarily cerebral or pulmonary in origin, or a mixture of both. Cerebral hypoxia or haemorrhage may be the primary cause of the respiratory symptoms.

The most common cause of dyspnoea in the newborn baby is the *respiratory distress syndrome* ('hyaline membrane syndrome'). This occurs under three main circumstances—when the baby is born prematurely, is born by caesarean section or is born from a diabetic mother. It is more common in boys than girls. Within the first hour of birth there is a rising respiration rate. The baby begins to make a grunting sound on expiration. There is indrawing of the lower part of the chest and sternum and there may be some cyanosis or cyanotic attacks. On examination there may be râles in the chest and dullness on percussion or signs of emphysema. There may be signs of heart failure with peripheral circulatory failure, cyanosis and muffled heart sounds. The X-ray of the chest shows a characteristic picture. Persistent pulmonary emphysema may follow the respiratory distress syndrome [22].

*Group B streptococcal infection* can mimic the respiratory distress syndrome. It occurs especially when there has been premature rupture of the membranes, and causes respiratory symptoms with shock in the first 24 hrs [1].

*Massive aspiration of amniotic fluid or meconium.* This occurs particularly in postmature babies and in babies delivered by forceps or breech, and after prolonged labour, placental insufficiency or prolapse of the cord, or a cord which has been tightly knotted round the neck. The child may be shocked as a result of hypoxia, and soon after birth, usually within 3 or 4 hrs, he becomes dyspnoeic. There may be associated signs of brain injury, such as a high-pitched cry or an absent or exaggerated Moro reflex. There may be complicating atelectasis, emphysema, pneumothorax or pneumonia.

*Transient tachypnoea of the newborn* occurs especially after caesarean section [8, 19]; it is more common in boys, in large babies and after prolonged labour. It may be due to surfactant deficiency [7].

Neonatal tachypnoea may be caused by *maternal fluid overload* during labour [21].

It is said that the symptoms may be a feature in the neonatal AIDS infection (p. 18).

Landman and his colleagues [14] showed that neonatal tachypnoea could be due to *rib fractures* in delivery.

Neonatal dyspnoea may be the result of drugs taken in labour (e.g. doxepin) [16] causing fetal respiratory depression. Dyspnoea in the newborn may be part of the *narcotic withdrawal syndrome* (p. 141).

*Intra-uterine pneumonia* may follow prolonged rupture of the membranes. The initial symptoms are non-specific. The child is ill at birth, shows little inclination to suck, and may vomit. The temperature is subnormal or raised. There are rapid often grunting respirations, usually without cough. The abdomen may be distended. It has to be distinguished from *staphylococcal pneumonia,* which develops later. The onset is usually insidious, the child becoming ill and toxic in appearance. He may develop an empyema or pyopneumothorax.

The *Wilson-Mikity syndrome* is a condition of uncertain aetiology, mainly in low-birth-weight babies with no known prenatal factors.

The symptoms begin a week or two after birth, sometimes after the respiratory distress syndrome. There is an insidious onset of cyanosis, wheezing and cough with rapid respirations, worsening in the next 3 or 4 weeks. It may last for several months before recovery.

*Bronchopulmonary dysplasia,* with cyanosis and dyspnoea, follows the treatment of respiratory distress by prolonged mechanical ventilation. It occurred in 21 per cent of 299 infants ventilated for the respiratory distress syndrome [17].

The rare *Joubert's syndrome* [13] consists of cerebral malformation with retinal dysplasia, presenting as tachypnoea, apnoeic attacks and defect of vision.

*Asphyxiating thoracic dysplasia* [18] consists of an abnormally small chest with short limbs and dwarfism. Achondroplasia and allied conditions [10] may have a similar chest anomaly.

*Atelectasis* may be associated with persistent cyanosis and feeble respiratory movements. The apex beat is deflected towards the affected side. Agenesis of the lung causes dullness and decreased breath sounds on the affected side with gross mediastinal displacement to the same side.

*Mediastinal emphysema and pneumothorax* are associated with dyspnoea, rapid shallow respirations and cyanosis. The chest may appear to be over-distended, and in the case of pneumothorax there will be decreased movement on one side, with displacement of the trachea and apex beat to the opposite side. In either case there will be hyper-resonance over the affected area, and in the case of mediastinal emphysema there may be a characteristic crunching sound with each heart beat (Hamman's sign). *A large air-containing cyst* cannot be distinguished clinically from pneumothorax.

*Obstructive emphysema* presents especially a week or two after birth, with increasing respiratory distress, tachypnoea, retraction of the chest with bulging on one side and sometimes an expiratory wheeze [26].

According to Chernick & Reed [3], a *pneumothorax* is more common in the newborn than at any other age. There is usually a history of fetal distress or difficult delivery, often with aspiration of meconium, followed by resuscitation; it may complicate the respiratory distress syndrome or pneumonia. They wrote that *pleural effusion* may be a manifestation of hydrops or Turner's syndrome or may follow pneumonia. The most common cause of pleural effusion in a neonate is chylothorax [24].

Mallard *et al.* [15] described the spread of a *pancreatic pseudocyst* bulging into the mediastinum, with resulting respiratory distress.

A *tracheo-oesophageal fistula* will cause dyspnoea if the diagnosis is delayed until after feeds are given, with resultant regurgitation or entry of milk into the trachea.

*Diaphragmatic hernia* is an acute emergency if the hernia is large. There are commonly cyanosis and dyspnoea from birth, though these may develop later. The chest may be overfilled while the abdomen may be flat. There is resonance or dullness. *Paralysis of the diaphragm* is most commonly associated with Erb's palsy. Respirations are rapid and there are decreased respiratory movements on the affected side with decreased sounds at the base.

*Severe anaemia* and *heart failure* are important though rare causes of dyspnoea, requiring immediate treatment. The symptoms of heart failure include feeding difficulties, rapid respirations and oedema. It may be caused by myocarditis, congenital heart disease, fibro-elastosis, glycogen storage disease, heart block, paroxysmal tachy-cardia, respiratory distress syndrome or septicaemia.

A *vascular ring* may cause dyspnoea and stridor with cyanosis during feeding.

The features of the various conditions may be summarized as follows (modified from Schaffer & Avery) [20]:

> Severe dyspnoea immediately after birth—suggesting a major malformation
>
> Violent respiratory efforts with no air entry—laryngeal atresia, choanal atresia
>
> Early dyspnoea—respiratory distress syndrome, diaphragmatic hernia, massive aspiration, intra-uterine pneumonia, group B *Streptococcus* infection
>
> Sudden dyspnoea after a few hours—pneumothorax, atelectasis
>
> Overfull chest—lobar emphysema, pneumothorax, diaphragmatic hernia
>
> Asymmetrical chest—diaphragmatic hernia, diaphragmatic paralysis, pneumothorax, air-containing cyst, lobar emphysema, pulmonary agenesis

Hyper-resonance—lobar emphysema, pneumothorax, air-containing cyst

Local dullness—atelectasis, tumour, diaphragmatic hernia

Wheeze—vascular ring, unilobular emphysema, mediastinal tumour

Stridor—see p. 159

Grunting respirations—respiratory distress syndrome, pneumonia

## References

1 Ablow RC, Driscoll SG, Effmann EL, *et al.* A comparison of early onset group B streptococcal neonatal infection and the respiratory distress of the newborn. *N Engl J Med* 1976; **294:** 65.
2 Butt W, Robertson C, Phelan P. Snoring in children: is it pathological? *Med J Austr* 1985; **143:** 335.
3 Chernick V, Reed MH. Pneumothorax and chylothorax in the neonatal period. *J Pediatr* 1970; **76:** 624.
4 Cotton WH, Davidson PJ. Aspiration of baby powder. *N Engl J Med* 1985; **313:** 1662.
5 Eriksson M. Whooping cough in infants. *Acta Paediatr Scand* 1979; **68:** 326.
6 Forsyth K, Farmer K, Lennon DR. High admission rate of infants and young children with whooping cough: clinical aspects and preventive implications. *Austr Paediatr J* 1984; **20:** 101.
7 Gross TL, Sokol RJ, Kwong MS, Wilson M, Kuhnert PM. Transient tachypnea of the newborn: the relationship to preterm delivery and significant neonatal morbidity. *Am J Obst Gynecol* 1983; **146:** 236.
8 Halliday HL, McClure G, McCreid M. Transient tachypnoea of the newborn: two distinct entities? *Arch Dis Child* 1981; **56:** 322.
9 Holbolth N, Buchman G, Sandberg LE. Congenital choanal atresia. *Acta Paediatr Scand* 1967; **56:** 286.
10 Hull D, Barnes ND. Children with small chests. *Arch Dis Child* 1972; **47:** 12.
11 Kattwinkel J. Neonatal apnea: pathogenesis and therapy. *J Pediatr* 1977; **90:** 342.
12 Kelly DH, Shannon DC. Periodic breathing in infants with near miss sudden death syndrome. *Pediatrics* 1979; **63:** 355.
13 King MD, Dudgeon J, Stephenson JBP. Joubert's syndrome with retinal dysplasia: neonatal tachypnoea as a clue to a genetic brain–eye malformation. *Arch Dis Child* 1984; **59:** 709.
14 Landman L, Homburg R, Sirota L, Dulizky T. Rib fractures as a cause of immediate neonatal tachypnoea. *Europ J Pediatr* 1986; **144:** 487.
15 Mallard RE, Stilwell CA, O'Neill JA, Karzon DT. Mediastinal pancreatic pseudocyst in infancy. *J Pediatr* 1977; **91:** 445.
16 Matheson I, Pande H, Albertsen AR. Respiratory depression caused by N. desmethyl doxepin. *Lancet* 1985; **2:** 1124.

17 Milner AD. Bronchopulmonary dysplasia. *Arch Dis Child* 1980; **55**: 661.

18 Oberklaid F, Danks DM, Mayne V, Campbell P. Asphyxiating thoracic dysplasia: clinical, radiological and pathological information on 10 patients. *Arch Dis Child* 1977; **52**: 758.

19 Rawlings JS. Transient tachypnoea of the newborn. 100 neonates. *Am J Dis Child* 1984; **138**: 869.

20 Schaffer AJ, Avery ME. *Disease in the newborn*. Philadelphia: Saunders, 1977.

21 Singhi SC, Chookang E. Maternal fluid overload during labour: transplacental hyponatraemia and risk of transient neonatal tachypnoea. *Arch Dis Child* 1984; **59**: 1155.

22 Stocker JT, Madewell JE. Persistent interstitial pulmonary emphysema: another complication of the respiratory distress syndrome. *Pediatrics* 1977; **59**: 847.

23 Sulayman RF, Thilenius OG. Complications of heart disease in children. Congestive heart failure, cyanotic spells and infective endocarditis. *Paediatrician* 1981; **10**: 99.

24 Sweet EM. Causes of delayed respiratory distress in infancy. *Proc Roy Soc Med* 1977; **70**: 863.

25 Taitz LS, Redman CWG. Ondine's curse with recovery. *Proc Roy Soc Med* 1971; **64**: 58.

26 Williams H, Phelan PD. *Respiratory illness in children*. Oxford: Blackwell Scientific Publications, 1975.

# Dyspnoea After the Newborn Period

Acute dyspnoea may be due to the following [6]:

Foreign body causing acute stridor (pp. 152, 159)

Pulmonary—pneumonia, asthma, asthmatic bronchitis, pneumothorax, mediastinal or obstructive emphysema, massive collapse of the lung, large air-containing cyst, pleural effusion, haemorrhage

Inhalation of smoke in a fire

Cardiovascular—heart failure, paroxysmal tachycardia, congenital heart disease

Of these conditions, those most likely to be missed are foreign body, pneumothorax or paroxysmal tachycardia. Confusion may occur if a foreign body causes only intermittent obstruction.

Pulmonary haemorrhage may be a feature of *hyperammonaemia* [5].

Mellins & Park [3] wrote that acute dyspnoea after exposure to smoke in a burning building is due to thermal burn of the airway, irritant gases (e.g. from burning plastic) or carbon monoxide.

Chronic dyspnoea may be due to the following conditions [5]:

Chest conditions

Asthma

Cystic fibrosis

Pneumothorax, air-containing cyst, emphysema, massive collapse, pleural effusion

Bronchopulmonary dysplasia (p. 142)

Pulmonary fibrosis, cor pulmonale, pulmonary agenesis, aspergillosis, farmers' lung, alpha$_1$ antitrypsin deficiency (p. 154), mediastinal mass

Diaphragmatic hernia

Severe chest deformity

Heart conditions

Congenital or rheumatic heart disease

Myocarditis. Kawasaki disease (p. 39)

Adherent pericardium

Hypertension

Anaemia

Obesity

Ascites

Renal failure

Overventilation

Drugs

It is one of the characteristic features of *asthma* that exertion causes wheezing and therefore dyspnoea. In severe cases the emphysema causes dyspnoea on exertion.

One has seen children referred for breathlessness with an unrecognized *pleural effusion* or *large diaphragmatic hernia*.

*Obstructive emphysema,* due to a tuberculous lymph node, a foreign body or other lesion, may cause symptoms and signs similar to those of a large air-containing cyst or pneumothorax.

Serious progressive dyspnoea results from *pulmonary fibrosis* and especially from *cystic fibrosis*. A common end result of cystic fibrosis or extensive bronchiectasis is cor pulmonale with severe dyspnoea. Another cause of severe extensive fibrosis is the *Hamman–Rich syndrome* [4]. The Hamman–Rich syndrome consists of diffuse interstitial fibrosis of the lungs, and leads to progressive dyspnoea and death. The diagnosis is made by X-ray. *Pulmonary aspergillosis* should be considered when there is asthma and eosinophilia. *Farmers' lung* is associated with the inhalation of the dust of mouldy vegetable material: it is associated with malaise, fever, febrile aches and pains and dyspnoea.

*Severe chest deformity,* such as that associated with kyphosis or severe degrees of funnel chest, may cause breathlessness. Severe anaemia or ascites are other causes. Renal failure with uraemia or hypertension are possibilities.

*Congenital heart disease,* especially pulmonary stenosis, is one of the main causes of chronic breathlessness in the first 3 or 4 years. After the age of 4 or 5, rheumatic carditis is a cause (mainly in developing countries). *Myocarditis* may be due to legionnaires' disease (p. 157), Kawasaki disease (p. 39), or several virus diseases. It may be due to *drug hypersensitivity* [2]; drugs responsible include amitriptyline, indomethacin, penicillin, phenytoin, sulphonamides and streptomycin. It is possible that the dyspnoea said to occur after dicyclomine [7] was a sensitivity reaction (or due to inhalation of the drug).

Other drugs may cause respiratory symptoms [1]. *Pulmonary eosinophilia* may be due to aspirin, imipramine, isoniazid, nitrofurantoin, penicillin, streptomycin or sulphonamides. *Pulmonary fibrosis* can be a side effect of cyclophosphamide, methotrexate, nitrofurantoin, sulphonamides or vincristine. Rifampicin may sometimes cause dyspnoea.

For over-ventilation see p. 148.

### References

1 Davies P. Drug-induced respiratory disease. *Medicine UK* 1976; **22**: 1074.
2 *Lancet.* Myocarditis due to drug hypersensitivity. Leading article. 1985; **2**: 1165.
3 Mellins RP, Park S. Respiratory complications of smoke inhalation in victims of fire. *J Pediatr* 1975; **87**: 1.
4 Pepys J. Hypersensitivity reactions in relation to pulmonary fibrosis. *La Medicina del Lavoro* 1965; **56**: 451 (in English).
5 Sheffield LJ, Danks DM, Hammond JW, Hoogenraad NJ. Massive pulmonary hemorrhage as a presenting feature in congenital hyperammonemia. *J Pediatr* 1976; **88**: 450.

6 Williams H, Phelan PD. *Respiratory illness in children*. Oxford: Blackwell Scientific Publications, 1975.
7 Williams J, Watkin-Jones R. Dicyclomine—worrying aspects associated with its use in some small babies. *Br Med J* 1984; **1:** 90.

# Over-ventilation

The causes of over-ventilation are mainly the following:

        Psychogenic over-ventilation
        Hypernatraemic dehydration
        Diabetic acidosis
        Uraemia
        Reye's syndrome (p. 80)
        Drugs

Three papers [1, 2, 3] described over-ventilation in a total of 132 children, many of them under the age of 8. The symptoms were episodes of chest pains (tightness or stabbing pains), head, limb or abdominal pains, breathlessness, paraesthesia, vertigo, dry mouth, choking feelings, palpitation, weakness, blurred vision or confusion. The over-breathing was not always a prominent feature. These symptoms all occurred in attacks or episodes, and were rarely persistent: they were thought to portend psychological symptoms in later years.

Over-ventilation is an important symptom in *hypernatraemic dehydration* of infancy. Diabetic acidosis is readily diagnosed by the smell of acetone in the breath and the finding of glycosuria.

*Drugs* which cause over-ventilation are acetazolamide, aminophylline, salicylates or sulthiame. Salicylate poisoning is of especial importance because of its frequency, and it must be considered, however firmly the parents deny that their child could have had access to drugs—because they do not wish to admit to carelessness, or because they deny that they have deliberately given the drugs (as a form of non-accidental injury), or because they genuinely do not believe that the child could have taken the drug. It is important that delayed-action preparations of salicylates may cause toxic symptoms later than other salicylate preparations (and a correspondingly later rise in the level of serum salicylate).

### References

1 Enzer NB, Walker PA. Hyperventilation syndrome in childhood. A review of 44 cases. *J Pediatr* 1967; **70**: 521.
2 Herman SP, Stickler GB, Lucas AR. Hyperventilation syndrome in children and adolescents: long-term follow up. *Pediatrics* 1981; **67**: 183.
3 Joorabchi B. Expressions of the hyperventilation syndrome in childhood. *Clin Pediatr (Phila)* 1977; **16**: 1110.

# Cough

The important conditions to consider include the following:

Acute cough
> Acute respiratory infections
> Colds, sore throats
> Acute bronchiolitis
> Asthma, asthmatic bronchitis
> Pneumonia, including legionnaires' disease, psittacosis
> Recurrent pneumonia
> Measles, pertussis
> Foreign body

Chronic cough
> Habit, tic. School phobia
> Smoking by parent or child
> Postnasal discharge. Chronic antrum infection. Adenoids
> Asthma, asthmatic bronchitis. Allergy
> Cystic fibrosis
> Overspill from hiatus hernia or chalasia
> Other congenital anomalies—laryngeal stenosis, cyst, angioma, neurofibroma, tracheomalacia, bronchomalacia, sequestrated lobe

Bronchiectasis. Collapse of the lung
Tuberculosis
AIDS
Immobile cilia syndrome
Immunological deficiency
Heart disease
Alpha$_1$ antitrypsin deficiency
Foreign body
Drugs [16]


## Acute cough

Cough is an unusual symptom in the newborn. There is usually little or no cough when the infant has the respiratory distress syndrome, atelectasis or pneumonia. Cough with choking in a newborn infant may be due to *tracheo-oesophageal* fistula or oesophageal atresia, congenital laryngeal cleft or perforation of the pharynx.

After the newborn period, the principal cause of cough is a *respiratory infection*. Acute respiratory infections include colds, pharyngitis, tonsillitis, laryngitis, tracheobronchitis, bronchiolitis, pneumonia, measles and whooping cough. I shall not discuss all those in which the diagnosis is obvious.

*Bronchiolitis* is predominantly a disease of infancy, especially in the first 6 months. It is usually due to the respiratory syncytial virus. It begins insidiously with a cold, and in a day or two the child may become severely dyspnoeic and often cyanosed. Respirations are rapid, with subcostal retraction, inspiratory crepitations and an expiratory wheeze. The inspiratory phase is short and expiration is prolonged. The temperature is usually but not always raised. It closely resembles bronchopneumonia, and an X-ray of the chest may be required to satisfy oneself about the diagnosis, but the wheeze supports the diagnosis of acute bronchiolitis. The distinction is important, because acute bronchiolitis, being a virus infection, does not respond to antibiotics. Bronchiolitis in infancy is commonly followed by asthma in later years. It is uncertain whether allergy predisposes to infection by the virus, or whether the bronchiolitis predisposes to asthma later [13].

Colds may be followed by *asthmatic bronchitis* or *asthma* (see p. 157).
I shall not discuss the usual forms of pneumonia, except to note that

bronchopneumonia is commonly diagnosed in error, when the true diagnosis is acute bronchiolitis or asthma; and that after infancy acute appendicitis may be diagnosed in error, when the true diagnosis is pain in the right iliac fossa referred from right lower lobe pneumonia.

Lobar pneumonia in older children is commonly due to mycoplasma. In a study of 108 children with mycoplasma pneumonia [19], 40 per cent wheezed in the attack—some never having wheezed before.

*Legionnaires' disease* [15, 24] commonly presents as a cough, dyspnoea and chest pain. There may be relative bradycardia, drowsiness, confusion, myalgia, haematuria, diarrhoea and vomiting. Rare complications include pneumothorax, myocarditis, pericarditis, polyneuritis, the Guillain–Barré syndrome, meningitis, arthritis, ileus or jaundice. Before the age of 9, legionnaires' disease commonly presents merely as a mild respiratory disease.

*Psittacosis* is usually a respiratory illness or atypical pneumonia, diagnosed by serological means.

The *drug* carbamazepine may cause a pneumonia-like illness.

Recurrent attacks of pneumonia suggest the possibility of cystic fibrosis, asthma, sick-cilia syndrome, a foreign body or immunodeficiency [7].

*Measles* is unusual in the first 6 months.

*Whooping cough* can occur at any age from the newborn period onwards. A cough which is worse at night and which repeatedly makes the child sick should be regarded as whooping cough until proved otherwise. For the first few days there is a non-specific cough, and then spasms develop with the characteristic long indrawing noise on inspiration after a series of coughs. The spasms may be precipitated by activity, excitement or feeds; there may be frequent sneezing and apnoeic attacks. The typical whoop may not be heard if the attack is a mild one or has been modified by partial immunization. The whoop is not specific for whooping cough; it occurs when there is inspissated mucus which is difficult for the child to cough up—as in cystic fibrosis. 'Whooping cough' can be caused by *Bordetella pertussis, B. parapertussis* or *B. bronchiseptica* and by several viruses. It is important that in uncomplicated whooping cough there are no abnormal physical signs on auscultation; there will be signs if there is a serious complication, such as bronchopneumonia or collapse of a lung.

Cough is *not* due to *teething*.

The possibility of a *foreign body* in the bronchus must be remembered, especially when there is a history of the sudden onset of a severe cough. This may be followed by a silent period and then by fever, cough and signs of infection in the obstructed lung. There may be a history of the child eating peanuts or playing with small objects which could have been inhaled. Whenever a child presents with a cough of sudden onset, without a preceding cold, or with collapse of a lobe of the lung, the diagnosis of a foreign body in the bronchus must be eliminated. In a review of 230 cases of inhaled foreign bodies, 46·5 per cent of all foreign bodies were nuts [17]. There is often a delay in the onset of signs and symptoms. One hundred and six of the children presented only with a wheeze without a cough. In a review of 200 cases, Blazer, Naveh & Friedman [2] reported that in twenty-four children there was no history of inhaling a foreign body. They emphasized that dyspnoea and stridor suggested laryngeal obstruction, while cough, wheezing or recurrent intractable pneumonia suggested a foreign body in the bronchus. The removal of one foreign body did not exclude the presence of another one. Peanuts frequently fragment.

It must be emphasized [23] that the triad of cough, wheezing and decreased breath sound is by no means always found; and a foreign body can complicate other lung conditions such as asthma or cystic fibrosis.

## Chronic cough

A cough may be due to a *habit, tic, attention-seeking device* [21], *imitation of others*, or *school phobia* [22].

Chronic coughing may be due to passive smoking (parents, siblings or friends), or to the child himself smoking, or to cannabis. Many studies have shown that children whose parents smoke suffer more bronchitis, asthma and pneumonia than children of non-smokers [3, 11, 12]. Children of mothers who smoked during pregnancy suffer more from bronchitis in their first year than do children of mothers who did not smoke in pregnancy [18]. It is of interest that parental smoking was shown to be significantly associated with admissions for acute bronchiolitis [8].

There have been several reports that *cannabis* smoking may cause even more bronchial irritation than cigarettes [5].

A common and troublesome cause of cough in a young child is a *postnasal* discharge. The usual cause of this is a cold. The child has little or no cough when up and about, but coughs continually as soon as he lies down. The postnasal discharge can be seen on inspection of the throat. The child may be helped by sleeping in the prone position.

*Adenoids* or *antrum infection* may cause a cough by the same mechanism. If a child has a postnasal obstruction and a postnasal discharge, with nasal speech and recurrent otitis media, the likely diagnosis is adenoids. If the ear, nose and throat specialist is unable to obtain a good view of the postnasal space in a young child, a lateral X-ray of the nasopharynx will show a pad of adenoids. If there is chronic antrum infection there will almost certainly be a history of a persistent purulent nasal discharge between colds, or of a postnasal discharge with cough. There may be an allergic basis. The diagnosis is confirmed by an X-ray. A chronic or frequently recurrent cough may be due to asthma, even though there is no wheeze [10].

*Cystic fibrosis* should be suspected when a child has a persistent or frequently recurring cough with pulmonary infections, except when the cough immediately follows an ordinary cold. For cystic fibrosis see p. 10, and for asthma and asthmatic bronchitis, see p. 157. Many children are referred on account of recurrent coughs and bronchitis when the correct diagnosis is asthma [9, 10].

When a child has an acute respiratory infection and fails to make the usual recovery, feeling tired and off-colour, the cough continuing, one suspects a *partial collapse of the lung*. There may be râles localized to one base, or even bronchovesicular breathing. Sometimes there are no definite signs, but the X-ray establishes the diagnosis.

When a young infant regularly coughs during feeds, the possibility of a *small tracheo-oesophageal fistula* has to be considered.

When an infant regurgitates a great deal and also has a cough, the cause could be *chalasia of the oesophagus* or *hiatus hernia*, with inhalation of some regurgitated material into the lung [4]. The presenting symptom may be a chronic cough, and it may be only on direct questioning that the history of regurgitation is obtained. Of eighty-two children with recurrent pneumonia and asthma, forty had gastro-oesophageal reflux [1].

Other congenital malformations include bronchomalacia, a sequestrated lobe or a bronchial cyst [14], laryngeal or tracheal stenosis, cysts or angioma.

*Bronchiectasis* is now rarely seen in British children. It would be suspected if the child had a persistent productive cough with clubbing of the fingers and an antrum infection. It may be due to an underlying congenital abnormality, or it may result from an adenovirus infection following measles.

*Pulmonary tuberculosis* is an unusual cause of cough in England. In primary tuberculosis without complicating bronchial obstruction, a cough is not to be expected. The diagnosis would be made on the history of exposure to an adult with tuberculosis (even if the tuberculosis were said to be healed), a positive tuberculin test, and an X-ray of the chest, and if necessary the culture of tubercle bacilli from stomach washings.

Chronic lymphoid interstitial pneumonia (CLIP) is said to be a characteristic feature of *AIDS* infection in children [20] (p. 18).

The *immotile cilia syndrome* is said to cause chronic obstructive bronchiolitis [6].

A chronic cough may be due to a *foreign body* in the bronchus, even though the X-ray of the chest does not show it.

Cough may be due to *congenital heart disease,* especially when there is a left-to-right shunt, or to *deficiency of alpha$_1$ antitrypsin* (p. 154), in which there are dyspnoea, chronic antrum and respiratory infections, emphysema and sometimes hepatosplenomegaly with jaundice.

Frequent severe respiratory illness should arouse the suspicion of an *immunological deficiency,* especially if there are also recurrent skin infections.

## References

1 Berquist W, Rachelefsky GS, Kadden M, *et al.* Gastro-esophageal reflux associated recurrent pneumonia and chronic asthma in children. *Pediatrics* 1981; **68:** 29.

2 Blazer S, Naveh Y, Friedman A. Foreign body in the airway. A review of 200 cases. *Am J Dis Child* 1980; **134:** 68.

3 Charlton A. Children's coughs related to parental smoking. *Br Med J* 1984; **1:** 1647.

4 Christie DL, O'Grady LR, Mack DV. Incompetent lower esophageal sphincter and gastro-esophageal reflux in recurrent acute pulmonary disease in infancy and childhood. *J Pediatr* 1978; **93:** 23.

5  Council on Scientific Affairs. Marijuana. Its health hazards and therapeutic potential. *JAMA* 1981; **246:** 1823.
6  Gerbeaux J. Immotile cilia syndrome in pediatric personal experience. *Acta Paediatr Japonica* 1985; **27:** 69.
7  Godfrey S. What is asthma? *Arch Dis Child* 1985; **60:** 997.
8  Hall CP, Hall WJ, Gala CL, Magill FB, Leddy JP. Long-term prospective study of children after respiratory syncytial virus infections. *J Pediatr* 1984; **105:** 358.
9  Hannaway PJ, Hopper GDK. Cough variant asthma. *JAMA* 1982; **247:** 206.
10  Konig P. Hidden asthma in childhood. *Am J Dis Child* 1981; **135:** 1053.
11  Lane SR. Passive smoking. *Clin Proc Children's Hospital Nat Med Center* 1980; **36:** 253.
12  Lenfant C, Marzetta B. (Passive) smokers versus (voluntary) smokers. *N Engl J Med* 1980; **302:** 742.
13  McConnochie KM. Bronchiolitis is a syndrome. *Am J Dis Child* 1983; **137:** 11.
14  Mellis CM. Evaluation and treatment of chronic cough in children. *Pediatr Clin North Am* 1979; **26:** 553.
15  Muldoon RL, Jaecker DL, Kiefer HK. Legionnaires' disease in children. *Pediatrics* 1981; **67:** 329.
16  Nicholi AM. The nontherapeutic use of psychoactive drugs. *N Engl J Med* 1983; **308:** 925.
17  Pyman C. Inhaled foreign bodies in childhood. A review of 203 cases. *Med J Austr* 1971; **1:** 62.
18  Rantakallio P. A follow-up study up to the age of 14 of children whose mothers smoked during pregnancy. *Acta Paediatr Scand* 1983; **72:** 747.
19  Sabato AR, Martin AJ, Marmion BP, *et al.* Mycoplasma pneumoniae: acute illness, antibiotics and subsequent pulmonary function. *Arch Dis Child* 1984; **59:** 1034.
20  Seale J. AIDS virus infection: prognosis and transmission. *J Roy Soc Med* 1986; **79:** 121.
21  Weinberg EG. Honking: psychogenic cough tic in children. *S African Med J* 1980; **57:** 198.
22  Williams HE. Chronic and recurrent cough. *Austr Paediatr J* 1975; **11:** 1.
23  Wiseman NE. The diagnosis of foreign body aspiration in childhood. *J Pediatr Surg* 1984; **19:** 531.
24  Woodhead A, Macfarlane JT. The protean manifestations of legionnaires' disease. *J Roy Coll Physns* 1985; **19:** 224.

# Wheezing

Wheezing is an extremely common symptom in childhood. It is commonly confused with 'ruttling'. Ruttling, heard readily without a stethoscope, is due to air bubbling through fluid in the trachea or bronchi: on auscultation coarse râles are heard. A wheeze is due to narrowing of the airway with the production of high-pitched rhonchi. In the young infant the wheeze is due largely to oedema of the mucosa: it is only later, when the smooth muscle has developed further, that bronchial spasm develops. A wheeze usually signifies asthma or asthmatic bronchitis [6]. In the first year, however, persistent 'ruttling' is commonly an early sign of asthma. Later, high-pitched râles develop and, gradually, as the infant gets older, there is a transition to rhonchi. In an older child a ruttle is usually a sign of bronchitis but not asthma.

A good review of wheezing was written by Godfrey [3]. Richards [7] listed ninety-four conditions which should be distinguished from asthma.

Wheezing has to be distinguished from laryngotracheobronchitis (p. 163), and the distinction can be difficult, partly because laryngeal stridor and bronchospasm may occur together [5].

The main causes of wheezing can be summarized as follows:

Asthma and asthmatic bronchitis

Acute bronchiolitis. *Mycoplasma pneumoniae*

Cystic fibrosis

Wilson–Mikity syndrome (p. 141), bronchopulmonary dysplasia (p. 142), congenital lobar emphysema, antitrypsin deficiency (p. 154)

Tracheal or bronchial obstruction. Tracheomalacia, tracheal web, stenosis or tumour

Tuberculous mediastinal lymph nodes. Mediastinal cyst or tumour

Vascular ring. Congenital heart disease

Foreign body

Inhalation of smoke from a burning house

Smoking and drugs

*Asthmatic bronchitis and asthma.* The diagnosis of asthma is commonly missed for a long time before the diagnosis becomes obvious. This may be due to the main or presenting symptoms being a cough rather than a wheeze, so that the incorrect diagnosis of recurrent bronchitis is made; but the cough fails to respond to cough medicine, antihistamine drugs and antibiotics. The three main components of asthma are infection, allergy and psychological stress. A virus infection commonly precipitates an attack of asthma, but being a virus infection it is useless to treat the infection with an antibiotic. The diagnosis of true asthma, rather than asthmatic bronchitis, may depend on the fact that the child with asthma wheezes at times when he has not just had a cold, but particularly on exertion or psychological stress; and a personal history of eczema, or a strong family history of significant allergy, help to make the diagnosis.

In the first 5 or perhaps 6 years many children respond to a cold by wheezing [4]. One to 3 days after the development of a typical cold the child becomes dyspnoeic and wheezes, and the attack is clinically indistinguishable from asthma. If the child only wheezes after a cold, and never at any other time, and did not have eczema, the prognosis is good, in that by the age of 5 or 6 he is likely to cease to respond to colds by wheezing, while others are likely to continue to have attacks for many years. Asthmatic bronchitis may be a mild form of asthma, the cold having lowered the threshold for the allergen to cause bronchial oedema or spasm but Butler & Peckham [1] claimed that the aetiological factors are different in the two conditions: in asthmatic bronchitis there is a lower incidence of eczema and hay fever in the family, but a higher incidence of migraine and sore throats in the child. It is significant that between attacks of asthmatic bronchitis there is no wheezing on exertion: the usual cause is the rhinovirus or respiratory syncytial virus. After the age of 5 the common organism concerned is *Mycoplasma*.

Attacks of asthma may be precipitated by drugs (see below). For allergy to cow's milk protein and soya see p. 13.

Children with acute bronchiolitis or with *Mycoplasma pneumoniae* infection often wheeze, so that asthma may be wrongly diagnosed.

Wheezing, and possibly true asthma, may be a feature of *cystic fibrosis*. Both asthma and cystic fibrosis can be complicated by aspergillosis, which may have some affinity with those conditions.

I have seen a known severely asthmatic child fail to respond to the usual treatment, and a peanut was then removed from the bronchus, despite a normal chest X-ray.

Some of the other, mostly rare, causes of wheezing have been listed above: but important causes are smoking and drugs. Smoking by parents, siblings or others was mentioned on p. 152; it may be an important factor in a child's attacks; and the child may himself smoke cigarettes or cannabis.

Drugs which may precipitate attacks of asthma include aspirin, propranolol and other beta-blockers. Some children, often those with nasal polypi, may react half an hour or so after taking aspirin with a profuse nasal discharge, vomiting, diarrhoea and wheezing. Similar reactions have resulted from non-steroidal anti-inflammatory drugs. Wheezing may also be caused by organophosphorous insecticides, as well as by many antibiotics, cromoglycate, lipiodol, meprobamate, vaccines (e.g. tetanus toxoid) and vitamin K.

Tartrazine, a yellow dye added to innumerable foodstuffs, fruit drinks and medicines, and soft drink preservatives [8] may cause hypersensitivity reactions, including asthma, wheezing, urticaria, dyspnoea, non-thrombocytopenic purpura, rhinitis, laryngitis, weakness, blurred vision, over-activity or anaphylactoid reactions [2].

A complaint that a child always has a cough and wheezing, or is allergic to numerous foodstuffs and other material may be part of the Munchausen syndrome by proxy (p. 33).

### References

1 Butler N, Peckham C. A national study of asthma in childhood. *J Epidemiol and Comm Health* 1978; **32:** 79.
2 *Drug and Therapeutic Bulletin.* Tartrazine—a yellow hazard. 1980; **18:** 53.
3 Godfrey S. What is asthma? *Arch Dis Child* 1985; **60:** 997.
4 Horn MEC, Reed SE, Taylor P. Role of viruses and bacteria in acute wheezy bronchitis in childhood. *Arch Dis Child* 1979; **54:** 587.
5 Lewis H, Hambleton G. Laryngeal stridor and bronchospasm. *Lancet* 1982; **2:** 1042.
6 Phelan PD. Wheezing in childhood. *Austr Paediatr J* 1972; **8:** 167.
7 Steinman HA, Weinberg EG. The effect of soft drink preservatives on asthmatic children. *South African Med J* 1986; **70:** 404.

# Stridor

As stated in the previous section, it is often difficult to distinguish acute laryngeal stridor from bronchospasm, particularly when they occur together. In order to consider the diagnosis it is necessary to distinguish chronic stridor from acute stridor. The commonest cause of chronic stridor in the very young infant is congenital laryngeal stridor. The usual cause of acute stridor in infants and young children is an acute infection, especially laryngotracheitis.

## Chronic stridor

The following are the main causes to consider:

Supraglottic causes
   Congenital laryngeal stridor
   Micrognathia. Macroglossia
   Down's syndrome
   Gross enlargement of tonsils and adenoids
   Lingual, aryepiglottic, thyroglossic or laryngeal cysts (rare)
   Supraglottic webs (rare)
Glottic causes
   Laryngeal web, polyp, papilloma
   Vocal cord paralysis
   Hydrocephalus
   Foreign body
   Dislocation of the cricothyroid or cricoarytenoid articulations
Infraglottic causes
   Congenital subglottic stenosis
   Tracheal obstruction or stenosis, haemangioma, neurofibroma
   Tracheomalacia
   Vascular ring
   Mediastinal tumour or thyroid (rare)
   Foreign body

The elucidation of the cause of stridor dating from birth can be a matter of considerable difficulty. It may also be a matter of great importance to the child, for some of the conditions which cause stridor may be fatal without surgical intervention. The danger of superadded upper respiratory tract infections may be considerable, and it is said by some that these children are more than usually prone to them. Hence it is important that the correct diagnosis should be known [5].

The first and most important observation which must be made in order to consider the diagnosis consists of the timing of the stridor. This is not always easy.

Stridor may be inspiratory or expiratory or both. *A purely inspiratory stridor is less likely to be of serious import than one which is both inspiratory and expiratory, or expiratory alone. On the other hand a purely inspiratory stridor can be due to a serious condition demanding surgical treatment.* It follows that, whatever the timing of the stridor, an accurate diagnosis should be established. Stridor which is entirely inspiratory is usually of supraglottic origin. Biphasic stridor may arise in the cervical trachea. Stridor which is largely expiratory usually arises from the trachea.

The second observation which must be made is the estimation of the quality of the voice [2]. If there is hoarseness or weakness of the voice, the glottis must be involved. Severe stridor with dyspnoea, but with a normal voice, may be subglottic or tracheal in origin. Stridor with a muffled cry is likely to arise from pharyngeal or supraglottic lesions. Inspiratory stridor with an abnormal cry may be due to weakness of the recurrent laryngeal nerve or to a laryngeal web or cyst.

A high-pitched stridor persisting through inspiration or expiration usually implies severe glottic obstruction. A low-pitched stridor usually points to a supraglottic cause.

Stridor with a deep barking or 'brassy' cough usually points to tracheal obstruction.

Hyperextension of the neck sometimes occurs when there is a *retropharyngeal abscess* or *obstruction of the trachea.*

Feeding difficulties sometimes occur with *congenital laryngeal stridor* or *a vascular ring.*

## Supraglottic causes

Supraglottic causes of stridor consist mainly of *congenital laryngeal stridor* (laryngomalacia) which is by far the commonest cause of stridor in infants. Other causes include *laryngeal* or *lingual cysts, supraglottic webs and micrognathia.*

*Congenital laryngeal stridor,* the commonest cause of stridor in infants, has also been termed laryngomalacia. It dates from shortly after birth, usually after the first week or two, and tends to get worse until the age of 3 to 6 months. There is usually no change between the age of 6 and 12 months, and thereafter it usually decreases, disappearing by 18 to 24 months; but according to Smith & Cooper [6] the symptoms may last considerably longer, with persistent inspiratory obstruction in later childhood. It is important to accept that so-called benign congenital laryngeal stridor, though usually benign, is not always so. It is due to abnormal collapse of the supraglottic tissues in inspiration. The epiglottis may be elongated or abnormally curved, or the arytenoepiglottic folds may be redundant. The stridor is mainly inspiratory but is sometimes partly expiratory [4]. Phonation is normal. The voice and cry are unaffected. It is commonly intermittent, disappearing during rest and sleep, but much increased by crying or feeding. It is reduced in the prone position and increased when the child lies supine. The stridor is of all degrees of severity, from the most trivial to the severe. In any but the trivial degrees, there is indrawing of the lower part of the chest on inspiration.

For reasons which are not altogether clear, infants with congenital laryngeal stridor are more liable to have feeding difficulties, such as regurgitation and choking on feeding, than are normal children. I have seen alarming cyanotic attacks in children with this condition.

*All patients with inspiratory stridor should be investigated: 90 per cent will prove to have congenital laryngeal stridor, but others will have a variety of conditions including haemangioma, neurofibroma or cleft larynx.*

*The micrognathic infant* is liable to have inspiratory stridor, probably because the hypoplasia of the mandible permits the base of the tongue to displace the epiglottis. *Macroglossia,* seen in cretinism and other conditions, may have the same effect.

Stridor is fairly common in *Down's syndrome.* The reason is not altogether clear. In some cases seen by me lateral X-rays of the airway have demonstrated an unexplained thickening of the tissues between the vertebral column and the airway.

When a child is older, stridor, worse when he is lying on his back, may be due to *gross enlargement of the tonsils and adenoids.* The obstruction may be so severe that it leads to cor pulmonale.

Inspiratory stridor may be due to a *thyroglossal cyst* at the base of the tongue, a *lingual thyroid* or a *dermoid cyst.* The epiglottis is pressed backwards and downwards, with the result that there is inspiratory stridor, a muffled cry and usually feeding difficulties. The condition can be demonstrated in a lateral X-ray of the airway.

A *supraglottic web* causes a marked inspiratory stridor, a subdued cry, hoarseness and chest retraction. *Laryngeal cysts* have the same effect.

## Glottic lesions

*Glottic lesions* include in particular *laryngeal webs, polypi* and *papillomata*. A laryngeal web is a serious condition and the treatment is difficult. The stridor is usually but not always inspiratory only, and occurs in all positions when the child is awake or asleep. The voice is usually abnormal and the cry weak. The diagnosis is made by laryngoscopy.

*Paralysis of both vocal cords* is seen in children with *hydrocephalus*, as a result of stretching of the vagi in the Arnold–Chiari malformation; though hydrocephalic infants are liable to have stridor due to other but undetermined causes. When there is a *bilateral vocal cord paralysis*, there is marked inspiratory stridor, chest retraction, a hoarse voice, a weak cry and choking in feeds.

Stridor may be due to *birth injury*, involving damage to the recurrent laryngeal nerve, or dislocation of the cricothyroid or cricoarytenoid articulations. In either case the diagnosis would be made by laryngoscopy.

## Subglottic causes

Stridor due to subglottic causes is more likely to develop only after a few weeks. *Subglottic causes* of stridor include in particular the *haemangioma* and *congenital subglottic stenosis*. The haemangioma causes serious obstruction, inspiratory or expiratory stridor or both, sometimes with a croupy or brassy cough. In only three of six cases described by Williams and his colleagues [7] was there a subcutaneous naevus to provide a clue to the diagnosis. I have seen a case due to a *subglottic neurofibroma*. The stridor is usually inspiratory, and the cry is usually weak, but not hoarse. The diagnosis should be made by laryngoscopy and lateral X-ray.

*Tracheal causes* of stridor include *tracheal stenosis, tracheal cysts* and *tracheomalacia*—a condition in which there is an absence of or a defect in the cartilaginous rings. The stridor is commonly expiratory only.

An important cause of stridor is the *vascular ring*, in which there is a double aorta or an abnormally placed subclavian artery. The presenting symptom is either regurgitation of food with cyanotic attacks or stridor. The stridor is commonly both inspiratory and expiratory, but may be either inspiratory only or expiratory only. It usually occurs in sleep as well as at rest. There is often opisthotonos, and flexion of the neck increases the dyspnoea. The cough in infants with a vascular ring is sometimes brassy or bitonal. There is unlikely to be a cardiac murmur on auscultation, or other abnormal physical signs on examination of the heart and chest. The diagnosis is made in the first place by exclusion of other cause by laryngoscopy and lateral X-ray of the airway. Some regard bronchoscopy as dangerous to these infants.

A *mediastinal tumour,* such as a thyroid, is a rare cause of stridor, but an enlarged thymus is not a cause.

## Acute stridor

The main causes of acute stridor are:

> Epiglottitis, laryngotracheobronchitis (croup)
> Trauma, corrosive, smoke
> Foreign body
> Diphtheria, rabies
> Retropharyngeal abscess
> Laryngeal spasm, tetany
> Angioneurotic oedema, allergy to cow's milk protein

Stridor of acute origin, commonly termed *croup,* is usually due to laryngeal involvement in an acute upper respiratory tract infection by the respiratory syncytial or other viruses. There are other causes such as epiglottitis, laryngeal oedema resulting from traumatic instrumentation, angioneurotic oedema or a foreign body. Diphtheria is now hardly seen in the United Kingdom. Rabies is a possible cause. In a review of acute stridor in the preschool child, Milner [3] wrote that the main differential diagnosis of acute stridor was acute viral croup, acute epiglottitis, staphylococcal laryngotracheitis, foreign body or angioneurotic oedema.

*Laryngotracheobronchitis* may be associated with a stridor which is inspiratory at first, and then both inspiratory and expiratory. There is indrawing of the lower part of the chest in severe cases. The air entry may be so poor that the stridor is not loud. It is by no means easy to distinguish it from asthma or acute bronchiolitis. If there is hoarseness the diagnosis of laryngotracheobronchitis is easy, but usually this is absent. One has to listen carefully in order to decide whether there is laryngitis or not. When one needs to know the diagnosis in order to decide the best line of treatment in a severely dyspnoeic child, laryngoscopy may be performed. The stridor of laryngitis could be confused with the noisy ruttle of an infant with *bronchitis* and tracheal exudate. Recurrent croup is frequently allergic in origin [1, 8].

*Acute epiglottitis* may be due to *Haemophilus influenzae, Staphylococcus* or *Pneumococcus*. It occurs predominantly in the 2- to 7-year-old group. Mild respiratory symptoms change in less than 24 hrs to a severe illness, often with dysphagia, and the child rapidly becomes ill, with increasing dyspnoea from obstruction of the airway. There is a low-pitched stertor, with a louder and lower-pitched coarse expiratory ruttle, resembling a snore, but the increasing dyspnoea may be more prominent than increasing stridor. There may be large cervical lymph nodes, dysphagia, drooling and an intensely sore throat. The inspiratory stridor decreases as respiratory efforts increase. The voice is muffled rather than hoarse, and is therefore unlike the voice of the child with viral laryngitis. On laryngoscopy, a swollen inflamed epiglottis will be seen, but *laryngoscopy, or even the use of a spatula is dangerous and should only be performed by the expert with equipment for tracheostomy at hand, for it may precipitate acute obstruction.* It is vital to distinguish acute epiglottitis from croup, but it can be difficult. In both there is inspiratory stridor. But the rapid deterioration with pallor, high fever, dyspnoea, dysphagia and salivation favour the diagnosis of epiglottitis, whereas hoarseness and a barking cough suggest croup.

A mild *laryngitis* following a cold does not usually occasion anxiety; there is often no fever, but if it occurs in a child already suffering from congenital laryngeal stridor there are serious grounds for anxiety, because the child may rapidly develop severe dyspnoea.

*Laryngeal oedema* may follow *trauma* resulting from instrumentation. It may follow contact with a *corrosive substance* or *inhalation of smoke* from a burning house.

*Laryngeal spasm* may occur in *tetany*, due to hypocalcaemia resulting from rickets, coeliac disease, hypoparathyroidism or renal failure.

There is a high-pitched inspiratory stridor, lasting usually for a few minutes or for a single inspiration.

A *retropharyngeal abscess* or *retropharyngeal lymphadenitis* commonly follow an upper respiratory tract infection. There is dysphagia, head retraction, mouth breathing and fever. The abscess may be seen in the back of the throat or even felt by the finger.

### Recurrent stridor

Recurrent stridor is usually due to recurrent attacks of laryngotracheitis; but it could be due to intermittent obstruction by a foreign body. If the baby is not old enough to get hold of a small object himself, his sibling may be responsible.

### References

1 Hide DW, Guyer BM. Recurrent croup. *Arch Dis Child* 1985; **60:** 585.
2 Ludman H. Hoarseness and stridor. *Br Med J* 1981; **1:** 715.
3 Milner AD. Acute stridor in the preschool child. *Br Med J* 1984; **1:** 811.
4 Phelan PD, Gillam GL, Stocks JG, Williams HE. The clinical and physiological manifestations of the infantile larynx. *Austr Paediatr J* 1971; **7:** 135.
5 Quinn-Bogard AL, Potsic WP. Stridor in the first year of life. *Clin Pediatr (Phila)* 1977; **16:** 913.
6 Smith GJ, Cooper DM. Laryngomalacia and inspiratory obstruction in later childhood. *Arch Dis Child* 1981; **56:** 345.
7 Williams HE, Phelan P, Stocks JG, Wood H. Haemangiomas of larynx in infants. *Austr Paediatr J* 1969; **5:** 149.
8 Zach M, Erben A, Olinksy A. Croup, recurrent croup, allergy and airways hyper-reactivity. *Arch Dis Child* 1981; **56:** 336.

# Hoarseness

Hoarseness in a newborn baby is likely to be due to trauma or to a congenital defect.

Hoarseness may result from prolonged crying and in the case of an older child from prolonged shouting, as in games.

The causes may be enumerated as follows:
  Newborn
    Trauma to the larynx by intubation
    Damage to the recurrent laryngeal nerve or vagus by traction
  Newborn or later
    Laryngeal web, cyst, tumour, stenosis
    Weakness of laryngeal muscles
      Myasthenia gravis, Werdnig–Hoffmann syndrome
    Cretinism
    Infection: laryngitis, especially viral, but also diphtheria,
      tuberculosis, syphilis
    Foreign body
    Mediastinal pressure by lymph nodes or tumour
    Cerebral tumour
    Rickets (laryngismus stridulus)
    Farber's disease (chronic granulomatous disease)
    Cannabis. Steroid aerosols

The history is essential in order to determine the duration of the hoarseness.

Generalized muscular weakness is most likely to be due to the Werdnig–Hoffmann syndrome; but in the newborn baby it could be due to myasthenia gravis if the mother has it.

Rickets used to be a cause of attacks of hoarseness under the name laryngismus stridulus. *Vincristine* may cause a recurrent laryngeal nerve palsy.

Williams *et al.* [2] described nine patients with hoarseness caused by inhaled steroids; there was bilateral adductor vocal cord deformity.

A rare finding in congenital heart failure is paralysis of the vocal cord related to traction on the left recurrent laryngeal nerve [1].

Hoarseness may be due to a foreign body.

Other causes of hoarseness, except that due to acute laryngitis, are diagnosed on laryngoscopy.

## References

1  Condon LM, Katkov H, Singh A, Helseth HK. Cardiovocal syndrome in infancy. *Pediatrics* 1985; **76:** 22.
2  Williams AJ, Baghat MS, Stableforth DE, Cayton RM, Shaenal PM. Dysphonia caused by inhaled steroids: recognition of a characteristic laryngeal abnormality. *Thorax* 1983; **38:** 813.

# Chest Pain

The most frequent cause of chest pain is stitch; this is a cramp-like pain on one side of the lower part of the chest or upper part of the abdomen, occurring on exertion after a meal. It is probably due to strain on the peritoneal ligaments attached to the diaphragm [1]. Chest pain is otherwise unusual in children [5]. It is often psychogenic [2]; it may be a feature of overventilation (p. 148).

*Pleural friction* or *pleural pain* causes a knife-like stabbing pain, worse on coughing and breathing. The usual causes are *lobar pneumonia* (rarely *Mycoplasma*) or *epidemic pleurodynia*, commonly due to the Coxsackie virus (Bornholm disease). This causes pleural pain, tenderness of chest and neck muscles and sometimes meningism. Any severe cough may cause pain in the chest. *Pneumothorax* may be associated with chest pain.

*Pericarditis* may result from rheumatic fever, tuberculosis, pyogenic organisms or virus infections. *Angina* is rare in children: it may result from aortic valve disease.

Chest pain may arise from a *hiatus hernia, oesophagitis* or *achalasia* (pp. 79, 153), or from disease or injury to a rib [3]. *Tietze's syndrome* (chondropathia costalis tuberosa [6] consists of pain in a rib due to a walnut-sized firm painful swelling in the anterior cartilaginous area of the ribs [2]. Pain is often intermittent, and may be aggravated by sneezing or movement. The swelling may last for months or years [4]. A similar condition is osteochondritis, in which there is minimal, if any swelling, but there is some tenderness on palpation. In Tietze's syndrome there is a single obvious visible swelling. *Osteitis* may occur in the rib.

Pain may be referred to the shoulder from various sources (p. 100) and to the chest from the spine or upper abdomen.

## References

1 Abrahams A. Stitch. *Practitioner* 1959; **182:** 771.
2 Asnes RS, Santulli R, Bemporad JR. Psychogenic chest pain in children. *Clin Pediatr (Phila)* 1981; **20:** 788.

3 Berquist WE, Byrne WJ, Ament ME, Fonkalsrud EW, Euler AR. Achalasia; diagnosis, management and clinical course in 16 children. *Pediatrics* 1983; **71:** 798.

4 Coleman WL. Recurrent chest pain in children. *Pediatr Clin N America* 1985; **31:** 1007.

5 Driscoll DJ, Glicklich LB, Gallen WJ. Chest pains in children. *Pediatrics* 1976; **57:** 648.

6 Weidemann H-R. Tietze's syndrome. *Helvet Pediatr Acta* 1972; **27:** 25.

# Haemoptysis

Haemoptysis is an unusual symptom in childhood. It is most unlikely to be due to tuberculosis. It hardly ever occurs in primary tuberculosis, but could occur in the adult type in the older child. It is unusual in lobar pneumonia.

It is frequently not easy to decide whether blood has been brought up from the chest or from the stomach (e.g. after a nose bleed).

Haemoptysis should be distinguished from red coloration of the sputum by *rifampicin.*

In the newborn baby, haemoptysis may be due to pulmonary haemorrhage, hypoxia, disseminated intravascular coagulation, cold injury, septicaemia, or respiratory distress syndrome. It could be the result of mechanical ventilation.

After the newborn period, causes include:

> Pneumonia
> Blood diseases
> Whooping cough. Tracheobronchitis
> Trauma (e.g. a broken rib)
> Foreign body in the lung
> Bronchiectasis
> Cystic fibrosis
> Rare
>> Bronchial polyp
>> Pulmonary abscess
>> Pulmonary haemosiderosis

>  Enterogenous cyst
>  Cardiac or renal failure
>  Malignant disease
>  Systemic lupus
>  AV malformation
>
> Drugs

The importance of blood diseases when there is unexplained haemoptysis must be emphasized.

Pulmonary haemorrhage is an occasional symptom in systemic lupus [1].

It is said that tolazoline, used for managing a persistent fetal circulation, may cause pulmonary haemorrhage.

## Reference

1 Miller RW, Salcedo JR, Fink RJ, Murphy TM, Magilavy DB. Pulmonary hemorrhage in pediatric patients with systemic lupus erythematosus. *J Pediatr* 1986; **108**: 576.

# Symptoms Related to the Nose

## EPISTAXIS

Epistaxis is rare in infancy but common in later childhood. Causes:

>  Nose picking, trauma
>  Foreign body (usually causing a unilateral sanguino-purulent
>      discharge)
>  Veins in nasal septum: telangiectasia (p. 363)
>  Acute coryza: measles and other virus infections
>  Whooping cough
>  Diphtheria, syphilis (both with serosanguineous discharge)
>  Tuberculosis
>  Blood diseases
>  Tumours and polyp
>  Terminal renal or hepatic disease
>  Atrophic rhinitis

## HALITOSIS

It is difficult to find papers on the causation of halitosis. Most of the textbooks seen by me, whether general or devoted to otorhinolaryngology, make no mention of the symptom. One article [1], which included halitosis in adults and children, listed sixty-three causes. They included putrefaction or sepsis in the mouth, nose, sinuses or lungs; severe disease of the alimetary canal, liver or kidney; drugs such as paraldehyde, alcohol, mercury, lead, iodides, bismuth; and foodstuffs such as garlic and onions.

Halitosis in an ill child may be due to acute tonsillitis, diphtheria or Vincent's infection.

Severe halitosis of recent origin, especially if there is a nasal discharge, would suggest a *foreign body in the nose*.

*Atrophic rhinitis* occurs predominantly at puberty or later, but may begin in early infancy [3]. It is almost entirely confined to girls. It often starts after some illness. In adolescence it is worse at the time of menstruation. The nasal cavity becomes widened and the halitosis is extreme. It is often a familial feature [2].

I consider that it is true to say that, if atrophic rhinitis and a foreign body in the nose have been eliminated, it is unlikely that one will find the cause of halitosis in an otherwise well child.

### References

1  Attia EL, Marshall KG. Halitosis. *Can Med Ass J* 1982; **126**: 1281.
2  *Drug and Therapeutics Bulletin*. Halitosis. 1969; **7**: 79.
3  Taylor M, Young A. Histopathological and histochemical studies on atrophic rhinitis. *J Laryngol Otol* 1961; **75**: 574.

## DISORDERS OF THE SENSE OF SMELL

For a full review of disorders of the sense of smell, see the articles by Schiffman [3]: conditions said to be associated with disorders of smell include severe disease of the liver, kidney, pancreas and adrenal glands; vitamin $B_{12}$ deficiency; hypothyroidism and Cushing's syndrome; Turner's syndrome, Sjögren's syndrome; and nasal or postnasal conditions including adenoids, allergic rhinitis or nasal polyposis. He listed twenty-six drugs which affect the sense of smell.

It has been shown [2] that nasal obstruction, especially if considerable, may affect smell sensation.

Drugs which may affect the sense of smell include amphetamine, antihistamines, anticonvulsants, baclofen, ethambutol, griseofulvin, metronidazole and tranquillizers.

*Kallman's syndrome* [1] consists of hypogonadism, anosmia, colour blindness, deafness, and renal or craniofacial anomalies.

### References

1 Evain-Brion D, Gendrel D, Bozzola M, Chaussain JL, Job JC. Diagnosis of Kallman's syndrome in early infancy. *Acta Paediatr Scand* 1982; **71:** 937.
2 Ghorbanian SN, Paradise JL, Doty RL. Odor perception in children in relation to nasal obstruction. *Pediatrics* 1983; **72:** 510.
3 Schiffman SS. Taste and smell in disease. *N Engl J Med* 1983; **308:** 1275, 1337.

## NASAL OBSTRUCTION AND MOUTH BREATHING

Not all mouth breathing is due to nasal obstruction. It may be due to habit: it is a common feature of mental subnormality.

Complete or partial nasal (really postnasal) obstruction in the newborn is likely to be due to *choanal atresia*. The infant is unable to breathe until he opens his mouth or an airway is inserted. I have seen three successive children in one family affected by it. When there is partial atresia a unilateral mucoid nasal discharge may occur.

After the newborn period the commonest causes are a foreign body in the nose, adenoids or allergic rhinitis.

Other causes of nasal obstruction [1] include malformations, dermoid, encephalocele, glioma, teratoma, angioma, polyp, the Torwal DT cyst (congenital, but not symptomatic until about 10 years of age), or deflection of the nasal septum.

Nasal congestion may be a side effect of phenothiazines.

### Reference

1 Myer CM, Cotton RT. Nasal obstruction in the pediatric patient. *Pediatrics* 1983; **72:** 766.

## COLDS AND NASAL DISCHARGE

The term *snuffles* refers to a clear mucoid nasal discharge sometimes seen in babies in their first few weeks. The reason for the discharge is uncertain. On microscopy there is no excess of polymorphonuclear white cells, such as would suggest infection, and no excess of eosinophils, such as would suggest allergy. The baby blows bubbles as he breathes and may have some difficulty in feeding because of blockage of the nose. It cures itself in a few weeks.

Even the youngest babies may develop a *cold,* and the common complication of otitis media may result. Other complications include laryngitis and bronchopneumonia. The baby may have difficulty in breathing because he does not open his mouth when the nose is obstructed. He may fail to gain weight or actually lose weight. Some babies develop diarrhoea when they have a cold. An ordinary respiratory infection in an infant or young child may lead to alarming dehydration requiring hospital treatment. Two of the most troublesome complications of colds in the young child are a postnasal discharge and asthmatic bronchitis (p. 157). Culture of the nasal discharge in a baby suffering from a cold may yield haemolytic streptococci.

*Allergic rhinitis* is commonly mistaken for colds in older infants and children. The persistence of nasal discharge, the fact that it is clear and mucoid, together with the continual sneezing, should alert one to the true diagnosis. If the child is never free from a nasal discharge, if the child's nose is running when there has been no history of exposure to infection, or if there is a strong family history of allergy, one would suspect allergic rhinitis rather than coryza. The presence of a wheeze would suggest allergy, though the difficulty of a cold precipitating an attack of asthmatic bronchitis is discussed on p. 157. When in doubt, a nasal smear should be examined under the microscope: if the proportion of eosinophils exceeds 3 per cent, one would think that allergic rhinitis is likely.

Rhinorrhoea sometimes occurs in an attack of migraine (p. 101).

When a child has a purulent nasal discharge between colds, he must be presumed to have an *antrum infection.* This can occur even in infancy. In making this diagnosis, which is confirmed by direct inspection of the nares and by X-ray of the antrum, one must distinguish the usual mucopurulent discharge at the end of a cold. An antrum infection is a common feature of bronchiectasis, and may complicate cystic fibrosis.

A unilateral purulent nasal discharge suggests a *foreign body* in the nose. When diphtheria was prevalent, a serosanguineous unilateral discharge suggested *nasal diphtheria*. A unilateral nasal discharge, with obstruction of the airway on the same side of the nose, may be due to *unilateral choanal atresia*.

A persistent nasal discharge is an early feature of Riley's syndrome (p. 46). Certain *drugs* may be responsible for nasal congestion or discharge. They include reserpine given to the mother during pregnancy, causing nasal congestion in the neonate, and in later childhood iodides, propranolol or trimeprazine.

## SNEEZING

Sneezing in the newborn may occur in the narcotic withdrawal syndrome if the mother is a drug addict (e.g. heroin) (p. 219).

Sneezing is a normal frequent event in young babies in the first 2 or 3 months, so that a mother is likely to think that her baby has a cold.

Older children and adults commonly sneeze at the beginning of a *cold*. Sneezing may be an early symptom of whooping cough.

Hay fever or other *allergic rhinitis* is by far the most likely cause of frequent sneezing.

A *foreign body* in the nose may possibly cause persistent sneezing.

*Intractable sneezing* is rare. The subject has been reviewed by Co [2]. Possible causes include, in particular, temporal lobe epilepsy or a sequel of encephalitis. In an older child intractable sneezing has been ascribed to psychological factors [1]; but I believe that investigation for organic causes is advisable.

### References

1 Bergman GE, Hiner LB. Psychogenic intractable sneezing. *J Pediatr* 1984; **105**: 496.
2 Co S. Intractable sneezing. Case report and literature review. *Arch Neurol* 1979; **36**: 111.

# Symptoms Related to the Mouth and Throat

## STOMATITIS AND GINGIVITIS

*Stomatitis* may be due to the following causes:

 Infection
 Allergy
 Avitaminosis
 Drugs
 The Stevens–Johnson syndrome
 Kawasaki syndrome
 Behçet syndrome
 Aphthous ulcers

*Infections* causing stomatitis include herpes, Vincent's infection, AIDS, the Coxsackie virus and monilia. It is probable that other viruses may cause it. Herpes causes vesicles on the tongue without necrosis, while Vincent's organisms cause necrotic ulcers on the tips of papillae and involve the gums and tonsils. Vincent's infection is confirmed by the smell and by a smear for spirochaetes. Coxsackie stomatitis closely resembles herpes, with small vesicles on the tongue and mucous membranes, but with more tendency to lymph node involvement. *Hand, foot and mouth disease* is usually due to Coxsackie virus: there are vesicles on the tongue, hands and feet—and occasionally on the knees. It clears spontaneously. Thrush infection resembles curds of milk on the tongue and buccal mucosa, but the white patches cannot be removed by a swab.

Oral *candidiasis* is very common in infancy. It may arise from the mother's vagina, or from the use of a dummy or pacifier, or for no apparent reason. It is commonly associated with a characteristic nappy rash. Other causes are T cell deficiency, AIDS infection (p. 18), Di George syndrome, and various serious diseases associated with severe wasting. It may result from the use of antibiotics and corticosteroid inhalers.

174

Other *drugs* which cause stomatitis include actinomycin D, cotrimoxazole, ethosuximide, gold, griseofulvin, lincomycin, meprobamate, 6-mercaptopurine, methotrexate, niclosamide, phenothiazines, tetracycline, troxidone and vincristine.

Stomatitis may be caused by *avitaminosis*, especially ariboflavinosis and other deficiencies of the vitamin B complex, particularly in children on synthetic diets without adequate vitamin supplements. Scurvy may cause it.

The *Stevens–Johnson syndrome* is more common in boys than girls. There is a severe stomatitis, with erythematous papular lesions, vesicles or bullae beginning on the extensor surfaces of the extremities, and spreading to the trunk, neck and scalp. There may be lesions on the conjunctivae, nares, anorectal junction, vulva and urethral meatus. The child is poorly and feverish, and may have kidney, joint or pulmonary involvement. The cause is not always known, but it may be due to anticonvulsants (barbiturates, carbamazepine, troxidone), aspirin, clindamycin, penicillin, quinine, rifampicin, or sulphonamides. Another cause is a *Mycoplasma* infection.

The Behçet syndrome [1] includes aphthous ulcers, keratoconjunctivitis, erythema nodosum, incontinentia pigmenti, diarrhoea, abdominal pain, encephalitis, ataxia, fits, memory loss, and even haematuria. Ammann [1] described six children with the syndrome age 2 months to 11 years.

Aphthous ulcers are not induced by virus infection [2]. They are the result either of delayed hypersensitivity or an auto-immune reaction induced by *Streptococcus sanguis*. The lesions characteristically involve the loose oral mucosa, while recurrent herpes is limited to the lip or attached oral mucosa.

Stomatitis may be a feature of Kawasaki disease (p. 39). It is a serious result of tobacco chewing.

*Gingivitis* may be due to the following causes:

Infection
Drugs
Avitaminoses
Dental caries
Overcrowding of teeth
Malocclusion
Mouth breathing
Familial type

The gums in gingivitis are red and boggy and bleed easily.

*Infections* which cause it include herpes, Vincent's infection, thrush and streptococcal and staphylococcal organisms. Herpes zoster or herpes simplex may cause vesicles on the gums with underlying inflammation. Vincent's infection and thrush have already been described. Staphylococcal gingivitis is usually found in children severely ill from another cause. The gums in streptococcal gingivitis are characteristically bright red and the child is ill.

The principal *drug* which causes gingivitis is phenytoin. The gingivitis subsides within 3 to 6 months of discontinuing the phenytoin. The severity of the gingivitis is related to the blood level of the drug.

Avitaminoses, especially scurvy, cause the gums to be inflamed and liable to bleed.

Gingivitis may be caused by dental decay and stagnating food between teeth, commonly related to overcrowding.

*Mouth breathing* causes gingivitis, but the gum trouble is more often due to a short upper lip providing an inadequate seal and so drying the gingivae.

There is a rare familial type of *fibromatous gingivitis,* resembling the gingivitis caused by phenytoin.

### References

1  Amman AJ, Johnson A, Fyfe GA, *et al.* Behçet syndrome. *J Pediatr* 1985; **107:** 41.
2  Becker DE. Aphthous ulcers in the mouth. *N Engl J Med* 1985; **313:** 330.

## ENLARGEMENT OF THE TONGUE

Englargement of the tongue is found in:

    Hypothyroidism

    Angioma, lymphangioma

    Rare diseases—Beckwith's syndrome, mucopolysaccharidoses, glycogenoses, amyloidosis, gangliosidosis, mannosidosis, Sandhoff's disease (ganglioside storage defect, with blindness, mental deterioration, fits, spasticity and hepatosplenomegaly)

*Beckwith's syndrome* [1] includes a large tongue, umbilical hernia, hypoglycaemia, congenital asymmetry, microcephaly, visceromegaly, facial naevus, renal dysplasia and a risk of Wilms' tumour.

### Reference

1 Cohen MM, Gorlin RJ, Feingold M, ten Bensel RN. The Beckwith–Wiedemann syndrome. *Am J Dis Child* 1971; **122:** 515.

## DISORDERS OF TASTE

For a full review of disorders of taste, see the articles by Schiffman [1]. Amongst the numerous conditions which he cited, the following were included: facial palsy; familial dysautonomia; severe disease of the liver, kidney, adrenal and pancreas; hyperthyroidism; Cushing's syndrome; Turner's syndrome; Sjögren's syndrome and zinc deficiency. He listed sixty-five drugs which may affect taste and smell. Another paper [2] reviewed drug-induced abnormalities of taste sensation.

*Cacogeusia* (an unpleasant taste) can be caused by various drugs—acetazolamide, antihistamines, carbimazole, ergotamine, ethambutol, griseofulvin, heavy metals, metronidazole, phenytoin and tranquillizers.

Penicillamine may reduce taste sensation for sweets and salt.

### References

1 Schiffman SS. Taste and smell in diseases. *N Engl J Med* 1983; **208:** 1275, 1337.
2 Willoughby JMT. Drug induced abnormalities of taste sensation. *Adverse Drug Reaction Bulletin* 1983; **No. 100:** 368.

## DRYNESS OF THE MOUTH

This may be due to *dehydration*, or a variety of *drugs*, including amphetamine, anticholinergic drugs, anticonvulsants, antihistamines, atropine, clonidine, codeine, cyclopentolate, ergotamine, fenfluramine, hyoscine, morphine, tranquillizers and vitamin A overdose. Cyclopentolate drops may cause an acute toxic psychosis, a dry mouth, ataxia and delirium. It is a feature of amphetamine addicts [1].

Dryness of the mouth may be due to mouth breathing or over-ventilation. It could be a psychological symptom.

Dryness of the mouth may be a feature of the *Mikulicz syndrome* (p. 51) or *Sjögren's syndrome* (p. 356).

### Reference

1 Adcock EW. Cyclopentolate toxicity in pediatric patients. *J Pediatr* 1971; **79**: 127.

## SALIVATION AND DROOLING

Most normal babies lack control of the flow of saliva until 12 months or so of age. Some seem to have more saliva than others, and their clothes are constantly wet. Salivation is a common sign of teething. Drooling sometimes continues for years without apparent reason. It is sometimes associated with mouth breathing. Mentally handicapped children, being late in all aspects of development, except occasionally sitting and walking, are late in controlling saliva, and this may be one of the troublesome features of mental handicap from the mother's point of view. Children with cerebral palsy, especially of the athetoid type, are particularly liable to 'drool' for several years, partly, perhaps, because of incoordination of the tongue and lips.

It seems likely that drooling is more often due to failure to swallow or retain saliva than to excessive salivation [1]. Hence it is a feature of *oesophageal atresia, perforation of the pharynx, bulbar palsy* (p. 183), *facial palsy, myotonia dystrophica, myasthenia gravis, polyneuritis* and *motor neurone disease*. It occurs in infections which interfere with swallowing—poliomyelitis, diphtheria, rabies and botulism.

Rare causes are familial dysautonomia (p. 46) and ataxia telangiectasia (p. 212).

Drooling may be associated with excessive salivation caused by *stomatitis*.

Many *drugs* may cause the symptom. Salivation may be a feature in the newborn baby born of a drug addict. Other drugs causing it include chlordiazepoxide, clonazepam, dicyclomine, ethionamide eye drops (anticholinesterase eye drops, containing phospholine iodide), fungi, haloperidol, organophosphorous insecticides and thallium.

### Reference

1  Smith RA, Goode RL. Sialorrhoea. *N Engl J Med* 1970; **283:** 917.

## TRISMUS

Trismus is an unusual symptom in children. Probably the commonest causes are mumps, anti-emetic drugs or trauma. It must be distinguished from a bony abnormality consisting of partial ankylosis or more commonly hypoplasia of the temporomandibular joint. A rare bony abnormality is myositis ossificans progressiva (p. 252).

The following conditions may cause trismus:

Mumps
Dental abscess: pericoronitis—around an incompletely erupted
  tooth
Peritonsillar abscess
Otitis media
Osteitis
Tetanus
Serum sickness (effusion into the joint)
Juvenile chronic arthritis
Costen's syndrome (see p. 206)
Epilepsy
Hysteria
Trauma, including dislocation
Drugs
Rare
  Myotonia atrophica
  Tumours
  Rabies

These are mostly self-explanatory. Perhaps the most important cause to eliminate is a dental abscess or inflammation around an unerupted tooth. *Drugs* which may cause trismus include particularly metoclopramide and the tranquillizing group, strychnine in an overdose, and antihistamines.

## THE TEETH

*Delayed dentition* is common in normal children. There are wide variations in the age at which the first tooth appears: these differences are commonly familial. Some babies are born with a tooth or teeth, while others may not cut the first tooth until after the first birthday.

The following are causes of abnormal delay in dentition and of teeth being missing:

*Supernumerary teeth,* particularly upper central and lateral incisors, impeding the eruption of the permanent ones.

*Overlong retention of deciduous teeth,* for unknown reasons.

*Crowding of the jaw*—as a result of the teeth being unduly large or the jaw being unduly small. These are often familial features.

*Delayed eruption of teeth* may occur in *hypothyroidism, hypoparathyroidism, cleidocranial dysostsis, the Gardner syndrome* (delayed teething, colonic polyposis, osteomata), and *vitamin D-resistant rickets* (X-linked recessive).

*Missing teeth,* apart from the usual loss of teeth, may be due to *ectodermal dysplasia.* There may be missing upper lateral incisors, lower third molars or premolars. The condition affects predominantly the permanent teeth and is familial. There are likely to be other signs of the disease—a dry skin, sparse hair and abnormal nails.

There is a rare form of *familial anodontia.*

*Premature loss of deciduous teeth* occurs in hypophosphatasia, vitamin-resistant rickets, hypoparathyroidism, cyclic neutropenia and histiocytosis X.

*Yellow staining* of the teeth is usually due to tetracycline (taken by the mother in pregnancy, or by the child): it may also be due to neonatal hyperbilirubinaemia.

## TOOTH GRINDING

Tooth grinding in sleep may occur in a normal child, but tooth grinding in a child who is awake is usually an indication of mental subnormality.

It is said to be an occasional side effect of fenfluramine and amphetamines.

## SNORING

The usual cause of loud snoring is adenoids.

The mechanism was discussed by Birch [1]: when the child is supine, and especially when mouth-breathing, the tongue falls back so that the soft tissue of the mouth and throat approximate, and vibrations in the posterior pillars of the fauces, and to a lesser extent in the soft palate, cause the characteristic noise on inspiration.

### Reference

1 Birch CA. Snoring. *Practitioner* 1969; **203**: 383.

## SORE THROAT

Infectious mononucleosis may cause pharyngitis or tonsillitis with exudate or membrane. Petechiae on the palate are said to be a common feature. It is not possible on inspection to distinguish a streptococcal tonsillitis from that due to viruses [1]. Vincent's infection may be suspected by the expert on account of the characteristic smell.

Diphtheria may be strongly suspected because of the membrane (which must be distinguished from the closely resembling membrane following tonsillectomy), but the diagnosis has to be confirmed in the laboratory. The possibility of agranulocytosis and other blood diseases has to be remembered.

Soreness of the throat often precedes by minutes other features of hay fever.

### Reference

1 Stewart D, Moghadam H. Diagnosis and treatment of throat infection in children. *Canadian Med Ass J* 1971; **105**: 69.

## DIFFICULTY IN SUCKING AND SWALLOWING

The diagnosis of the cause of sucking and swallowing problems in infancy is liable to be a matter of great difficulty. I have reviewed the subject fully elsewhere [1]. I suggested the following classification:

1   Gross congenital anatomical defects
> Palate—cleft
> Tongue—macroglossia, cysts, tumours
> Retronasal space—choanal atresia
> Mandible—micrognathia
> Temporomandibular joint—ankylosis, hypoplasia
> Pharynx—cyst, diverticulum
> Oesophagus—atresia, fistula, stenosis, web
> Thorax—vascular ring
> Laryngeal cleft

2   Neuromuscular defects
> Rumination, tongue thrusting
> Delayed maturation—normal variation, prematurity, mental subnormality
> Cerebral palsy
> Cranial nerve nuclei or tracts
> Bulbar or suprabulbar palsy
> Congenital laryngeal stridor
> Achalasia (p. 75)
> Muscular dystrophy
> Hypotonias
> Rare
>> Myotonia dystrophica
>> Myasthenia gravis
>> Syndromes of Möbius, Cornelia de Lange, Riley and Prader–Willi

3   Acute infections—stomatitis, oesophagitis, poliomyelitis, diphtheria, tetanus, botulism, rabies

4   Effect of drugs

Space will not permit a full discussion of all these numerous conditions, and I propose to mention a few only. Even an expert is liable to find the establishment of the diagnosis a matter of considerable complexity.

For the most part the group consisting of gross congenital anatomical defects is not difficult to diagnose.

A *submucous cleft* may be missed. Pointers to it include a bifid uvula, or a palpable V-shaped notch at the midline posterior border of the hard palate, replacing the normally palpable posterior nasal spine. Sometimes there is a translucent membrane replacing the median raphé, with a short palate. There is likely to be nasal speech and nasal regurgitation of fluid.

Swallowing difficulties are common in *micrognathia*, whether or not it is associated with a cleft palate (Pierre Robin syndrome). The receding chin fails to support the tongue in its normal forward position, impinges against the posterior wall of the pharynx, obstructing respiration and causing feeding difficulties and cyanotic attacks.

Obstructive lesions in the *oesophagus* or impacted foreign body may be suggested by the story that the child can swallow liquids but not solids.

The *vascular ring* is discussed on p. 163. An abnormally placed subclavian artery ('dysphagia lusoria', the game of nature), frequently causes no symptoms, but in some cases it causes difficulty in swallowing.

*Choanal atresia* is discussed on pp. 139, 171.

A *congenital laryngeal cleft* causes feeding difficulties with stridor and choking, and closely simulates a tracheo-oesophageal fistula.

The differential diagnosis of the large group of neuromuscular defects is much more difficult. Delayed maturation of the swallowing mechanism is commonly the principal difficulty. This occurs in mentally subnormal children, with or without cerebral palsy, and may occur for no apparent reason—and is thus termed 'birth injury'—but with no firm evidence. It is normal for the small preterm infant to have difficulty in sucking and swallowing, and therefore the mentally subnormal child, being late in all aspects of development, may have the same difficulties as that of the preterm baby. There is incoordination of the relevant muscles—that of the palate and pharynx in particular. The normal infant displays the tongue-thrusting reflex if solid material is placed on his tongue in the early weeks, but loses this response as he matures, and so is able to take solids by 6 or 7 months: but the mentally subnormal child is later in losing this response, and in addition is late in learning to chew.

It is not known why some infants have delayed development of the bulbar centres necessary for the swallowing mechanism. In some there is transient palatal, pharyngeal or cricothyroid incoordination or defective tongue movements. Some apply the term suprabulbar paresis for this condition. These difficulties may last only a few weeks or months, followed by full recovery. They are almost always found in children with Riley's syndrome of familial dysautonomia (p. 46) and in the Prader–Willi syndrome (p. 23): they occur in the Cornelia de Lange syndrome, in children with severe hypotonia, and in the Möbius syndrome (congenital facial diplegia) and the similar condition of myotonia dystrophica. The child with cerebral palsy, in addition to the commonly associated mental subnormality, has stiffness and incoordination of the muscles concerned with swallowing. In some of these children there are other cranial nerve palsies.

It is not clear why many children with *congenital laryngeal stridor* have swallowing difficulties.

*Infections* which may cause swallowing difficulties include stomatitis and oesophagitis—viral or monilial, diphtheria (causing polyneuritis) and poliomyelitis (bulbar palsy). Swallowing difficulties are commonly seen in *tetanus, botulism* and *rabies*. Johnson, Clay & Arnon [2], studying ten cases of *infant botulism*, found that early symptoms were constipation and weakness, followed by difficulty in sucking and swallowing, hypotonia, lethargy, ptosis and weakness of facial and extra-ocular muscles, with diplopia and blurring of vision. The infection is from food or wounds, mostly compound fractures [3]. The condition may resemble poliomyelitis, the Guillain–Barré syndrome or myasthenia.

*Drugs* which may cause dysphagia include haloperidol, metoclopramide and clonazepam. Maternal heroin addiction or phenothiazines taken in late pregnancy may be a cause.

The exact diagnosis can be difficult. The first stage is to observe the facial and limb movements and to examine the cranial nerves for signs of spasticity or weakness. One watches the child take a drink of water, and offers the baby a finger to suck in order that one can determine whether he is able to suck. The tongue is examined for wasting and fasciculation, as in anterior horn cell lesions. The movements of the palate are observed for signs of bulbar palsy, and the configuration of the palate for signs of a submucous cleft. Other signs of cerebral palsy and mental subnormality are looked for.

Special investigations necessary include laryngoscopy, oesophagoscopy, cineradiography and a lateral X-ray of the neck for delineation of the airway and soft tissue masses.

## References

1 Illingworth RS. Sucking and swallowing difficulties in infancy. Diagnostic problems of dysphagia. *Arch Dis Child* 1969; **44:** 655.
2 Johnson RO, Clay SA, Arnon SS. Infant botulism, diagnosis and management. *Am J Dis Child* 1979; **133:** 586.
3 Keller MA, Miller VH, Berkowitz CD, Yoshimori RN. Wound botulism in pediatrics. *Am J Dis Child* 1982; **136:** 320.

# Symptoms Related to the Eye

## SUSPECTED VISUAL DEFECT

It is easy to make the mistake of thinking that a baby is blind, because he shows no interest in his surroundings, when his lack of interest is due to *mental subnormality*; as he matures it becomes clear that he can see. The optic discs of normal babies are pale, and one can readily and wrongly diagnose optic atrophy—and assume that one's suspicion of a visual defect has been confirmed. The absence of a roving nystagmus should help to prevent such a mistake. *Infantile autism* may lead to the same mistake, because of the child's lack of responsiveness and his gaze aversion.

## DELAYED VISUAL MATURATION

An otherwise normal child, who is developmentally normal, may for the first weeks or months appear to be blind; yet there is no roving nystagmus, such as one would expect if he were blind, and on ophthalmoscopy no abnormality is found [1, 2, 3, 4]. A high proportion of cases described had been born preterm or small for dates. It is difficult to decide whether in the early weeks they are unable to see or are unable to interpret what they see (visual agnosia). It seems likely that the delay corresponds with delayed maturation in other fields— such as walking, talking, sphincter control or reading.

**References**

1  Cole GF, Hungerford J, Jones RB. Delayed visual maturation. *Arch Dis Child*
     1984; **59:** 107.
2  Harel S, Holtzman M, Feinsod D. Delayed visual maturation. *Arch Dis Child*
     1983; **58:** 298.
3  Illingworth RS. Delayed visual maturation. *Arch Dis Child* 1961; **36:** 407.
4  *Lancet*. Delayed visual maturation. Leading article. 1984; **1:** 1158.

## RISK FACTORS FOR A VISUAL DEFECT

The following conditions increase the risk that a child will have a visual defect:

> In pregnancy—rubella, cytomegalovirus, toxoplasmosis; chickenpox (rarely)
>
> Drugs—antimitotics, chloroquine, phenothiazines, quinine, radioactive iodine, thalidomide, warfarin
>
> Prematurity (retinopathy, myopia, squint)
>
> Mental subnormality, cerebral palsy, hydrocephalus, craniostenosis, congenital anomalies
>
> Fixed squint
>
> Delayed treatment of squint or cataract
>
> Juvenile chronic arthritis, prolonged corticosteroid treatment
>
> Rare metabolic diseases—cystinosis, galactosaemia, homocystinuria, Lowe's syndrome (eye and kidney abnormality)

### Congenital defects causing blindness

Some of these are implicit in the section on risk factors. The subject is a massive one, and it would not be profitable to review the whole subject here. A useful source of information is the fourteen-volume text by Duke-Elder [1].

Congenital cortical blindness may be diagnosed by the suspicion of blindness, the absence of opticokinetic nystagmus, with normal optic fundi and normal pupil reflex. There would not be the roving nystagmus found in other examples of serious visual defect [3]. Whiting and colleagues [4] described fifty children with permanent cortical visual blindness. It is said that optic nerve hypoplasia is fairly often found [2]; the defect may be bilateral, and may be associated with other abnormalities. For Joubert's syndrome, see p. 142.

### References

1 Duke-Elder S. System of ophthalmology. London: Kimpton, 14 volumes (various dates).
2 Fielder AR, Levene MI, Trounce JQ, Tanner MS. Optic nerve hypoplasia in infancy. *J Roy Soc Med* 1986; **79:** 25.
3 Ronen S, Nawratzki I, Yanko L. Cortical blindness. *Ophthalmologica* 1983; **187:** 217.
4 Whiting S, Jan JE, Wong PK, Flodmark O, Farrell K, McCormick AG. Permanent cortical visual impairment in children. *Dev Med Child Neurol* 1985; **27:** 730.

## BLURRING OF VISION

Temporary blurring of vision may be due merely to exudate from an infection on the eyelids.

Unless it is recent, it may be due to an error of refraction.

Blurring of vision may be a premonitory symptom of migraine (p. 101). It may be due to over-ventilation or malingering.

The symptom may result from diphtheria or botulism.

Drugs which cause blurring of vision [1] include acetazolamide, antibiotics, anticonvulsant drugs, antihistamines, atropine, barbiturates, chloroquine, digoxin, ergotamine, isoniazid, nalidixic acid, non-steroidal anti-inflammatory drugs, paracetamol, PAS, piperazine, tartrazine and tranquillizers. It may result from solvent sniffing.

### Reference

1 McFane PA. The adverse effect of some drugs on the eye. *Prescribers' Journal* 1973; **13:** 68.

## DETERIORATION AND LOSS OF VISION

Significant deterioration of vision may be due to papilloedema, optic neuritis, optic atrophy, iridocyclitis, glaucoma, cataract, retinitis pigmentosa, demyelinating diseases or drugs.

*Papilloedema* may be due to a space-occupying lesion, such as subdural effusion or tumour, hypertension, meningo-encephalitis, hydrocephalus, degenerative disease or drugs (notably cortico-steroids, imipramine, nalidixic acid, tetracycline or vitamin A excess).

Unilateral optic atrophy or papilloedema suggests a cranio-pharyngioma [5] (p. 340).

*Optic neuritis* may be due to multiple sclerosis, neuromyelitis optica, or drugs (notably barbiturates, chloramphenicol, clioquinol, diodoquin, ethambutol, isoniazid, non-steroidal anti-inflammatory drugs, streptomycin or sulphonamides).

*Multiple sclerosis* may occur in childhood. In a study of five affected children [2], the age ranged from 2 to 9 years. It may present as optic neuritis, encephalitis, focal neurological signs or focal convulsions with mental deterioration.

*Optic atrophy* is usually a sequel to papilloedema, but occurs in a variety of degenerative diseases (e.g. Leber's hereditary optic neuropathy, progressive visual failure, possibly related to faulty detoxification of cyanide).

*Drugs* which cause optic atrophy, apart from the above, include arsenic, methanol, penicillamine, quinine, streptomycin and thallium. It may result from solvent sniffing. Short-lasting loss of vision may be a premonitory symptom of migraine.

*Sudden loss of vision.* Sudden loss of vision may result from trauma, acute hypoxia (cardiac arrest, cardiac surgery, vertebral angiography) or carbon monoxide poisoning [1, 3].

Taylor *et al.* [6] described four cases of sudden blindness due to infarction of the optic nerve head caused by a too rapid reduction of blood pressure in children with malignant hypertension.

Blindness may be due to infections—toxoplasmosis, toxocara, ophthalmia neonatorum, and in the tropics trachoma, onchocerciasis or keratomalacia.

# References

1 Barnet AB, Manson J, Wilner E. Acute cerebral blindness in children. *Neurology* 1970; **20**: 1147.
2 Bye AM, Kendall B, Wilson J. Multiple sclerosis in childhood: a new look. *Dev Med Child Neurol* 1985; **27**: 215.
3 Duffner PK, Cohen ME. Sudden bilateral blindness in children. *Clin Pediatr (Phila)* 1978; **17**: 705.
4 Duguette P, Murray TJ, Pleines J, *et al.* Multiple sclerosis in childhood. *J Pediatr* 1987; **111**: 359.
5 Garfield J, Neil-Dwyer G. Delay in diagnosis of optic nerve and chiasmal compression presenting with unilateral failing vision. *Br Med J* 1975; **1**: 22.
6 Taylor D, Ramsay J, Day S, Dillow M. Infarction of the optic nerve head in children with accelerated hypertension. *Br J Ophthalmol* 1981; **65**: 153.

## CATARACT

The following are some causes of cataracts in children:
Congenital
Rubella syndrome
Down's syndrome
Trauma
Juvenile chronic arthritis
Diabetes mellitus
Head-banging
Syndromes of Niemann–Pick, Rothmund–Thomson (p. 364), Fabry, Fanconi, Lowe, Zellweger (hepatorenal), Alport (deafness), Marfan, Marchessani (short fingers, glaucoma, short stature, mental subnormality)
Myotonia congenita
Metabolic conditions—galactokinase deficiency, galactosaemia, hypoparathyroidism, hypophosphatasia, mucopolysaccharidoses, abetalipoproteinaemia, homocystinuria, Wilson's disease
Skin conditions—congenital ichthyosis, incontinentia pigmenti, ectodermal dysplasia
Skeletal conditions—craniofacial dysostosis, punctate epiphysial dysplasia
Drugs

An opacity due to toxocara can resemble that due to retinoblastoma in infancy.

Apart from the *genetic forms* of cataract, the common congenital form is that due to the *rubella syndrome*: but in the rubella syndrome the cataract may develop after birth, during the first year. The virus has been isolated from a surgically removed cataract as late as 2 years after birth.

About 10 per cent of children with Down's syndrome develop cataracts, usually after the first 10 years or so, but sometimes earlier.

About 10 per cent of children on continuous *corticosteroid* therapy for a year or more develop a cataract. Such prolonged therapy is sometimes (unwisely) used for *juvenile chronic arthritis*, which may itself cause iridocyclitis and a lens opacity. *Diabetes mellitus* only rarely causes a cataract in childhood.

It is said that prolonged *head-banging* may cause a cataract to develop after a few years [2]. Other causes are *maternal galactosaemia* or *galactokinase* deficiency [1].

Various *drugs*, other than corticosteroids, may cause lens opacities: they include antimitotic drugs, carbamazepine, chlorambucil, chloroquine, indomethacin and the phenothiazines. Isoniazid may cause *keratitis*.

### References

1 Sidbury JB. Some inferences from galactokinase deficiency. *Pediatrics* 1974; **53:** 309.
2 Spalter HF, Bemporad JR, Sours JA. Cataracts following head-banging in children. *Arch Ophthalmol* 1970; **83:** 182.

## NYSTAGMUS

*By far the commonest cause of nystagmus in an infant is a defect of vision such as optic atrophy.* This should be considered to be the diagnosis until proved otherwise. The nystagmus in such children is often but not always of the roving type, unlike the finer nystagmus due to other conditions. Roving eye movements and nystagmus may follow an intraventricular haemorrhage in the newborn [1].

The following are the main causes of nystagmus:

Sitting in a moving vehicle
Defect of vision and astigmatism
Congenital nystagmus
Anti-epileptic and other drugs
Albinism
Spasmus nutans (p. 230)
Friedreich's ataxia, ataxia telangiectasia (p. 212)
Cerebellar ataxia, tumour, abscess
    Infratentorial tumours
Hypothyroidism
Drugs—anticonvulsants, colistin, diphenoxylate, salicylates

Nystagmus is almost invariable in *albinism,* and it is usual in *spasmus nutans* in which there are jerky head movements, ceasing when the child concentrates on an object.

Nystagmus may be caused by various diseases of the cerebellum or cerebellar tracts—such as Friedreich's ataxia, congenital ataxia, tumour or abscess. *Friedreich's ataxia* is a progressive hereditary disease, whose features include ataxia, absence of the knee jerks, plantar extensor responses and pes cavus with rombergism. Schulman & Crawford [2] described four cases of congenital nystagmus associated with hypothyroidism.

## References

1 Dubowitz LMS, Levene MI, Morante A, Palmer P, Dubowitz V. Neurologic signs in neonatal intraventricular hemorrhage: a correlation with real-time ultrasound. *J Pediatr* 1981; **99:** 127.
2 Schulman JD, Crawford JD. Congenital nystagmus and hypothyroidism. *N Eng J Med* 1969; **280:** 708.

## DIPLOPIA

Diplopia is caused usually by muscle imbalance, due to weakness of an external ocular muscle. It may result from a variety of neurological diseases, encephalitis, Guillain–Barré syndrome, meningitis, diphtheria, botulism, myasthenia, increased intracranial pressure, tumour or trauma.

*A blow-out fracture of the orbit* in children is an important cause of diplopia [1]. A blow on the eye may cause a swelling, haemorrhage and increased intra-orbital pressure. There may be enophthalmos, downward displacement of the eye, ptosis, limited vertical gaze, with diplopia following 4 or 5 days after the 'black eye'. An important physical sign is loss of sensation in the area supplied by the infra-orbital or superior dental nerves.

Other eye conditions causing diplopia include cataract, dislocation of the lens and iridocyclitis.

A variety of *drugs* may cause diplopia: they include anticonvulsants, antihistamines, non-steroidal anti-inflammatory drugs, chloroquine, cytotoxic drugs, fenfluramine, quinine, tranquillizers and vitamin A excess.

*Unilateral diplopia* may be caused by a meibomian cyst on the eyelid; mucus or exudate alters the refraction of the eye and leads to blurring. Unilateral diplopia could also be caused by dislocation of the lens or by corneal lesions.

### Reference

1 Illingworth CM. *The diagnosis and primary care of accidents and emergencies in children.* Oxford: Blackwell Scientific Publications, 2nd edn, 1982, p. 74.

## STRABISMUS

It is essential that a squint should be diagnosed shortly after the age of 6 months, because if left untreated the child will develop amblyopia as a result of suppressing the squinting eye. In the same way if a congenital cataract is not removed sufficiently early, the eye will remain blind: and a child with marked asymmetry of refraction or visual acuity may suppress vision in one eye.

It is normal for some degree of strabismus to occur before the age of 6 months, but a fixed squint at any age is abnormal, so that the child should be referred to an ophthalmologist as soon as possible. An important and treatable condition which causes a fixed squint in the first few weeks is the *retinoblastoma*.

A *fixed squint* is commonly found in cerebral palsy, microcephaly and hydrocephalus. The sudden development of a squint could be due to *ophthalmoplegic migraine* [2]; manifestations include third nerve palsy, headache and vomiting. Other causes include *trauma, cerebral tumour* or *haemorrhage, encephalitis, tuberculous meningitis, botulism, myasthenia, cavernous sinus thrombosis, cerebral vascular abnormalities,* and the *Guillain–Barré syndrome.*

Squints are due to imbalance of muscle, as a result of weakness or maldevelopment of the muscle or faulty innervation; to differences in the refraction of the two eyes; to hypermetropia or to a visual defect in one eye—such as that due to a corneal opacity or the retinopathy of prematurity [1]. A squint is an unusual side effect of *nalidixic acid* and of *tricyclic antidepressants.*

When the squint is of the paralytic type (non-comitant), due to paralysis of muscle, the eyes are straight except when moved in the direction of the paralysed muscle, when diplopia occurs.

When the squint is concomitant (non-paralytic), as it usually is, all muscles move the eyes normally, but they do not work in conjunction. The two eyes are in the same relative position to each other whatever the direction of the gaze. There is no diplopia.

In young infants one can determine whether there is a squint by noting the position of the light reflex on each cornea when a torch is held in front of the child. The reflex should be in the centre of the pupil or at a corresponding point on the two corneas.

In testing an older child, one covers one eye while with the other he looks at an auriscope light 32–37 cm in front of him. When the card is slowly moving away, the eyes should not move if the eyes are straight. When the fixating eye is covered the other eye should not move unless a squint is present. If there is a convergent squint, there will be a lateral movement: if there is a divergent squint, there will be a medial movement. The examiner watches the eye which is being uncovered.

A false appearance of a convergent squint is caused by *epicanthic folds*: the examiner should pinch the nose in such a way that the folds disappear—when it will be easier to see whether there is or is not a squint.

### References

1 Phelps DL. Vision loss due to retinopathy of prematurity. *Lancet* 1981; **1:** 606.
2 Raymond LA, Tew J, Fogelson MH. Ophthalmoplegic migraine of early onset. *J Pediatr* 1977; **90:** 1035.

## MYOPIA

The following are the known causes of myopia [1]:

    Congenital and familial. Myopia is commonly a familial feature. There may be other congenital conditions, such as colobomata or albinism.

    Maternal toxaemia or hypertension. A history of these conditions is frequent when myopia is severe.

    Rubella syndrome

    Malnutrition *in utero*. Prematurity and particularly dysmaturity are proper precursors. Retrolental fibroplasia may result in myopia.

    Social. Myopia is more common in the poor than in the well-to-do

    Marchesani syndrome (p. 189)

    Degenerative conditions usually commence after the age of four. They may lead to retinal degeneration or detachment of the retina

    The effect of drugs (rare). These include acetazolamide, corticosteroids, sulphonamides and tetracycline

### Reference

1 Gardiner P, James G. Myopia. *Brit J Ophthalmol* 1960; **44:** 172.

## PHOTOPHOBIA

Photophobia may be due to hysteria. It is experienced by some children with migraine (p. 101). It may be associated with blepharospasm resulting from a corneal or conjunctival irritant. Other causes include:

    Meningitis
    Foreign body in the eye
    Iridocyclitis, phlyctenular conjunctivitis
    Corneal ulcer
    Measles
    Albinism

Drugs—atropine eye drops, ethosuximide, mercury (pink disease), PAS, troxidone

Vitamin A deficiency

Rare

Congenital glaucoma

Acrodermatitis entropathica (p. 362)

Cystinosis

Botulism

Retinitis pigmentosa

It is a troublesome symptom in phlyctenular conjunctivitis, which is usually due to tuberculosis; there are white or grey papules 1–2 mm in diameter on the cornea or bulbar conjunctiva, with injection of the surrounding sclera and profuse lachrymation.

Photophobia is sometimes an early symptom in *congenital glaucoma*.

## LACHRYMATION AND EPIPHORA

The newborn baby does not usually shed tears when he cries, and often does not do so until he is 4 to 6 weeks old, unless there is injury to the eye. Some normal babies (not babies with Riley's syndrome) may not shed tears for several weeks. When babies begin to shed tears, the eyes may water (epiphora) if the nasolachrymal duct has not completely opened: this opens spontaneously in almost all cases in a few weeks or months [1]. Other causes of lachrymation are as follows:

Maternal heroin addiction

Malposition of the punctum as a result of facial palsy, chronic blepharitis or trauma

Trauma: eyelash in the canaliculus

Other foreign bodies

Pain in the eye (mainly injury or iridocyclitis)

Infection—conjunctivitis, including phlyctenular conjunctivitis due to tuberculosis, corneal ulcer

Migraine

Measles

Bad smells

Eyestrain

Hay fever

Thyrotoxicosis

Facial palsy

Drugs—amphetamine, arsenic, bromides, iodides, mercury, nitrazepam

Conjunctivitis does not usually cause pain: if there is pain one should suspect that there is iritis.

Tartrazine sensitivity may cause lachrymation (p. 158).

### Reference

1 Muller K, Burse H, Osmers F. Anatomy of the nasolacrymal duct in newborn: therapeutic considerations. *Eur J Pediatr* 1978; **129**: 83.

## PAIN IN THE EYE

Pain in the back of the eye is a frequent symptom accompanying the general aches and pains of any fever. It may be a feature in migraine.

Pain in the eye may be due to a foreign body, ingrowing eyelashes, iridocyclitis or corneal lesions. It may occur in retrobulbar neuritis.

Rare causes in children include glaucoma, herpes, ethmoiditis, sinusitis, orbital periostitis and Kawasaki disease (p. 39).

It can be caused by drugs.

## COLOUR VISION

Colour vision may be affected by ethambutol. Loss of colour vision occurs in retinitis pigmentosa and in night blindness. White vision may result from troxidone.

Yellow vision may be due to barbiturates, digoxin, streptomycin, sulphonamides or thiazide diuretics.

Blue or purple vision may be due to nalidixic acid.

## PTOSIS

In *congenital ptosis* there is a defective development or absence of the levator palpebrae superioris or a defect in the superior rectus. It occurs in the *fetal alcohol syndrome.*

Rare causes include:

Horner's syndrome—a disturbance of the cervical sympathetic chain, with unilateral miosis, apparent enophthalmos, ptosis, absence of facial sweating and heterochromia of the iris. It may occur in association with Klumpke's paralysis.

Myotonic dystrophy (p. 207) and congenital facial diplegia (Möbius syndrome). In both there is an immobile face and open mouth

Myotubular myopathy

Myasthenia gravis

Dystrophic ophthalmoplegia. This may start at any time from infancy to adult life, usually with ptosis as the first symptom. It is slowly progressive, and is confined to the levators of the eyelid and external ocular muscles. Later there is weakness of the lateral and vertical eye movements

Ophthalmoplegic migraine

Marcus Gunn phenomenon—ptosis until the mouth is opened, when the eyelid is simultaneously raised

Smith–Lemli–Opitz syndrome (ptosis, syndactyly, cryptorchidism)

Tumours—rhabdomyosarcoma, neuroblastoma

Abetalipoproteinaemia

Encephalitis. Wernicke's encephalopathy

Botulism

Syndromes of Leigh (p. 16), Noonan (p. 22), Aarskog (p. 24)

Porphyria

Trauma: blow-out fracture of orbit (p. 191)

Drugs—sulthiame or vinicristine

## PROPTOSIS

Proptosis is an uncommon symptom [2].
  Rare causes are:
      Thyrotoxicosis
      Craniostenosis, craniofacial dysostosis
      Tumours—neuroblastoma, angioma, rhabdomyosarcoma,
          retinoblastoma, teratoma, glioma, neurofibroma,
          osteoma, histiocytosis X
      Cysts or cystic swellings—dermoid, orbital encephalocele,
          anterior meningocele, mucocele of the paranasal sinus
      Orbital cellulitis, ethmoiditis
      Cavernous sinus thrombosis, arteriovenous aneurysm
      Haemorrhage—blood diseases, pertussis
      Trauma—fractured base of skull
      Cystic fibrosis (rare) [1]
  For orbital cellulitis, cavernous sinus thrombosis and ethmoiditis,
see p. 50.
  Proptosis may occur in *orbital periostitis* or *osteitis of the frontal bone*.

### References
1 Strauss RG, West PJ, Silverman FN. Unilateral proptosis in cystic fibrosis.
    *Pediatrics* 1969; **43**: 297.
2 Vanselm JL. Proptosis in paediatrics. *S African Med J* 1980; **57**: 662.

# Symptoms Related to the Ear

## EAR PAIN AND EAR DISCHARGE

### Pain

The usual cause of ear pain is *acute otitis media*, especially if the
temperature is raised. [1]. Other causes are as follows [2]:
      The pinna—injury, boil, herpes

External auditory meatus—boil, foreign body, herpes, otitis externa, injury

Referred pain—from lower molar teeth, temporomandibular joint, throat, possibly cervical spine, mumps

## Discharge

When a mother complains that her child's ear discharges she usually refers to wax. A purulent discharge is usually due to otitis media but it could be due to a foreign body or boil in the external auditory meatus, or to otitis externa. A clear watery discharge after a head injury suggests cerebrospinal fluid in association with a fracture of the skull. Blood from the ear may be due to insertion of a foreign body by the child, or to injury by a parent (child abuse or Munchausen syndrome by proxy) [1].

## References

1 Bourchier D. Bleeding ears; case report of Munchausen syndrome by proxy. *Aust Paediatr J* 1983; **19:** 256.
2 Smyth GDL. *Diagnostic ear, nose and throat.* London: Oxford University Press, 1978.

## DEFECTIVE HEARING

A child may appear to be deaf because he does not listen—perhaps because he is engrossed in an interesting occupation, or because of indiscipline or bad manners. A mentally handicapped infant is likely to be slow to respond to sound and to be wrongly suspected of deafness.

A child with infantile autism may appear to be deaf because of lack of social responsiveness.

If a parent suspects deafness it is likely that her fears are well founded, and a full testing should be carried out by an expert.

It is a routine practice to check the hearing of all children with delayed or defective speech. A child may appear to be deaf when he has delayed auditory maturation—a condition similar to delayed visual maturation (p. 185) [2].

Conditions liable to be associated with deafness include the following:

Important congenital conditions

Genetic (familial) deafness

Prenatal—rubella, cytomegalovirus, syphilis, chickenpox, drugs (quinine, streptomycin, kanamycin, gentamicin, neomycin, vancomycin, thalidomide)

Mental subnormality

Cerebral palsy

Cleft palate, Pierre Robin syndrome

Down's syndrome [1]

Hypothyroidism

Rare congenital syndromes

Syndromes of Alport, Lowe, Waardenburg, Treacher Collins, Klippel–Feil, Kallman (p. 183), Pendred (goitre), Hurler, Refsum (p. 212), Netherton (p. 356)

Surcardiac syndrome (p. 245)

Xeroderma pigmentosum (p. 359)

Multiple lentiginoses (p. 358)

Retinitis pigmentosa

Albinism

Osteogenesis imperfecta. Osteopetrosis

Acquired conditions

Neonatal hyperbilirubinaemia

Extreme prematurity. Severe hypoxia or acidosis at birth

Prolonged nasotracheal intubation

Recurrent otitis media, glue ear, adenoids

Meningitis, measles, mumps, mumps vaccine, infectious mononucleosis (p. 48)

Trauma

Repeated exposure to loud noise

Acoustic neuroma

Drugs

Before other factors are considered one should examine the ears with an auriscope in order to eliminate blockage of the meatus by wax.

About 30 per cent of children born to mothers who had *rubella* in the first 3 months of pregnancy will have some defect of hearing. It should be noted that this may be only partial or it may be confined to one ear, or it may develop in the early years after infancy. In making a diagnosis (which is essential for genetic counselling) one must not be misled by the absence of a history of rubella in pregnancy. In a survey of 732 cases [8], 47 per cent of mothers gave a history of a rubella-like illness, 15 per cent contact only, 12 per cent a non-specific fever, while 25 per cent were well throughout the pregnancy, with no history of contact, rash or illness. Prenatal cytomegalovirus may cause progressive deafness. Deafness may result from mumps whether or not there is parotitis (p. 14).

*Cerebral palsy and mental subnormality* are strongly associated with deafness. Some 20 to 25 per cent of all children with cerebral palsy have some degree of deafness. Children with athetosis are more likely to have a hearing defect than those with the spastic form of cerebral palsy.

*Hyperbilirubinaemia* in the newborn period, whether due to prematurity, haemolytic disease or other causes, predisposes to deafness. In the fully developed case there are other signs of kernicterus such as athetosis. A history of severe jaundice in the newborn period should alert one to the possibility of deafness in later months and years. There is some association between deafness and extreme prematurity, severe perinatal hypoxia, acidosis and prolonged assisted ventilation.

It is said that there is an increased incidence of deafness in children with preauricular tags [5].

Delayed auditory maturation, not associated with mental subnormality or other defects, has been described [2].

Most children with a *cleft palate* develop deafness.

Some infants with *hypothyroidism* have a hearing defect. Balkany *et al.* [1] found a significant hearing loss in two thirds of 103 children with *Down's syndrome*—a factor which would add to their mental handicap.

*Meningitis and recurrent otitis* are important causes of deafness. The danger that recurrent attacks of otitis may cause deafness, particularly if perforation of the drum is allowed to occur, is an important reason for the prompt treatment of otitis media. The development of deafness in association with a mass of adenoids is a strong indication for adenoidectomy.

The so-called *'glue-ear'* or *serous otitis media* may be a sequel of repeated and usually inadequately treated otitis media. Grommets may damage the drum [3, 7, 9] by causing scarring, permanent perforation or tympanosclerosis.

*Congenital syphilis,* now rare in Britain, is an important cause of deafness in some countries.

Repeated or prolonged exposure to *loud noise,* as in discos, is liable to cause permanent deafness.

A variety of *drugs* cause deafness [6]. Some of these may affect the child when given to the pregnant woman. The main ones are actinomycin, aminoglycosides, ampicillin, non-steroidal anti-inflammatory drugs, chloroquine, cotrimoxazole, erythromycin lactobionate, ethacrynic acid, framycetin, frusemide, medroxyprogesterone, nortriptyline, propranolol, quinine, rifampicin, salicylates and vincristine. [1] Neomycin-containing aerosols applied to broken skin have caused many cases of deafness.

Of the many rare congenital syndromes associated with deafness, *Waardenburg's syndrome* is probably the most common. It consists of a white forelock, heterochromia of the iris and congenital deafness.

## Conclusion

There are many possible causes of deafness and many factors which increase the likelihood of deafness. These 'risk' factors should alert one to the possibility of deafness. It must be remembered that the child born with defective hearing cannot know that he does not hear well. It is our responsibility to make the diagnosis. *Every child with delayed or defective speech must have his hearing tested by an expert.*

The method of clinical diagnosis has been described in detail in my book [4]. Suitable test sounds are the crinkling of paper, a small hand bell, the sound of PS or PHTH (for high tones) and OO (for low tones), on a level with the ear and 30–45 cm away, out of sight of the baby. In the first 3 months the baby may respond by a startle reflex, by blinking the eyes, by momentarily stopping sucking his dummy, by crying, or by quieting if he is already crying. At between 3 and 4 months he responds by turning his head to sound.

## References

1 Balkany TJ, Downs MP, Jafek BW, Krajicek MJ. Hearing loss in Down's syndrome. *Clin Pediatr (Phila)* 1979; **18:** 116.
2 Fisch L. Integrated development and maturation of the hearing system. *Br J Audiology* 1983; **17:** 137.
3 Fox AM. Grommets don't work. *Pediatrics* 1980; **65:** 1198.
4 Illingworth RS. *Development of the infant and young child, normal and abnormal.* Edinburgh: Churchill Livingstone, 9th edn, 1987.
5 Kankkunen A, Thiringer G. Hearing impairment in connection with pre-auricular tags. *Acta Paediatr Scand* 1987; **76:** 143.
6 Miller JJ. Drug-induced ototoxicity. *Hospital Update* 1983; **9:** 555.
7 Narula AA, Bradley PJ. Glue ear: the new dyslexia. *Br Med J* 1985; **2:** 411.
8 Smithells RW, Sheppard S, Holzel H, Dickson A. Communicable diseases: national congenital rubella surveillance programme. July 1971 to 30 June 1984. *Br Med J* 1985; **2:** 40.
9 Stickler GB. The attack on the tympanic membrane. *Pediatrics* 1984; **74:** 291.

## HYPERACOUSIS

Hyperacousis, or undue sensitivity to sound, is usually a normal and common reaction of small children to loud noise. True hyperacousis is sometimes a feature of Bell's palsy.

## TINNITUS

The complaint of buzzing in the ears (tinnitus) may be psychological. It may precede an attack of migraine or an epileptic fit.

Tinnitus may be caused by antihistamines, carbamazepine, quinine, salicylates, non-steroidal anti-inflammatory drugs and methylphenidate.

The symptom may originate from an acoustic nerve tumour.

A rare cause is an intracranial arteriovenous communication. It is worthwhile looking for distended veins on the face and scalp, and auscultating the skull for a continuous bruit.

## VERTIGO

Vertigo is such a subjective symptom that it is not easy to assess it in children [2]. The young child cannot describe what he feels; and the fact that he is experiencing vertigo may not be recognized. Vertigo commonly precedes a faint or fit, or occurs with a change of posture when he has been ill or is anaemic. It could be a *psychological symptom*, and may be due to *over-ventilation* (p. 148).

The causes of vertigo include:

>Benign paroxysmal vertigo
>Epidemic vertigo and vestibular neuronitis
>Epilepsy
>Hypoglycaemia
>Migraine (premonitory symptom)
>Drugs
>Rare
>>Cerebellar lesions
>>Cerebral tumours
>>Labyrinthitis after mumps
>>Sequela of meningitis or head injury
>>Chronic otitis media
>>Ramsay Hunt syndrome
>>Occlusive disease of the vertebrobasilar vessels
>>Multiple sclerosis

*Benign paroxysmal vertigo* [1] is a mysterious but distressing condition, occurring mainly at about 1 to 3 years of age, in which there is a sudden attack of severe vertigo lasting for seconds or minutes, sometimes with nystagmus or vomiting. The child is terrified, becomes pale and sweats and may cling to the parents, fall, stagger or cry for help. The attacks may recur after an interval of days or months, ceasing after a period varying from 4 months to 4 years. Vestibular caloric tests always show absence or short duration of the normally induced nystagmus. The CSF and EEG are normal. It was suggested by Koehler [3] that it could be a migraine equivalent. It is most important to distinguish these attacks from epilepsy; the most important distinguishing feature is the retention of consciousness in benign paroxysmal vertigo.

Vertigo may be a manifestation of *epilepsy* especially when there is a focus in the temporal lobe, and it may be a premonitory symptom of *migraine* or a symptom of *hypoglycaemia*.

*Epidemic vertigo and vestibular neuronitis* (which may or may not be the same thing) occurs usually a few days after an upper respiratory tract infection, with recurring attacks of vertigo without neurological signs, but with abnormal labyrinthine responses to hot and cold. They are thought to be of virus origin and are infectious. The child recovers in days or weeks.

Rare causes of vertigo include *cerebellar tumour and abscess*, and the *acoustic neuroma, labyrinthitis* complicating mumps, a *posterior fossa tumour, chronic otitis media* and the *Ramsay Hunt syndrome* (facial palsy with herpes of the external auditory canal), *multiple sclerosis* [4] and *occlusive disease of the vertebrobasilar vessels*. In the latter condition there are attacks of vertigo, followed later by the development of ataxia. Diagnosis is by vertebral angiography.

Vertigo may be due to certain *drugs*, especially acetazolamide, alcohol, aminophylline, antibiotics, anticonvulsants, antihistamines, betablockers, cimetidine, clonidine, fenfluramine, isoniazid, nasal decongestant drops, metronidazole, non-steroidal anti-inflammatory drugs, pethidine, piperazine, quinine, salicylates and thiazides. It may be due to solvent sniffing; and it may be a reaction to monosodium glutamate (Chinese restaurant disease) (p. 102).

## References

1 Dunn DW, Snyder H. Benign paroxysmal vertigo in childhood. *Am J Dis Child* 1976; **130:** 1099.
2 Eviatar L, Eviatar A. Vertigo in children: differential diagnosis and treatment. *Pediatrics* 1977; **59:** 833.
3 Koehler B. Benign paroxysmal vertigo in childhood, a migraine equivalent. *Eur J Pediatr* 1980; **134:** 149.
4 Molteni RA. Vertigo as presenting symptom of multiple sclerosis in childhood. *Am J Dis Child* 1977; **131:** 553.

# Face Pain

Pain in the face may arise from a molar tooth, an acute antrum infection, a boil in the ear, or osteitis. Pain from herpes is rare in childhood.

Pain may be due to the *Costen temporomandibular syndrome* [1]. There is muscle spasm over the joint with a tender point in the temporalis muscle. The pain may be due to asymmetry of the bite, tooth grinding or gum chewing: it is rare before adolescence. Other causes are injury, mumps, recurrent parotitis or stone in the parotid duct.

### Reference

1  Sutcher HD, Lerman MD. Temporomandibular syndrome. *JAMA* 1973; **225:** 1248.

# Facial Palsy

It is not always easy to decide which side is normal and which abnormal when an infant or young child has a facial palsy [3, 9]. It was suggested that the abnormal side is indicated by the side on which the lip is pulled lowest.

The following are the usual causes of facial palsy:

    Newborn babies

        Pressure *in utero* against the facial nerve

        Injury by forceps

        Nuclear agenesis (rare)

        Möbius syndrome (rare) or myotonia dystrophica (rare)

        Congenital hypoplasia of the depressor anguli oris

    Older children

        Bell's palsy

        Post-ictal

        Mastoiditis

Infectious mononucleosis

Virus infection. Lyme disease

Cerebral tumour, leukaemia

Trauma

Rare

Sarcoid

Facioscapulohumeral type of muscular dystrophy

Hypertension

Melkersson's syndrome

Cardiofacial syndrome

Guillain–Barré syndrome

Increased intracranial pressure

Anaphylactoid purpura

Drugs—vincristine, vitamin E deficiency

The facial palsy of the newborn infant usually clears up in a few weeks. Though facial palsy is usually ascribed to pressure by forceps, it is known that almost all are of antenatal origin and are caused by pressure *in utero* against the facial nerve [5]. When the facial palsy does not improve, one suspects the more serious agenesis of the facial nucleus.

The *Möbius syndrome* is also termed congenital facial diplegia. There is striking immobility of the face with hardly any movement, so that the child does not smile and shows little expression when crying. Though the level of intelligence is usually below the average, these children are liable to be considered severely handicapped when in fact they are only slightly subnormal or even within normal limits. The cause is probably a failure of development of the facial and extra-ocular muscles. *Myotonia dystrophica* (sometimes called dystrophia myotonica) gives a similar facial appearance. It is characterized by hypotonia, mental retardation, myotonia, progressive muscle wasting, baldness, cataracts and gonadal atrophy. Early weakness in the facial muscles is followed by weakness in the neck, forearm extensors, hand, vasti, quadriceps and ankle dorsiflexors. The mouth tends to hang open and there is a droopy immobile face. There is myotonia, and wasting of the sternomastoid muscle. The mother is affected, but not the father. There may be a history of fetal movement and hydramnios. The EMG is characteristic.

Facial palsy developing in the older child is usually *Bell's palsy*: or it can result from mastoid infection or from herpes of the external auditory meatus (Ramsay Hunt syndrome). Other virus infections have been implicated. They include poliomyelitis, chickenpox and infectious mononucleosis. In a Scandinavian study [10] of seven children with peripheral facial palsy, six showed cerebrospinal fluid pleocytosis. Facial palsy has occurred in the spirochaetal infection Lyme disease [6] (p. 278). It may occur in mumps without parotitis [1]. There may be facial weakness for a few hours after a fit (Todd's paralysis).

Facial palsy of supranuclear type may be due to a *cerebral tumour*, especially a glioma of the pons [7].

Weakness of the facial muscles may develop in infancy or early childhood in the *facioscapulohumeral type of muscular dystrophy*.

Facial palsy may be associated with *hyerptension* [11]. The facial palsy is of lower motor neurone type. It was found in 20 per cent of thirty-five severely hypertensive children, possibly as a result of haemorrhage into the facial canal.

*Melkersson's syndrome* consists of facial palsy, chronic or recurrent oedema of the face and a furrowed tongue.

Cayler [2] described the association of transient facial palsy with *congenital heart disease* and other defects (cardio-facial syndrome).

Bilateral facial palsy occurs in the *Guillain–Barré syndrome*.

It may occur in *anaphylactoid purpura* [8] and in increased intra-cranial pressure. It can be caused by vincristine. It has resulted from vitamin E deficiency [4]; features include ataxia, chronic liver disease, areflexia, sensory loss, paralysis of gaze and facial weakness.

## References

1 Azimi PH. Mumps meningoencephalitis in children. *JAMA* 1969; **207**: 509.
2 Cayler GC. Cardiofacial syndrome. *Arch Dis Child* 1969; **44**: 69.
3 Evers K, Groneck P. Asymmetric crying facies, which is the right-wrong side? *Pediatrics* 1983; **71**: 144.
4 Guggenheim MA, Jackson V, Lilly J, *et al*. Vitamin E deficiency and neurologic disease in children with cholestasis. *J Pediatr* 1983; **102**: 577.
5 Hepner WR. Some observations on facial paresis in the newborn infant. *Pediatrics* 1951; **8**: 494.
6 Lycka BAS. Lyme disease in Canada. *Can Med Ass J* 1986; **134**: 48.
7 May M. Facial paralysis in children. *Head Neck Surgery* 1981; **89**: 841.
8 Meadow R. Schönlein–Henoch syndrome. *Arch Dis Child* 1979; **54**: 822.
9 Monreal FJ. Asymmetric crying facies: an alternative interpretation. *Pediatrics* 1980; **65**: 146.

10 Sandstedt P, Hyden D, Odkvist LM, Kostulas V. Peripheral facial palsy in children. *Acta Paediatr Scand* 1985; **74**: 281.
11 Trompeter RS, Smith RL, Hoare RD, Neville BG, Chantler C. Neurological complications of arterial hypertension. *Arch Dis Child* 1982; **57**: 913.

# Clumsiness and Ataxia

It seems to me to be irrational to write separate sections on the clumsy child and ataxia, because there are all gradations between the slight clumsiness of innumerable 'normal' children and severe disabling ataxia, with overlapping of the causes [3].

The causes of clumsiness and chronic ataxia are mainly as follows:

Normal variations
Delayed motor maturation: often familial
Emotional factors
Visual defect
Migraine
Mental subnormality
Minimal cerebral palsy of the spastic, ataxic or athetoid types
Visuospatial defects
Chorea
Muscular dystrophy
The effect of drugs: lead or mercury poisoning
Solvent sniffing and other drug addiction
Post-traumatic, postencephalitic
Cerebral tumour
Mirror movements
Hypothyroidism
Rare
  Degenerative diseases of the CNS. Multiple sclerosis, leucodystrophies
  Lipoidoses
  Huntington's chorea (p. 230), Wilson's disease
  Syndrome with chronic liver disease
  Ataxia telangiectasia

Basilar artery migraine

Abetalipoproteinaemia

Metachromatic leucodystrophy (p. 259) and other organic acidurias

Pyruvate carboxylase deficiency and vitamin E deficiency [4]

Xeroderma pigmentosum (p. 359)

Cerebral gigantism (p. 289)

Syndromes of Cogan (oculomotor apraxia), Klippel–Feil, Riley (p. 46), Von Hippel–Lindau (retinal changes, cerebellar ataxia), Pelizaeus–Merzbacher, Refsum, Sjögren (p. 51), Rett

The child who was late in learning to walk is usually late in learning to walk steadily, and falls more than others of the same age who learnt to walk sooner. I have frequently seen ataxia diagnosed in such cases.

Mothers commonly complain that one of their children falls a great deal, always has bruises on his legs, or seems awkward with his hands. The teacher complains that the child writes badly, holds his pencil in an odd way and is poor at physical training. Such children may have difficulty in tying shoelaces or buttoning coats. They may swing the arms in an odd way, bump into furniture, misjudge distance (as in going through a doorway) and frequently break objects. They find needle-threading a hopeless task: they are awkward in dressing, drawing, writing or feeding themselves. They tend to write with the whole body, with the tongue protruding and the paper at an unusual angle, while the free hand roams. They sometimes have difficulty in distinguishing right from left. They cannot throw a ball properly. These children often concentrate badly and are over-active and impulsive. They find reading difficult and may indulge in mirror writing. They may have difficulties in spatial appreciation. All the symptoms are made worse by scolding. Affected children commonly present as behaviour problems. They get into constant trouble at school, for teachers are apt to think that they are just naughty, dull, lazy or awkward. They may present as truancy. They often hate games because they are so bad at them and may be unpopular and ridiculed by their fellows. They may develop manifestations of insecurity, such as stuttering, excessive shyness, silly behaviour or bed-wetting.

On superficial examination these children look normal and intelligent. They may have an IQ well above the average, though some are merely average or below average. On neurological examination abnormal signs may be found. Whereas a normal child of 3 can stand for a few seconds and at 4 quite steadily on one foot, many of the clumsy children at the age of 5, 6 or 7 are unsteady when standing on one foot. They cannot jump like a 3-year-old or hop like a 5-year-old. When building a tower of ten cubes they have some tremor of the hand and may knock the tower down accidentally before it is completed. In timed tests of fine manipulation, such as the placing of small pegs into a peg board or bead-threading, they are far below the average in performance. They are poor at placing shaped objects through holes or at making designs with blocks or at copying letters. In the various tests performed by the psychologist, the performance is much inferior to the verbal tests.

There are wide normal variations in children, and these variations are often familial. Sometimes they are of emotional origin and are related to insecurity, yet many 'clumsy' children, though regarded as 'normal' but 'naughty' by their teachers, are not really normal—they show evidence of organic disease.

Mentally handicapped children tend to be more clumsy with the hands and other movements than normal children. It is said that small-for-dates children are more likely to be clumsy than children who were of average birth weight.

The term 'minimal brain dysfunction' or 'minimal brain damage' is applied by some to this condition. (See also 'over-activity', p. 215.) In some of these children there were minimal signs of cerebral palsy of the spastic or athetoid types.

Clumsiness may be related to myopia, visual defect or visuospatial difficulties. In some there is merely ataxia; they are examples of 'congenital ataxia'. Some have a slight tremor which interferes with fine hand movements [7].

Awkwardness and clumsiness with poor writing and emotional disturbance are common features of early *chorea*, and should alert one to this if the child had been normal previously. *Muscular dystrophy* may be the cause of the clumsiness (p. 209). There is a rare form of congenital myopathy which is manifested by persistent clumsiness.

Numerous *drugs* cause mild to severe clumsiness or ataxia; probably the commonest is phenytoin and other anticonvulsant drugs. A variety of other drugs may be responsible, in particular, antihistamines, colistin, cyclopentolate, diphenoxylate, indomethacin, niclosamide, piperazine, polymyxin, sedatives and tranquillizers, streptomycin, sulthiame and vincristine.

*Solvent sniffing* and *alcohol* may cause severe ataxia (p. 218).

Some children are clumsy because of *mirror movements*. When one hand tries to get a button through a buttonhole, the opposite free hand makes the same movements. As a result of these mirror movements the child finds it difficult to tie shoelaces and to carry out innumerable daily tasks.

Some children with the *Klippel–Feil* syndrome have a similar difficulty. They cannot let go of something with one hand while grasping with the other. This makes it difficult to climb a ladder.

Ataxia may occur in *hypothyroidism* [5]. Macfaul *et al.* [9] described neurological abnormalities in thirty patients where treatment started before the age of 2. Ten were clumsy, sixteen had a squint, three had nystagmus, six had speech defects and fifteen had minor motor abnormalities.

Rendle-Short, Appleton & Pearn [11] described the features of *Cogan's syndrome* of congenital oculomotor apraxia: the children are unable to turn the eyes in a horizontal position when asked to do so, and may be thought to be blind in early weeks. There may be jerky movements of the head, difficulty in changing direction suddenly when running, lateness in walking and mild mental subnormality.

A wide variety of *degenerative diseases of the nervous system* and *metabolic diseases* cause clumsiness.

*Ataxia telangiectasia* is a hereditary condition. The telangiectases appear at about 4 to 6 years of age, first on the bulbar conjunctiva, and then on the ear, on the face in a butterfly distribution, and later on the palate and sternum. There are frequent and sinus respiratory infections due to defective humoral and cellular immunity. Mental deterioration ensues, with dysarthria, drooling and athetosis. There may be ovarian hypoplasia, and a risk of the development of lymphoma.

In *Hartnup disease* there are episodes of ataxia with pellagra-like skin lesions. In *maple syrup urine* disease there are episodes of ataxia and convulsions, and the urine smells of maple syrup. The *Pelizaeus–Merzbacher* syndrome is a sex-linked slowly degenerative disease with nystagmus, ataxia, tremors and spasticity. *Refsum's* syndrome is characterized by ichthyosis, the development of nerve deafness, peripheral neuropathy, retinitis pigmentosa, ataxia and mental deterioration [10].

. In Rett's syndrome [2, 6, 8] a girl develops normally in the first year, then develops ataxia, repetitive hand movements, mental deterioration, autism and hypotonia proceeding later to rigidity (see autism, p. 305). Pyruvate carboxylase deficiency [1] is a progressive neurological disease with ataxia, peripheral nerve disease, weakness of eye movements, and episodes of increased weakness or ataxia. Ataxia is sometimes a feature of *paroxysmal torticollis* (p. 229).

*Acute ataxia.* Acute ataxia could be due to hysteria. It may be caused by *alcohol, acute labyrinthitis* (p. 205), *encephalitis, cerebral tumour* or *trauma*.

### References

1 Evans OB. Pyruvate carboxylase deficiency. *J Pediatr* 1984; **105:** 961.
2 Gillberg C, Wahlström J, Hagberg B. Infantile autism and Rett's syndrome. *Lancet* 1984; **2:** 1094.
3 Gubbay SS. *The clumsy child.* Philadelphia: Saunders, 1975.
4 Guggenheim MA, Jackson V, Lilly J. Vitamin E deficiency and neurologic disease in children with cholestasis; a prospective study. *J Pediatr* 1983; **102:** 577.
5 Hagberg B, Westphal O. Ataxic syndrome in congenital hypothyroidism. *Acta Paediatr Scand* 1970; **59:** 323.
6 Hagberg B, Aicardi J, Dias K, Ramos O. A progressive syndrome of autism, dementia, ataxia and loss of purposeful hand use in girls: Rett's syndrome. *Ann Neurol* 1983; **14:** 471.
7 Henderson SE, Hall D. Concomitants of clumsiness in young school children. *Dev Med Child Neurol* 1982; **24:** 448.
8 Kerr AM, Stephenson JBP. Rett's disease in the West of Scotland. *Br Med J* 1985; **2:** 579.
9 Macfaul R, Dorner S, Brett EM, Grant DB. Neurological abnormalities in patients treated for hypothyroidism from early life. *Arch Dis Child* 1978; **53:** 611.
10 Poulos A, Pollard A, Mitchell JD, Wise G, Mortimer G. Patterns of Refsum's disease. *Arch Dis Child* 1984; **59:** 222.
11 Rendle-Short J, Appleton B, Pearn J. Congenital ocular motor apraxia; paediatric aspects. *Austr Paediatr J* 1973; **9:** 263.

# Abnormal Gait

Abnormality of gait may be due to any of the causes of ataxia (p. 209). Other causes include:

Hysteria (older children, after about 7 years of age)

Hip conditions such as subluxation commonly cause a waddling gait. The same gait is seen in cases of muscular dystrophy involving the muscles around the hip. Other diseases of the hip, such as Perthes' disease, cause a limp

Cerebral palsy of the spastic type causes a characteristic gait: its nature depends partly on the distribution of the cerebral palsy—hemiplegia or diplegia. The hemiplegic child walks with a limp, partly because of the shortening of the affected leg, and he characteristically carries the affected arm adducted, partly across the abdomen

Hypotonia causes a characteristic gait. The causes include benign congenital hypotonia, poliomyelitis and rarely peripheral neuritis (p. 256)

# Paraesthesiae

Paraesthesiae are difficult to assess in children. The obvious cause of paraesthesiae in the legs is sitting with the legs crossed, or pressure of the edge of a chair against the back of the thigh.

Paraesthesiae may be one of the premonitory symptoms of *migraine* or a feature of *temporal lobe epilepsy*.

*Tetany* may result from hysterical over-ventilation, sulthiame, or hypoparathyroidism, and lead to paraesthesiae.

The symptom may be due to *drugs*—acetazolamide, amitriptyline, chlorothiazide, cotrimoxazole, ergotamine, imipramine, kanamycin,

metronidazole, nalidixic acid, nitrofurantoin, niclosamide, piperazine, polymyxin, streptomycin, sulthiame, trimethoprim, thiabendazole, or vincristine. Ergotamine may cause tingling, numbness
and chilling of the extremities.

Paraesthesiae may be a symptom in the Chinese restaurant disease
(p. 102), in which there is a sensitivity reaction to monosodium
glutamate.

# Over-activity

It is difficult to define the term over-activity with precision [6]. Many
mothers think that their children are 'over-active', and complain that
they are always on the go and never sit still, when in fact they are
normal. This sort of behaviour is usual in the child from 5 to 10 or so.
The healthy 6-year-old is always on the go: he does not walk, he runs;
when his mother holds one hand, he skips and hops. That which is
normal at one age, however, is not normal at another. As children
mature they lose much of this excess activity. In this section I shall
discuss what one may term 'unusual over-activity'. This is commonly
accompanied by a lack of concentration, ready distractability and
short attention span. The children tend to be impulsive, clumsy,
excessively talkative and even destructive. Their movements are more
purposeless than just increased in amount. These children wear their
mothers out and exhaust their teachers. The condition is more
common in boys. The term *'minimal brain dysfunction'* or *'attention
deficit disorder'* is applied by some to this condition—and to
clumsiness and some hundred other symptoms—though there is no
laboratory or psychological test which indicates that there was brain
damage [2, 5, 6]. It is now becoming recognized that the condition of
'minimal brain damage' is a myth, and that the term should be
abandoned [2, 9]. There may be a biochemical basis for the problem,
involving biogenic amines [4, 7]. There may be an underlying variant
in monoamine metabolism.

The main causes of 'unusual over-activity' may be summarized as follows:

> Normal variation
> Delayed maturation
> Heredity
> Prenatal hypoxia, alcohol, toxaemia, maternal smoking, other drug addictions
> Neonatal hyperbilirubinaemia
> Personality, insecurity, excessive restraint, boredom, poor teaching or motivation
> Mental handicap
> Allergy or hypersensitivity
> Autism
> Temporal lobe epilepsy
> Lead poisoning
> Drugs

Unusual over-activity may be a *familial* trait. It may be partly a matter of an inherited personality characteristic. It must not be assumed that an over-active child has suffered 'brain injury' without first enquiring about the behaviour of the mother or father at that age.

*Mental subnormality* is a common cause of unusual over-activity in the young child, partly because mentally subnormal children mature more slowly than normal ones. As a result they are late in growing out of over-activity. Over-activity is often a feature of *autism* or *temporal lobe epilepsy*.

Certain *drugs* may be responsible for over-activity. They include chlordiazepoxide, clonazepam, phenobarbitone, phenytoin, primidone and the tricyclic antidepressants. Children taking theophylline [1] may experience insomnia, depression, irritability and over-activity.

Allergy to cow's milk protein or certain other foodstuffs, or hypersensitivity to tartrazine or other food additives, may sometimes be a factor [8]. Drugs of addiction taken by the mother in pregnancy [3], or later taken by the child himself, may be responsible.

## References

1 Brumback RA, Wilson H, Staton RD. Behavioural problems in children taking theophylline. *Lancet* 1984; **1:** 958.

2 Carey WB, McDevitt SC. Minimal brain dysfunction and hyperkinesis. *Am J Dis Child* 1980; **134:** 926.

3 Olofsson M, Buckley W, Anderson GE, Friis-Hansen B. Investigation of 89 children born to drug dependent mothers. *Acta Paediat Scand* 1983; **72:** 403, 407.

4 Rapoport JL, Ferguson HP. Biological validation of the hyperkinetic syndrome. *Dev Med Child Neurol* 1981; **23:** 667.

5 Rie HL, Rie ED. *Handbook of brain dysfunctions.* New York: John Wiley, 1980.

6 Safer D, Allen RP. *Hyperactive children: diagnosis and management.* Baltimore: University Park Press, 1976.

7 Shaywitz SE, Cohen DJ, Shaywitz BA. The biochemical basis of minimal brain dysfunction. *J Pediatr* 1978; **92:** 179.

8 Stare FJ, Whelan EM, Sheridan M. Diet and hyperactivity. Is there a relationship? *Pediatrics* 1980; **66:** 521.

9 Wender PH, Wender EH. Minimal brain dysfunction myth. *Am J Dis Child* 1976; **130:** 900.

# Symptoms of Drug Addiction

I have no personal experience of patients with drug addiction, and this brief summary is based entirely on the work of others, especially those mentioned in the reference list. I have introduced this section in order to emphasize the wide diversity of symptoms which may result from drug abuse and therefore the importance of considering the possibility of drug abuse, especially when symptoms are bizarre and otherwise not explained. Owing to the frequent practice of combining drugs of addiction, there is much overlap in the grouping below.

## The newborn

The nature and timing of withdrawal symptoms depend in part on the drugs taken by the mother [7, 10]. For instance, withdrawal symptoms in the case of barbiturates commonly begin 2 to 14 days after birth, consisting largely of irritability, vomiting, sweating, hiccoughs and increased appetite, while those with other drugs mostly tend to occur earlier.

Symptoms or signs commonly found [8] are low birth weight, especially with opiates or nicotine, salivation, sneezing, grunting, nasal stuffiness, tachypnoea or respiratory distress, irritability, high-pitched cry, excessive crying, hypertonia, coarse flapping tremor, convulsions (less often with heroin), feeding difficulties, fever, vomiting or diarrhoea.

## Older children

General symptoms [3, 5, 6] include deterioration in behaviour and school performance, defective memory and concentration, confusion and hallucinations. Results of addiction include hepatitis or AIDS by injection, and criminal behaviour to obtain the drugs.

Cannabis [1, 3, 4, 5] may cause defective concentration and memory, slow thought, reduced perception of time and space (leading to road accidents), loquacity, euphoria, sleepiness, ataxia, hallucinations, rapid respirations and pulse, bronchial irritation and wheezing. It may delay secondary sexual characteristics.

Amphetamine may cause mental deterioration, paranoia, bruxism, dry mouth, hallucinations, tremor, depression, aggressiveness, fatigue, dysarthria, sweating and tremors.

Heroin may lead to mental deterioration, drowsiness, euphoria, constipation, polyneuritis, muscle weakness, lacrymation, convulsions, increased intracranial pressure, transverse myelitis, slow pulse and slow respirations.

Cocaine may cause euphoria, decreased fatigue, depression, increased motor activity, paranoia, hallucinations, anorexia, hypertension and fever. It is probably the most addictive of all the drugs of addiction.

LSD and other hallucinogens may cause exhilaration, unpredictable behaviour, incoherence, depression, panic reactions and suicide.

Barbiturates cause irritability, aggressiveness, depression and fits.

Solvent sniffing causes a wide variety of symptoms, because there are so many solvents in use. They may cause primarily liver, kidney, blood and bone marrow damage, or neurological symptoms, including ataxia, encephalomyelitis, loss of concentration, impaired judgement, coma, polyneuritis, loss of inhibitions, vertigo, confusion, diplopia and hallucinations.

Lead poisoning may result from inhaling lead-containing petrol [9].

I have mentioned alcohol and tobacco addiction elsewhere (p. 152). *Tobacco chewing* [2] is a dangerous practice. It may lead to stomatitis and oral cancer.

*Withdrawal symptoms* in older children include tremors, insomnia, cramp, vomiting, diarrhoea, fever, depression, convulsions, coma, lachrymation and insomnia.

## References

1 Council on Scientific Affairs. Marijuana. *JAMA* 1981; **246:** 1823.
2 Council on Scientific Affairs. Health aspects of smokeless tobacco. *JAMA* 1986; **255:** 1038.
3 Friedman JJ. Drug abuse problems in the pediatric age group. *Paediatrician* 1972; **1:** 8.
4 Kolansky H, Moore WT. Marihuana, can it hurt you? *JAMA* 1975; **232:** 923.
5 Litt IF. Substance abuse during adolescence. In: Behrman RE, Vaughan VC (eds). *Nelson's textbook of pediatrics.* Philadelphia: Saunders, 12th edn, 1983.
6 Nicholi AK. The nontherapeutic use of psychoactive drugs. *N Engl J Med* 1983; **308:** 925.
7 Olofsson M, Buckley W, Andersen GE, Friis-Hansen B. Investigation of 89 children born to drug-dependent mothers. *Acta Paediatr Scand* 1983; **72:** 403, 407.
8 Reddy AM, Harper RG, Stern G. Heroin withdrawal in the newborn. *Pediatrics* 1971; **48:** 353.
9 Seshia SS, Rajani KR, Boeckx RL, Chow PN. The neurological manifestations of chronic inhalation of leaded gasoline. *Dev Med Child Neurol* 1978; **20:** 323.
10 Zelson C. Infant of the addicted mother. *N Engl J Med* 1973; **288:** 1393.

# Undue Excitement, Aggressiveness, Irritability

Undue irritability in the newborn baby may be due to perinatal hypoxia, cerebral oedema or cerebral damage. It may be due to drugs taken by the mother in pregnancy, such as tricyclic antidepressants, barbiturates or phenothiazines, to smoking in pregnancy, or to other drugs of addiction.

A young baby's excessive irritability may be due to *phenylketonuria* or to *coeliac disease* (when given cereals).

In the older child, undue excitement, aggressiveness and irritability are usually behaviour problems, without organic disease. Like most behaviour problems, they result largely from a conflict between the child's personality and developing mind with that of the personalities and attitudes of his parents, friends and teachers. But all these symptoms could be due to disease, biochemical changes, epilepsy or drugs. Any debilitating disease, such as anaemia, may have a bad effect on a child's behaviour. The difficult and dangerous cases are those in which there is a combination of organic disease and behaviour problems. For instance, a *cerebral tumour* may cause a variety of personality changes.

Irritability and loss of appetite or energy can be due to *urea-cycle disorders* with hyperammonaemia.

Undue excitement or aggressive behaviour may be due to *hypoglycaemia*. When a child comes home in a bad temper, it may be due to hypoglycaemia, responding rapidly to a meal. Otherwise he may have been bullied at school by a teacher or child.

The most likely cause of persistent undue irritability in a well older child is *insecurity*, due probably to lack of love, excessive strictness, punishment or domestic friction. The irritability may be a familial personality trait. It may be due to lassitude, boredom, anaemia, infection or other illness.

A *wide variety of drugs* affect behaviour. In a review I included ninety of them in a table [1]. One of the worst offenders is a barbiturate—often with a paradoxical effect of causing insomnia and irritability, particularly in mentally subnormal children.

220

Drugs which cause undue excitement or irritability include the following: acetazolamide, aminophylline, amphetamine, anti-depressants, antihistamines, carbamazepine, ephedrine, fenflur-amine (on withdrawal), mepacrine, methimazole, nitrofurantoin, sulthiame, theophylline, thyroxine and troxidone. The symptoms can also be caused by alcohol, solvent sniffing and other drugs of addiction.

Cyclopentolate, cycloserine, ethionamide, hyoscine and fenflur-amine may cause a psychotic reaction. Various nose drops [3] may cause excitement, hallucinations, drowsiness or convulsions.

*Pink disease,* due to mercury in teething powders or other sub-stances, was characterized by irritability, constant crying, pinkness and peeling of hands and feet, excessive sweating and photophobia.

Sudden seriously aggressive behaviour with minimal provocation may occur in temporal lobe epilepsy or 'the episodic dyscontrol syndrome' [2].

### References

1 Illingworth RS. Developmental variations in relation to minimal brain dysfunction. In Rie HE, Rie HD (eds). *Handbook of minimal brain dysfunctions.* New York: Wiley, 1980.
2 Nunn K. The episodic dyscontrol syndrome in childhood. *J Child Psychol Psychiatr* 1986; **27**: 439.
3 Söderman P, Sahlberg D, Wiholm B. CNS reaction to nose drops in small children. *Lancet* 1984; **1**: 573.

# Confusion and Hallucinations

A short-lasting *confusional state* may be a premonitory symptom of *migraine* (p. 101); there may be partial aphasia at the time.

The symptoms could be due to *head injury, hypoglycaemia, temporal lobe epilepsy* or *heat stroke. Reye's syndrome, severe disease of the liver or kidney,* or *malaria* could be responsible.

Various drugs may be responsible, in particular alcohol, amphetamine, antibiotics, anticonvulsants, antihistamines, corticosteroids, cyclopentolate, digoxin, fenfluramine, food additives, griseofulvin, hyoscine, mepacrine, non-steroidal anti-inflammatory drugs, nose drops [1], phenmetrazine, piperazine, salbutamol, theophylline and tranquillizers.

*Hallucinations* may be a feature of *temporal lobe epilepsy* or *schizophrenia*. They may result from bites, various poisons, carbon monoxide or drugs of addiction including solvent sniffing.

### Reference

1 Drennal P. Visual hallucinations in children receiving nasal decongestants. *Br Med J* 1984; **1:** 1688.

# Delirium and Coma

*Delirium* may be defined as a state of confusion, disorientation, irrational speech or excitability. It is commonly due to lobar pneumonia or other acute infections, but may result from head injury, drugs and poisons.

*Coma* may be defined as prolonged profound unconsciousness. The most important causes to consider are diabetes or hypoglycaemia, head injury, drugs or cerebral haemorrhage.

Both delirium and coma have to be distinguished from hysteria.

Causes of coma include the following:

Metabolic conditions

Diabetes mellitus, hyperglycaemia, hypoglycaemia, hypoxia, hyponatraemia, hypernatraemia, dehydration, heat stroke, hyperpyrexia

Addison's disease

Liver or kidney failure

Hyperammonaemia

Porphyria

Inborn errors of metabolism—glycine encephalopathy, urea cycle disorders, organic acidurias, mucopolysaccharidoses, leucodystrophies

Infections and other encephalopathies
  Acute viral encephalitis (p. 224). Postinfectious or allergic
    encephalomyelitis
  Vaccine 'damage'
  Meningitis. Cerebral abscess
  Typhoid fever, malaria, rabies, poliomyelitis, herpes,
    mumps, measles. Insect-borne illness in the tropics.
    Fungus infections in immunosuppression
  Reye's syndrome (p. 80)
  Rett's syndrome. Leigh's syndrome
  Toxic shock syndrome (p. 92)
  Kawasaki disease
  Haemolytic uraemic syndrome. Disseminated intravascular
    coagulation
  Burn encephalopathy (p. 247)
  Cerebral vascular problems. Stokes—Adams syndrome.
    Acute infantile hemiplegia. Hypertension
  Trauma. Child abuse and shaking the child
  Epilepsy—postconvulsive. Status epilepticus
  Drugs and poisons. Munchausen syndrome by proxy (p. 33)
    Aluminium toxicity

A less usual cause of diabetic coma is the *non-ketotic hyperosmolar form* with hyperglycaemia, dehydration and convulsions, but with no significant ketosis. An important cause of hypoglycaemic coma is *alcohol poisoning*.

*Hyponatraemia* and *dehydration* or *heat stroke* are important causes of coma, especially in mentally subnormal children when they have a respiratory or alimentary tract infection. Over-ventilation would support the likelihood of the *hypernatraemic* type of dehydration. Hypernatraemia may also be caused by errors in the constitution of feeds—either by making them too concentrated, or by carelessly adding salt instead of sugar to feeds [7]; it could be due to over-clothing in hot weather causing hypernatraemia.

*Infective hepatitis* can be acute and lead to coma in a few hours. The Kussmaul breathing of uraemia should point to renal failure.

*Hyperammonaemia* may be caused by any of five inborn errors of metabolism involving the urea cycle. It is manifested in infancy or early childhood by vomiting, irritability, lethargy, fits, and often hypertonia and hepatic enlargement. Acute episodes may be precipitated by infection, anaesthetics or surgical procedures.

The symptoms of *encephalitis* include drowsiness, coma, convulsions, high-pitched cry, cranial nerve palsies, and mixed sensory and motor neurological abnormalities. There are numerous causes and they cannot all be discussed separately. For a comprehensive review of encephalitis, see the chapter by Ross & Bellman [5]. The main group of causes consists of infections, mainly viral. Encephalitis has been ascribed to pertussis vaccine, but there is no evidence for this [3, 4]. Focal fits with fever and increasing drowsiness may be due to herpes simplex encephalitis [1].

Postinfectious encephalomyelitis may occur in any of the acute infectious diseases, and may precede the rash in the exanthems or the parotid swelling in the case of mumps. The encephalitic symptoms may occur without the rash or the parotid swelling. Subacute sclerosing panencephalitis (SSPE) is usually related to a slow virus of measles; it begins with fits and is followed by sudden rhythmical convulsive movements, with slowly progressive dementia and death.

*Head injury,* including that due to child abuse, may be responsible. This may be due to shaking the child in anger. Minutes to an hour or more after what was thought to be minimal head injury, the child may become pale, sleepy and irritable and may vomit. Recovery may be complete, but it can progress to severe brain damage [2].

Coma may follow a severe *epileptic convulsion*: but, when a known epileptic presents in coma, one should remember that he might have taken an overdose of anti-epileptic drugs.

*Numerous drugs* and *poisons* may cause coma, and clinical examination may provide vital clues [3]. A hot dry skin may suggest belladonna poisoning. Perspiration may suggest salicylates, LSD or organophosphates. Nystagmus may suggest poisoning by phenytoin or barbiturates. Over-ventilation suggests salicylates, paraldehyde, methyl or ethylene glycol. Needle marks point to narcotics. Small pupils suggest narcotics, barbiturates or phenothiazines. Dilated pupils suggest belladonna, amphetamine or antihistamines.

Drugs and poisons which may cause coma include acyclovir, alcohol, amphetamine, aminophylline, antibiotics, anticonvulsants, antihistamines, atropine group, betablockers, carbon monoxide, cimetidine, cyclopentolate, digoxin, diphenoxylate, fenfluramine, iron, lead, mepacrine, mushroom poisoning, non-steroidal anti-inflammatory drugs, opiates, organophosphates, paracetamol, piperazine, salicylates, thallium, theophylline and tranquillizers.

Aluminium toxicity may occur in chronic renal failure with long-term dialysis [6]. The symptoms include personality change, encephalopathy, deterioration in school work, dysarthria, convulsions and myoclonus.

Coma may be due to solvent sniffing or other drugs of addiction.

The parents' statement that the child could not have had access to drugs must never be taken to eliminate poisoning (pp. 8, 148). Sometimes one strongly suspects narcotic poisoning but evidence is lacking; a therapeutic test of naloxone may provide that evidence.

### References

1 Brett EM. Herpes simplex encephalitis in children. *Br Med J* 1986; 2: 1488.
2 Bruce DA. Delayed deterioration of consciousness after trivial head injury in childhood. *Br Med J* 1984; 2: 715.
3 Maragos GD. The unconscious child. *Paediatrician* 1978; 7: 142.
4 Prensky AL. Pertussis vaccination. *Dev Med Child Neurol* 1974; 16: 539.
5 Ross EM, Bellman M. Encephalitis and encephalopathy. In Rose FC (ed.) *Paediatric neurology*. Oxford: Blackwell Scientific Publications, 1979, p. 522.
6 Sedman AH, Wilkening G, Warady BA, *et al*. Encephalopathy in childhood secondary to aluminium toxicity. *J Pediatr* 1984; 105: 836.
7 Stern GM, Jones RB, Fraser ACL. Hyperosmolar dehydration in infancy due to faulty feeding. *Arch Dis Child* 1972; 47: 468.

# Drowsiness

Undue drowsiness may be due merely to *fatigue* or *lack of sleep* if the child is otherwise well.

It may be due to any *serious illness*, including febrile conditions, meningitis, diabetic acidosis and uraemia.

A variety of *drugs* cause drowsiness. They include the anticonvulsant drugs, antihistamines, diphenoxylate, fenfluramine, indomethacin, methimazole, nalidixic acid, nose drops, PAS and the tranquillizing drugs. *Poisons* should be considered. As in the case of coma, drugs may be administered by the mother as child abuse or Munchausen syndrome by proxy.

Drowsiness may be due to *dehydration* including *heatstroke*. It may be due to hypernatraemia caused by the baby's feeds being made up too concentrated. It is sometimes an early symptom of *hypoglycaemia*.

In newborn babies *cold injury* may cause drowsiness, loss of appetite, oedema of the extremities, facial erythema, sclerema, haematemesis and pulmonary haemorrhage. Convulsions, due to hypoglycaemia, may result from over-rapid rewarming.

Drowsiness and apathy are a feature of severe malnutrition and kwashiorkor.

# Depression

Depression in childhood may present in a variety of symptoms—loss of appetite or excessive eating, insomnia or hypersomnolence, loss of energy, poor concentration, deteriorating school performance, school phobia, enuresis, drug-taking, suicidal thoughts, or a mixture of somatic and psychological symptoms, such as abdominal pain [1, 3, 5, 6]. There is commonly a family history of depression.

Depression is a major sequel of sexual abuse [2].

The *Kleine–Levin syndrome* has been described in a 10-year-old [4]. Features include significant episodic depression, weeping, hypersomnia, lethargy and over-eating; it is more common in boys.

Drugs which may cause depression include amphetamine, barbiturates, betablockers, chloroquine, cimetidine, clonidine, corticosteroids, digoxin, fenfluramine, indomethacin, isoniazid, nalidixic acid, nitrofurantoin, phenytoin, propranolol, reserpine, sulphasalazine, sulthiame, theophylline and tranquillizers.

## References

1 Aylward GP. Understanding and treatment of childhood depression. *J Pediatr* 1985; **107**: 1.
2 Barrett ML, Kolvin I. Childhood depression and sexual abuse. *Br J Hosp Med* 1985; **34**: 51.
3 Brumbach RA, Dietz-Schmidt SG, Weinberg WA. Depression in children referred to an educational diagnostic centre: diagnosis and treatment and analysis of criteria and literature review. *Dis Nervous System* 1977; **38**: 529.

4 Ferguson BG, Kleine–Levin syndrome: a case report. *J Child Psychol Psychiatr* 1986; **27**: 275.
5 Herzog, DB, Rathbun JM. Childhood depression. *Am J Dis Child* 1982; **136**: 115.
6 Kashani JH, Husain A, Shekim WO, *et al*. Current perspectives on childhood depression: an overview. *Am J Psychiatry* 1981; **138**: 143.

# Childhood Obsessional Behaviour

In a review of obsessional and compulsive behaviour in children, Rapoport [1] noted that about half of all adult cases begin by the age of 15; she described thirty cases in children with an onset between 3 and 14 years of age. It is associated with depression, the Tourette syndrome (p. 229), anorexia nervosa (p. 67) and a history of temporal lobe epilepsy.

### Reference

1 Rapoport JL. Childhood obsessive compulsive disorder. *J Child Psychol Psychiat* 1986; **27**: 289.

# Involuntary Movements

A wide variety of involuntary movements of differing types and severity may occur at any age in childhood. Below is a summary of the causes.

All normal infants exhibit the *Moro* and *startle reflexes* in the first three months. These reflexes may be exaggerated when there is cerebral irritability. The Moro reflex consists of a sudden abduction of the arms at the shoulder, with extension of the elbows and opening of the hands, followed by adduction as if in an embrace. It is probably due to vestibular reflexes set up by movement of the neck. The startle reflex results from a loud noise; it differs from the Moro reflex in that there is flexion of the elbows and the hands remain closed.

Normal children when asleep in the first few weeks have *sudden jerky movements* resembling the startle reflex.

Many newborn infants show a rapid *jittery movement* of the limbs. It occurs particularly in the presence of hypocalcaemia; for distinction from convulsions, see p. 234.

## Tremors

All normal infants in the early weeks display '*jaw trembling*'. In older children mild tremors are normal, but they are more often seen in clumsy or mentally subnormal ones. Tremor may be familial.

Tremors in the young baby may be related to maternal drug addiction, especially addiction to alcohol, and tremors in the fetal alcohol syndrome may persist for several weeks. Other drugs taken by the mother in pregnancy and which may cause tremors in the baby include amphetamine, diphenhydramine, heroin, pentazocine and tranquillizers. Drugs taken by the baby which may cause tremors include aminophylline, anticonvulsants, betablockers, cimetidine, lithium, metoclopramide, piperazine, salbutamol, terbutaline and tranquillizers. Other causes of tremor are thallium and solvent sniffing. Tremors may occur in the monosodium glutamate 'Chinese restaurant' syndrome (p. 102).

Other causes of tremors include Wilson's disease (p. 231), cerebellar lesions, encephalitis, hypoglycaemia and thyrotoxicosis.

## Hiccoughs

Hiccoughs occur in the normal fetus *in utero*. Young babies frequently hiccough after a feed. It is said that hiccoughs must not be assumed always to be benign [3]; they may immediately precede an apnoeic attack.

Other causes of hiccoughs include a subphrenic abscess, diaphragmatic pleurisy, cerebral tumour, peritonitis or uraemia. Epidemic hiccough may follow encephalitis. It may follow a respiratory infection, and last up to a week.

Hiccoughs may be a side effect of ethosuximide.

## Tics

Tics are extremely common in children. They usually consist of blinking of the eyes, twitching of the face, inappropriate opening of the mouth, shrugging the shoulders, sniffing or clucking the tongue. They are usually single repeated movements, but may be multiple and complex, and then resemble chorea; but in chorea the movements are always complex, and one never knows which movement is going to occur next. The characteristic hand movement of the child with chorea, when he is asked to hold the hands out pronated, help to establish the diagnosis of chorea.

Tics are more common in girls [20]. The onset is most often at around 7 years of age, and 90 per cent begin before the age of 10. They often disappear at puberty, but may persist throughout life. One tic usually lasts several months. Insecurity is often a factor.

Tics may be a side effect of amphetamine, antidepressants, carbamazepine or methylphenidate [9, 16]. Tics are related to dopamine metabolism, and are inhibited by dopamine antagonists, such as haloperidol and phenothiazines, and caused by dopaminergic drugs, which may also cause the Tourette syndrome, which usually begins between 2 and 15 years of age, with tics, head jerkings and later complex movements with involuntary noises—barking, grunting, hissing or uttering of obscenities [8], the symptoms waxing and waning.

## Spasmodic torticollis

Spasmodic torticollis consists of recurrent sudden single lateral movements of the neck. It may be a form of tic. A paroxysmal form can occur in infancy [5, 10], with two or three attacks a year, associated with crying, pallor, ataxia, nystagmus and vomiting on rotation of head. The attacks last 10 min to 14 days, with spontaneous recovery by the age of 5. It could be a vestibular neuronitis or a precursor of migraine. There is often a familial factor.

*Sandifer's syndrome* [23] consists of oesophagitis, with or without hiatus hernia, with dystonic movements or episodes of body stiffening and torticollis, resembling fits—sometimes preceded by eating, coughing or sneezing.

Torticollis is a frequent side effect of haloperidol, methylphenidate, metoclopramide or phenothiazines.

## Torsion spasm (Dystonia musculorum deformans)

Torsion spasm begins between the ages of 5 and 10, with hypertonus of the calf muscles, leading to inversion and adduction of the foot, and later a fixed flexion and adduction of the hip with lordosis, torticollis and involuntary twisting movements.

## Spasmus nutans

Spasmus nutans [11] occurs in infants usually aged 3 to 24 months, with rhythmical jerking movements of the neck, usually in the lateral or horizontal direction, ceasing when the child concentrates on something. He has a characteristic way of looking at objects out of his eye corner, and may tilt his head to one side. The movements disappear in sleep. There is usually nystagmus. The movements are increased by holding the head; they disappear spontaneously by the age of 3 or 4.

Some cases of spasmus nutans have been associated with an optic glioma [1] or the diencephalic syndrome [7].

## Chorea and choreo-athetosis

Rheumatic chorea (Sydenham's chorea), like rheumatic fever, is no longer seen in Britain, but rheumatic fever continues to occur in developing countries. I used to see children thought to have chorea, when the diagnosis was simply over-activity—or rarely hysteria. A benign familial form of chorea has been described [18].

*Huntington's chorea* may first show itself by isolated chorea [4, 6]. Fits are often an early feature, followed by slowness of movement, dysarthria, rigidity, ataxia, tremors and mental deterioration. Only about 3 per cent begin before the age of 15.

*Athetosis* constitutes 10–15 per cent of all cases of cerebral palsy. It may be familial; it may be due to hypoxia *in utero* or in the perinatal period—and possibly to a prenatal malformation. The slow writhing movements of athetosis disappear in sleep.

*Choreo-athetoid movements* occur in many degenerative diseases of the nervous system. They include *Wilson's disease* of hepatolenticular degeneration [19], sometimes with an onset resembling acute hepatitis, but later developing ataxia, dysarthria, dysphagia, rigidity, involuntary movements and haemolysis; the *Hallervorden–Spatz* and *Creutzfeld–Jakob* syndromes with progressive dementia; the *Lesch–Nyhan* syndrome of hyperuricaemia, self-mutilation, choreo-athetosis, and mental subnormality, mostly in boys; the *Pelizaeus–Merzbacher* syndrome, *ataxia telangiectasia, Lowe's syndrome* (cataract, renal tubular defect, rickets and mental deterioration), *Rett's syndrome* (p. 213) and *disseminated lupus; paroxysmal choreo-athetosis* [12, 18]—a non-progressive condition in which choreiform movements are precipitated by startling or anxiety; and *xeroderma pigmentosum* (p. 359).

Choreo-athetoid and other involuntary movements have resulted from acute infantile striatal necrosis, encephalitis, tumours, vascular malformations, tuberous sclerosis, methylmalonic acidaemia, glutaric acidaemia, juvenile Batten's disease, cytomegalovirus and *Toxoplasma* infection, or poliomyelitis.

*Kernicterus* used to be a common cause of athetosis: in Britain it is rarely seen, because the hyperbilirubinaemia of prematurity or rhesus incompatibility are largely prevented; but kernicterus may still occur as a result of fulminating neonatal septicaemia. It is said to be relatively common in Chinese children, and Yeung [24] described 152 full-term cases—53 per cent with non-haemolytic conditions, including cephalhaematoma, and 44 per cent with glucose-6-phosphate dehydrogenase deficiency; thirty had ABO incompatibility without obvious haemolysis.

*Tardive dyskinesia,* and other forms of extrapyramidal type of movements, are caused by many drugs, including amphetamine, anticonvulsants, antihistamines, cephalosporins, chloroquine, diazoxide, fenfluramine, metoclopramide, pimozide (in USA) and tranquillizers. It may result from carbon monoxide poisoning, methaqualone poisoning, and narcotic withdrawal. There are involuntary, repetitive and purposeless movements [15, 17], with tongue protrusion, lip-smacking, chewing, myoclonic jerks, facial grimacing or athetoid movements, exaggerated by stress, usually absent in sleep. They occur especially on discontinuing a drug; they may decrease in time, or remain static indefinitely.

## Miscellaneous

*Hemiballismus* is a rare form of violent involuntary movement, thought to be due to degenerative changes in the corpus luysi in the subthalamus [21, 22]. There are continuous, large-amplitude, unilateral hitting or beating movements of the arm, beating the thigh and possibly bruising it and excoriating the skin. It is continuous during the day but does not occur in sleep.

In *Rett's syndrome* (p. 213) there is often a continuous rubbing of the hands or hand clapping, often with extrapyramidal movements.

In *infantile autism* (p. 305) a child often continuously flicks his fingers in front of his eyes, for hour after hour.

Bizarre movements may occur in *hysteria* in older children.

Coarse flapping tremors may be an important feature of the narcotic withdrawal syndrome (p. 219).

## Myoclonus

Benign myoclonic jerks may occur in sleep in child or adult. They closely resemble the startle, twitching of the face in sleep, or tetany. They can begin as early as 2 weeks of age. There is a familial form of benign myoclonus.

For myoclonus in the *Lennox–Gastaut syndrome*, see p. 242.

Myoclonic jerks can be a side effect of *tricyclic* antidepressants. They may occur in *aluminium toxicity*.

Irregular myoclonic jerks of the limbs, with coarse nystagmoid movements, ataxia and tremors, are features of *Kinsbourne's syndrome* of myoclonic encephalopathy of childhood, also called the 'dancing eye syndrome' [13]. The onset is usually between 1 and 3 years of age. The condition is associated with neuroblastoma. Other causes of myoclonus include certain storage diseases and spinocerebellar degenerative diseases.

Myoclonus, choreo-athetosis, tremors and hemiballismus may complicate bacterial meningitis [14].

## References

1 Albright AL, Sclabassi RJ, Slamovits TL, Bergman I. Spasmus nutans associated with optic gliomas in infants. *J Pediatr* 1984; **105:** 778.

2 Blennow G. Benign infantile nocturnal myoclonus. *Acta Paediatr Scand* 1985; **74**: 505.

3 Brouilette RT, Thach BT, Abu-Osba YK, Wilson SL. Hiccups in children: characteristics and effects on ventilation. *J Pediatr* 1980; **96**: 219.

4 Caviness VS. Huntington's chorea. *Dev Med Child Neurol* 1985; **27**: 826.

5 Deonna T, Martin D. Benign paroxysmal torticollis in infancy. *Arch Dis Child* 1981; **56**: 956.

6 Folstein S, Abbott M, Moser R, *et al.* Hereditary disorders of dystonic movement. *The Johns Hopkins Hosp Med J* 1981; **148**: 104.

7 Garty B, Weitz B, Mimouni M, Bauman B. Spasmus nutans as a presenting sign of the diencephalic syndrome. *J Pediatr* 1985; **107**: 484.

8 Gillies DRN, Forsythe WI. Treatment of multiple tics and the Tourette syndrome. *Dev Med Child Neurol* 1984; **26**: 781.

9 Gualtieri CT, Evans RW. Carbamazepine induced tics. *Dev Med Child Neurol* 1984; **26**: 546.

10 Hanukoglu A, Somekh E, Fried D. Benign paroxysmal torticollis in infancy. *Clin Pediatr (Phila)* 1984; **23**: 272.

11 Hoefnagel D, Biery B. Spasmus nutans. *Dev Med Child Neurol* 1968; **10**: 32.

12 Kinast M, Erenberg G, Rotner AD. Paroxysmal choreoathetosis: report of 5 cases and review of the literature. *Pediatrics* 1980; **65**: 74.

13 Kinsbourne M. Myoclonic encephalopathy of infancy. *J Neurol Neurosurg Psychiatr* 1962; **25**: 271.

14 Lancet. Involuntary movements and bacterial meningitis. Leading article. 1987; **1**: 142.

15 Moore A, O'Donohoe NV, Monaghan H. Neuroleptic malignant syndrome. *Arch Dis Child* 1986; **61**: 793.

16 Neglia JP, Glaze DG, Zion TE. Tics and vocalisation in children treated with carbamazepine. *Pediatrics* 1984; **73**: 841.

17 Singer S. Tardive dyskinesia; a concern for the pediatrician. *Pediatrics* 1986; **77**: 553.

18 Sleigh G, Lindenbaum RH. Benign (non-paroxysmal) familiar chorea. *Arch Dis Child* 1981; **56**: 616.

19 Slovis TL, Dubois RS, Rodgerson DO, Silverman A. The variable manifestations of Wilson's disease. *J Pediatr* 1971; **78**: 578.

20 Torup E. A follow-up study of children with tics. *Acta Paediatr Uppsala* 1962; **51**: 261.

21 Vinken PJ, Bruyn GW. *Handbook of clinical neurology.* Amsterdam: North Holland, 1982, Vol. 1, p. 288.

22 Walton J. (ed.) *Brain's diseases of the nervous system.* London: Oxford University Press, 1977, p. 623.

23 Werlin SL, D'Souza BJ, Hogan WJ, Dodds WJ, Arndorfer RC. Sandifer syndrome: an unappreciated clinical entity. *Dev Med Child Neurol* 1980; **22**: 374.

24 Yeung CY. Kernicterus in term infants. *Austr Paediatric J* 1985; **21**: 273.

# Convulsions

Convulsions occur in about 7 per cent of all children in the first 5 years and about 1 per cent of all newborn babies. They occur in about 20 per cent of mentally subnormal children, except those with Down's syndrome, in whom convulsions are rare; they occur in about 35 per cent of all children with cerebral palsy—50 per cent of those with spastic hemiplegia, 40 per cent of those with spastic quadriplegia but in fewer of those with diplegia. They occur in about 10 per cent of athetoids, but rarely in those with congenital ataxia.

It is often difficult to decide whether an infant or child has had a convulsion or not. Unless one is able to witness the episode oneself, accurate history-taking is essential. It may be impossible to diagnose without witnessing the episode, and even then it may be difficult.

Non-convulsive epilepsy is a confusing group of conditions, including the Lennox–Gastaut syndrome (especially age 1 to 7, p. 242) and petit mal ('absence epilepsy', especially after the age of 7). There may be episodes of prolonged periods of slowness of thought, speech or movement, ataxia, abnormal behaviour and salivation, progressing to severe mental deterioration if it is not recognized and treated [25, 35].

A convulsion in a newborn baby rarely presents as an obvious major fit [31]. It may consist of mere twitching of a limb, limb posturing, repetitive chewing, an abnormal cry or fluttering of the eyelids. The twitchings may migrate from one limb or part of the body to another. Conjugate deviation of the eyes would be a vital indication of a fit, as would hypertonus in a twitching limb. Convulsive movements have to be distinguished from the normal sudden jerks in sleep or awakening, and from the tremulousness of a baby when hungry.

The jittery movements were described by Bergman *et al.* [6] as rhythmic alternating movements of equal amplitude, whereas the clonic activity of seizures is of unequal amplitude. Jittery movements may be precipitated by a stimulus, and stopped by flexion of the limb or restraint, while clonic movements cannot be stopped in this way. The jittery movements, unlike seizures, are not usually accompanied by conjugate deviation of the eyes or sucking movements in the mouth.

234

Because of the difficulties in diagnosis, non-specialized units are likely to report a lower incidence of fits in the newborn than do special centres which can employ continuous cerebral function monitoring [16]. In a study of eighty-seven newborn infants in an intensive care unit, twenty-six infants, with no clinical indications except perhaps some limpness or quietness, showed electrographical signs of repeated seizure activity.

Many conditions may be confused with epilepsy. Snyder [34] discussed twenty diseases which in his experience have led to erroneous diagnoses.

*Apnoeic or cyanotic attacks* (p. 138) may be a form of convulsion, or the result of one. One has seen a convulsion wrongly diagnosed because of the attacks of pallor and shock in *intussusception*. The rigidity, flushing and staring eyes of a *masturbating* older infant or child may wrongly suggest an epileptic fit, as may sudden attacks of *paroxysmal vertigo* (p. 204). A child with *spastic hemiplegia* may have twitching of the affected limbs without loss of consciousness so that the diagnosis of a convulsion may be missed. The distinction from *faints* can be difficult (p. 244), as may be the distinction from *hysterical convulsions* or *tetany* (p. 237). The diagnosis of *temporal lobe epilepsy* may be missed because of the bizarre symptoms, such as sudden outbursts of rage without apparent reason.

When obtaining the history about episodes in an older child which might be convulsions, probably the most important question to ask is whether the mother has noticed anything unusual in the eyes during an episode: conjugate deviation of the eyes—lateral or vertical— would be conclusive evidence of a convulsion.

It is useful to ask a mother to imitate the child's movements of 'twitching' in the episode. Special investigations, such as the EEG, may or may not help, for in grand mal epilepsy the EEG is frequently normal between attacks.

Convulsions are the end result of a wide variety of pathological processes. From the nature of the convulsions one can rarely make a diagnosis of the cause; for most convulsions, with the exception of petit mal and infantile spasms, look alike. Every effort must be made to establish the correct diagnosis, because only then can appropriate treatment be prescribed; hence hospital investigation is always necessary. It is particularly important to determine whether the child is well between convulsions: if he is not well between attacks, or has symptoms such as personality changes, one should strongly suspect that the diagnosis is more serious than ordinary epilepsy.

The common causes vary with age. The commonest causes in a newborn baby are *hypoxia, hypoglycaemia, hypocalcaemia* and *infection*, but there are numerous rare *metabolic diseases* which may cause convulsions in the newborn period [12, 23]. In some developing countries *tetanus* is the commonest cause. *Febrile convulsions* are rare in the first 6 months. From 6 months to 5 years the commonest diagnosis will be *benign febrile convulsion*, though *breath-holding fits* are common. After the age of 2 or 3, epileptic fits become common and after the age of 5 the usual diagnosis will be *epilepsy*. Petit mal is very rare below the age of 3. Fits due to hysteria or malingering are confined to the older age group.

## Fits in the newborn period

Fits in the newborn period are most likely to be due to:

Cerebral defects or malformation

Hypoxia

Cerebral haemorrhage

Hypoglycaemia, hypocalcaemia, hyponatraemia, hypomagnesaemia, hypernatraemia

Narcotic withdrawal syndrome

Infection

Kernicterus

Adrenal haemorrhage

Rare metabolic syndromes

An unusually small cranial circumference would point to a cerebral malformation, but that sign is not invariable.

Fits due to hypoxia or intraventricular haemorrhage are most likely to occur within the first 2 days [11, 36] and may follow hypoxia *in utero*, prolonged labour, intra-uterine growth retardation or other adverse prenatal or perinatal factors. The child may have a fit, deep stupor, respiratory depression, cyanotic attacks or vomiting. Thalamic haemorrhage may occur 7 to 10 days after normal delivery [37]. Around 20 per cent of neonatal convulsions are due to intracranial haemorrhage or infarction of a major cerebral artery [20]. Signs include bulging of the fontanelle, undue separation of the sutures, or retinal haemorrhage—though retinal haemorrhages are often found in normal babies.

*Neonatal hypoglycaemia.* Neonatal hypoglycaemia occurs particularly in babies who are small in relation to the duration of gestation, in babies of toxaemic mothers, in boys rather than in girls, in the smaller of twins and in babies of diabetic mothers. It follows birth injury or cold injury, and may be associated with the respiratory distress syndrome, kernicterus, Beckwith's syndrome (umbilical hernia with macroglossia and hypoglycaemia), adrenocortical hyperplasia, infections and glycogenoses. The symptoms begin a few hours after birth in most babies, but a few develop them up to 5 or 6 days later. They consist of twitches, cyanotic attacks and convulsions. It is important to establish the diagnosis promptly in order that appropriate treatment can be given.

*Neonatal tetany.* Neonatal *hypocalcaemia* is most often seen about the fifth to the seventh day, and is due mainly to the inability of the newborn baby to handle the high phosphorus content of cow's milk. It is also related to physiological hypocalcaemia, which occurs particularly between the third and the fifth or sixth days. It may occur when the mother has suffered from hyperparathyroidism or diabetes in pregnancy. There may be associated *hypomagnesaemia*. The symptoms are convulsions which are indistinguishable from other convulsions. The typical carpopedal spasm of tetany in older children is rarely seen. A positive Chvostek's sign does not establish the diagnosis because it occurs in normal babies. It is important that the correct diagnosis should be made in order that treatment can be given. The prognosis is better for this condition than it is for other causes of convulsions in the newborn period.

Less frequently hypocalcaemia occurs on the first day or two in low-birth-weight babies and after placental insufficiency. Causes include mainly cerebral malformations, hypoxia, birth injury and maternal diabetes or infection. The prognosis is then not so good. Neonatal tetany occurs in the *Di George syndrome*, in which there is thymic aplasia, hypoparathyroidism, failure to thrive, frequent virus and fungal infections, with congenital anomalies of the mouth, neck and great vessels.

*Hyponatraemia* or *hypernatraemia* may cause convulsions. Hyponatraemia may result from the mother being given large quantities of intravenous sodium-free fluid (e.g. 5 per cent dextrose) in labour [2].

Important *infections* which may cause convulsions in the newborn period include particularly septicaemia due to group B *Streptococcus,*

*Staphylococcus* and Gram-negative bacteria, and pyogenic meningitis. In *neonatal meningitis* there is usually no neck stiffness or other sign of meningitis, and there may be no bulging of the fontanelle. The baby is just ill and no good reason is found for it until a lumbar puncture reveals the diagnosis. Other infections include otitis media and pneumonia. *Neonatal tetanus* is common in certain countries abroad in which goat or cow dung, mud or other undesirable materials are applied to the umbilicus at birth. The first symptom is usually difficulty in sucking at the age of 5 or 6 days, followed by stiffness of the jaws and generalized spasticity. Twitchings develop and spasms occur spontaneously or in response to stimulation. The child lies stiffly with flexed extremities or opisthotonos, with a risus sardonicus, stiff jaws, or a stiff upper lip on feeding, and short spasms accompanied by little snorts or grunts.

*Rare infections* which may cause convulsions include toxoplasmosis, generalized herpes, cytomegalovirus and malaria in tropical countries.

For *kernicterus,* which may be accompanied by convulsions, see p. 73. For the *narcotic withdrawal syndrome,* see p. 219.

*Adrenal haemorrhage* may result in shock, pallor, lethargy, cyanosis, respiratory distress and convulsions, with a palpable mass.

All other causes of convulsions in the newborn period, mainly metabolic, are rare [6]. They include pyridoxine dependency, faulty carbohydrate metabolism (galactosaemia, fructosaemia, lactic acidosis, lactose intolerance, glycogenoses) and a wide variety of inborn errors of metabolism, mostly with abnormal amino-aciduria [23, 29]. They include isovaleric acidosis, arginosuccinic-aciduria, citrullinaemia, propionic acidaemia, methylmalonic acidaemia, hyperglycaemia, hyperammonaemia; oast house syndrome, carnosinaemia, hyperprolinaemia, beta-alaninaemia, Leigh's disease and maple syrup urine disease.

## Convulsions after the newborn period

> Benign febrile convulsions
> Breath-holding convulsions
> Epilepsy, infantile spasms
> Faints, syncope, surcardiac syndrome
> Cerebral trauma. Subdural effusion. Brain defects

Acute infantile hemiplegia

Hypertension, haemolytic uraemic syndrome, nephritis, disseminated intravascular coagulation

Sickle cell crisis

Infections. Toxic shock. Kawasaki disease

Metabolic conditions—hypoglycaemia, hypocalcaemia, hypoparathyroidism, hyponatraemia, hypernatraemia, dehydration, heat stroke, cold injury, Di George syndrome, Reye's syndrome. Phenylketonuria and other inborn errors of metabolism

Burn encephalopathy

Migraine

Fused cervical vertebrae

Shuddering spells

Hysteria, over-ventilation

Munchausen by proxy

Drugs and poisons

After the first week of life, and up to the age of 4 or 5 years, the commonest cause of fits is the so-called *benign febrile convulsion*. This is a bad term, which has led to much confusion, because fever may precipitate fits in an epileptic child (or adult), so that the term 'febrile convulsion' in the minds of some includes both the benign form and the epileptic form. Livingston and Pauli [21, 22] in Baltimore have repeatedly laid down the criteria necessary for the diagnosis of the benign febrile convulsion:

1 Benign febrile convulsions are definitely unusual before the age of 6 months, and they should not be diagnosed before the age of 5 years. The peak age incidence is 18 months.

2 They only occur with a rapid rise of temperature, and there must be a history of the child having been off colour and probably off his food for a few hours before the fit occurred.

3 Fits occurring more than 12 hrs after the onset of an illness are almost certainly not benign febrile convulsions, unless there is a complication such as otitis media developing after a sore throat, and causing a new rise in temperature.

4 The fits should not last more than 10 min.

5 They should be general and not focal.

6 There must be no history of fits without a precipitating infection.

7 There is normally only one fit with the rapid rise of temperature:

rarely there may be another fit, but it should not be more than 12 to 18 hrs after the first [22].

**8** There must not be residual weakness of a limb (Todd's paralysis) after a fit.

**9** The EEG between fits is normal.

I should be particularly cautious about diagnosing a benign febrile convulsion if the child were mentally subnormal or had cerebral palsy, because epileptic fits are so common in those conditions [1]. Accurate diagnosis is important: fewer than 3 per cent satisfying these criteria will have fits later, while 97 per cent of children with other fever-precipitated fits will later have epilepsy.

There are some important difficulties with regard to the diagnosis. Firstly, fever may precipitate fits in epileptics. Hence the criteria above must be satisfied. In particular there must be no history of fits between the 'febrile convulsions'. Secondly, any severe convulsion may cause a rise of temperature. Hence the finding of an elevated temperature following a fit does not prove that an infection caused the fit.

If a child has an infection which caused both an elevation of temperature and a fit, the temperature may have dropped in transit to the hospital. Hence the finding of definite infection together with the appropriate history may be more important for the diagnosis than the finding of an elevated temperature. If a convulsion were focal, or occurred at a time other than the beginning of an infection, with the rapid rise of temperature, the diagnosis of epilepsy would be likely to be correct.

A family history of benign febrile convulsions is very common, whereas in fever-precipitated fits in epilepsy there is a family history in only 3 per cent. If one were in doubt as to whether a child had a benign febrile convulsion or a fever-precipitated fit with epilepsy, a close family or a personal history of epilepsy would make one doubt-ful about the diagnosis of a benign febrile fit. It is said [19] that virological studies indicate a viral cause for the great majority of febrile fits. A febrile convulsion may occur with the rapid rise of temperature within a few hours of pertussis vaccine, or 6 to 12 days after measles vaccine.

The differentiation of benign febrile convulsions from convulsions precipitated by fever in epilepsy is important, because of the major difference in the outlook for future development of non-febrile epileptic fits [3].

An extremely important source of error is *pyogenic meningitis* in the infant or young child, for in about 15 per cent the onset is with fever and a convulsion, and in half of these presenting in that way there is no meningism—no neck stiffness, no Kernig sign or other indication of meningitis.

*Breath-holding convulsions* may occur at any age between about 6 months and 5 years, and very rarely after that age. The usual age of onset is 6 to 18 months. The child when thwarted or hurt may cry, hold his breath in expiration, or cry 'till all the air has gone out of his lungs', as one parent said. The child rapidly becomes blue and, if he holds the breath for a further 10 or 15 seconds, he will have a major convulsion indistinguishable from epilepsy. There is often opisthotonos, and occasionally vomiting or wetting. The basic cause of the attack is reduced cardiac output resulting from reduced cardiac return as a result of the increased intrathoracic pressure from breath-holding. It is said that there is often a hypersensitive oculocardiac reflex—slowing of the heart on compression of the eyeball. It is important to note the exact sequence of events, for this sequence helps one to distinguish the attacks from epileptic fits. In a typical epileptic fit the child has a sudden convulsion, becoming stiff first, then twitches and becomes blue. There is no aura and no preceding stimulus (pain or thwarting). If there is a cry it is synchronous with the tonic phase; this is followed by the clonic phase. Cyanosis occurs late in the epileptic fit, not at the beginning, as it does in a breath-holding attack. A fit following anger or a fright is unlikely to be epilepsy.

Toronto neurologists [24] have described a pallid type of breath-holding attack usually following pain or fright; in it there is rapid loss of consciousness with pallor but without preceding cyanosis. This is a form of syncope, and is likely to be precipitated by a sudden unexpected unpleasant stimulus [7]. In both types there is commonly a family history of similar fits.

Many make the mistake of thinking that breath-holding attacks are merely a behaviour problem, occurring only when the child cannot get his own way. In fact they commonly occur when the child has a fall or other injury. It has been suggested that there is some association with hypochromic anaemia. Anticonvulsant drugs do not affect the frequency of the attacks—a useful therapeutic test when one is in doubt. The EEG is normal and no other investigation is necessary.

*Infantile spasms.* The so-called infantile spasms have also been termed 'salaam spasms', 'myoclonic seizures' and 'hypsarrhythmic attacks'. They consist of sudden rapid flexion of the trunk, lasting a fraction of a second. In 70 per cent of cases the attacks begin during the first 6 months, particularly at about 4 to 6 months of age. They usually cease by the age of 18 months, but are commonly replaced by major convulsions. They are not examples of petit mal epilepsy, with which they are commonly confused.

The attacks may result from a wide variety of causes [26], including gross *brain malformations or damage, hypoxia, subdural effusion, phenylketonuria, syphilis, meningitis* and *intracranial infections, hypoglycaemia, neurodermatoses* (e.g. tuberous sclerosis, neuro-fibromatosis, the Sturge–Weber syndrome of facial port-wine stain with mental subnormality), *cerebral palsy and fits, Tay–Sach's disease,* viruses and other causes. In a third no cause can be found. One of the known causes is *Aicardi's syndrome* [41] of agenesis of the corpus callosum, mental subnormality and chorioretinopathy. It was at one time thought that they could be caused by pertussis or other vaccine, but it is now thought that the apparent association was purely coincidental, in that infantile spasms characteristically begin at the very age at which pertussis vaccine is administered [13, 32, 38]. Matsumoto *et al.* [26] in their analysis of 200 causes of infantile spasms noticed a high incidence of laughing attacks—as in Wilson's disease or temporal lobe epilepsy.

The EEG in cases of infantile spasms is characteristic: it shows hypsarrhythmia—sudden peaks of electrical activity.

Infantile spasms have to be distinguished from petit mal, which occurs in the older age group. Strangely, infantile spasms have been confused with 'colic'.Infantile spasms (West's syndrome), when the infant passes his first year or so, may be replaced by another form of epilepsy, the *Lennox–Gastaut syndrome,* which commonly begins at 2 to 7 years of age. In this condition there are very frequent myoclonic jerks, commonly causing many falls each day and associated with mental handicap.

The most common cause of fits after the fifth year is *epilepsy.* Many children are thought to have *petit mal* when in fact they have *grand mal.* The distinction is important for the treatment of the two conditions is different.

Petit mal (absence epilepsy) consists of brief lapses of conscious-ness, lasting up to 20 seconds, without a preceding aura, without convulsive movements and not followed by sleep. The attacks are commonly called 'dizzy spells' or 'fainting turns'. The child may stop, stand and stare. There may be flickering of the eyelids and a momentary upward deviation of the eyes, but there is no twitching of the limbs. Not more than 5 per cent of affected children fall in an attack. There is no change of colour. The child may drop an object held in the hand and may wet himself. The attacks can usually be precipitated by forced over-ventilation.

Petit mal is distinguished from infantile spasms by the following features:

**1**  The age incidence. Infantile spasms occur mainly at 4 to 6 months and cease by 3 years. Petit mal is rare before 3, occurs predominantly between the ages of 4 and 8 years, usually ceasing by puberty (when it may be replaced by grand mal).

**2**  The duration of the attacks. The duration of petit mal is longer than that of infantile spasms, which consist of a sudden jack-knife flexion lasting a fraction of a second.

**3**  Infantile spasms are almost always associated with mental handicap, while in 95 per cent of children with petit mal the IQ is normal.

**4**  The EEG is different. The EEG in infantile spasms shows sudden peaks of electrical discharge: that of petit mal shows 3 per second spike and wave activity.

Petit mal is distinguished from grand mal by the following points:

**1**  The rarity of petit mal. Petit mal is a relatively rare form of fits in children. It occurred in 2 to 3 per cent of 15 102 epileptics seen at the Johns Hopkins Hospital at Baltimore.

**2**  The nature of the fit. Convulsive twitching in limbs suggests grand mal. A fall usually signifies grand mal, for a change in posture is rare in petit mal. Stiffness in an attack signifies grand mal. A change of colour is against the diagnosis of petit mal.

**3**  The duration of the fit. Grand mal can be momentary, but it usually lasts longer. A petit mal attack lasts not more than 20 seconds, but there may be a rapid succession of petit mal attacks.

**4**  Petit mal attacks can usually be precipitated by over-ventilation. The child is instructed to blow 100 times a piece of paper 30 cm away.

**5**  Grand mal attacks are commonly followed by sleep and sometimes by vomiting. This does not apply to petit mal.

**6**  The EEG is different. The EEG is abnormal in children with petit mal, showing the 3 per second spike and wave activity. It is often normal in children with grand mal.

There are many different kinds of epileptic fit. In *temporal lobe epilepsy* there may be aurae consisting of hallucinations of smell, taste, sight or hearing. There may also be feelings of fear or abdominal pain. Chewing and odd movements may occur. There may be sudden tachycardia, blanching followed by blushing, paroxysmal confusion, meaningless words, senseless laughter, delusions or hallucinations, and catastrophic rage, with violent unexplained outbursts of temper. It may follow hypoxia, pyogenic meningitis, encephalitis, head injury, a long fit of any cause, Schilder's disease, tuberous sclerosis or phenylketonuria [28]. Epileptic fits may be precipitated not only by flashing lights, but by video games [10].

*Psychomotor epilepsy* may show itself by sudden unexplained temper tantrums. These should be considered when an epileptic child has unexplained outbursts of temper and screaming. *Epileptic automatism* occurs in children—leading to sudden irrational acts, such as walking fully clothed into a lake

By no means all epileptic children have tonic and clonic phases in a fit. Some have unexplained falls and are limp when picked up, without twitching.

A sudden instantaneous onset of headache or of abdominal pain, lasting a few minutes only and followed by sleep may be a manifestation of epilepsy. For *narcolepsy*, see p. 299.

Migraine may be confused with epilepsy, when in the latter condition there are sudden attacks of severe headache of instantaneous onset lasting for a few minutes followed by sleep, but without convulsive movements. Many children go to sleep after an attack of migraine. In the initial vasoconstriction phase of migraine, a convulsion may occur; and the occasional neurological features of migraine, such as hemiplegic symptoms, may further confuse the diagnosis.

It can be difficult to distinguish *faints* from fits. Faints or syncopal attacks are definitely rare in a young child, but from early puberty to adolescence they are common. A faint usually occurs on change of posture or on prolonged standing (as in school prayers), while a fit may occur at any time (particularly on awakening or on going to sleep). If a mother tells me that her child 'faints' when sitting in a chair I would certainly say that her diagnosis was incorrect, an epileptic fit being far more likely. Likewise if a child suddenly 'faints' when playing it is far more likely to be an epileptic fit. Loss of colour or limpness can occur with either faint or fit. Loss of consciousness is more gradual in a faint than in a fit and is commonly associated with preceding pallor and sweating. Sweating may follow recovery from a fit [15]. Convulsive movements can occur during a faint: they do not definitely point to the diagnosis of epilepsy. In a study of 362 blood donors who became faint when blood was withdrawn, forty-seven lost consciousness; twenty-five of these (53 per cent) had a convulsion during the period of unconsciousness. An EEG is normal in many cases of grand mal epilepsy, and a fit resembling a faint would be grand mal, not petit mal.

Syncopal attacks occur in various cardiac conditions, such as Fallot's tetralogy, the 'sick sinus' syndrome [33], heart block, aortic stenosis, paroxysmal tachycardia, pulmonary stenosis, prolonged Q–T interval without deafness, and in the surcardiac syndrome [30]— an autosomal recessive condition consisting of a prolonged Q–T interval with deafness and fainting or syncopal attacks. *Cough syncope* has occurred in asthma.

A *severe head injury*, a cerebral abscess or a subdural effusion may be followed in months or years by convulsions. In 10 per cent or more of children in whom convulsions follow cerebral injury or abscess, the first fit may not occur till 10 years or more after the injury. *Child abuse* is one of the causes of head injury by shaking or a fractured skull.

*Brain defects*, such as cerebral agenesis, are an important cause and are commonly associated with mental subnormality, cerebral palsy or hydrocephalus. They occur in various neurodermatoses, especially tuberous sclerosis: facial lesions on the mother's face, or hypo-pigmented areas on the child's skin seen under a Wood's light, point to the diagnosis.

For acute infantile hemiplegia, see p. 264. For migraine, see p. 101.

Convulsions may be a feature of hypertension, the haemolytic uraemic syndrome (p. 57), disseminated intravascular coagulation and sickle cell crises.

Convulsions (apart from benign febrile fits) may occur in many acute infections, including encephalitis (p. 224), meningitis, toxic shock syndrome (p. 92), Kawasaki disease (p. 39) and Reye's syndrome (p. 80). An unusual cause of convulsions is that of focal fits associated with subclinical measles [27].

*Tetanus* causes spasms which may be confused with epileptic fits. The excessive muscle tone and stiffness between convulsive movements, and their occurrence with the slightest stimulus after a history of trauma, point to the diagnosis. Fits may occur in *malaria* and in *pertussis*.

A convulsion following *immunization* may be due to one of several causes. The injection may cause a breath-holding attack, faint or syncope. The rise of temperature which commonly follows within a few hours of pertussis immunization, or between 6 and 12 days after measles vaccine, may cause a benign febrile convulsion, or a fit in an epileptic (or in a child who is particularly liable to have a fit as a result of mental subnormality or cerebral palsy). There is no convincing evidence that pertussis immunization causes encephalitis: but an allergic encephalomyelitis may follow certain other vaccines (such as that against rabies).

*Hypoglycaemia.* Convulsions may be due to hypoglycaemia, other than that due to insulin overdosage. It is of vital importance that the diagnosis should be established, because recurrent hypoglycaemic attacks with convulsions cause irreparable brain damage. The fit is commonly preceded by weakness, tremors, pallor and sweating. Proper history-taking is important: a history of fits occurring only in the early hours of the morning, or a long time after a meal, should suggest the need to perform a fasting blood sugar estimation to eliminate hypoglycaemia.

Hypoglycaemia may be due to hyperplasia or tumour of the islets of Langerhans, hypopituitarism, adrenocortical insufficiency, glycogenoses, hepatic disease or carbohydrate intolerance. With regard to the latter, an example is fructose intolerance, in which the child has hypoglycaemic symptoms such as vomiting, malaise and tremors on eating sweets (p. 12). Investigation for these conditions is laborious and should be carried out in hospital.

The symptoms of ketotic hypoglycaemia commonly begin after the first birthday, especially in low-birth-weight babies who have remained small and thin. The symptoms may be drowsiness in the morning before eating or at other times of food deprivation.

*Hypocalcaemia* after the newborn period is due to a variety of causes, including rickets, steatorrhoea, alkalosis, hypopara-thyroidism or damage to the parathyroid glands following thyroidectomy for thyrotoxicosis. In older children hysterical over-ventilation may cause tetany. Tetany due to rickets occurs especially between the age of 4 months and 3 years. The clinical diagnosis of rickets is made by the thickened epiphysis of the wrist and the enlarged costochondral junctions. There is commonly some anaemia and hypotonia. The diagnosis can only be suspected on clinical grounds, but it must be confirmed by X-ray of the wrist or costochondral junctions and the serum alkaline phosphatase. Owing to the relative frequency of resistant rickets in Britain, one must not be misled by the history that adequate doses of vitamin D have been given, though tetany in resistant rickets is rare.

Fits due to tetany are commonly indistinguishable from other major convulsions. Occasionally, however, one may see the typical thumb posture of tetany—the thumb drawn into the palm of the hand, the hands abducted with the wrists flexed, the fingers flexed at the metacarpophalangeal joints and extended at the distal joints.

For Di George syndrome, see p. 237.

Fits may be due to *hypoparathyroidism*. There may be a history of late teething, muscular pains, a dry skin and mental deterioration. There may be moniliasis of nails and oral mucosa, loss of hair and cataracts.

Fits due to *hyponatraemia* have resulted from the ingestion of large quantities of fluid by infants who have been given swimming lessons [5, 14]. The symptoms included vomiting, polyuria or oliguria, weakness, fits and coma.

*Dehydration* following gastro-enteritis and sometimes respiratory tract infections may be accompanied by convulsions. The causes are varied, and include electrolyte disturbances such as hyponatraemia, hypernatraemia and hypocalcaemia; hydraemia as a result of over-hydration; hyperthermia; and cerebral thrombosis. It may result from giving too much fluid without sufficient sodium or from hydrating too rapidly.

Convulsions may be a manifestation of *heat-stroke* [4].

In the first 48 h after a *burn*, but not necessarily a severe one, a child may begin to vomit and then develop fluctuating levels of con-sciousness, twitching, hypertension or respiratory arrest (burn encephalopathy). It may be due to cerebral oedema [39].

An unusual cause of sudden unconsciousness, sometimes with a fit, is sudden extension of the neck in the presence of fused cervical vertebrae [18].

'*Shuddering spells*' have to be distinguished from convulsions. They can occur in infants and older children [17] and present as spasms or bilateral tremors, sometimes with stiffening of the arms, without alteration in consciousness. They may occur many times a day, and seem to be benign. The EEG is normal in the attacks. For the shuddering in the Chinese restaurant syndrome, see p. 102.

*Hysteria* and *hysterical over-ventilation tetany* are unusual in young children (p. 148). Hysteria is confined to older children—after the age of 6 or 7 years. The fit can be difficult to distinguish from epilepsy if one is unable to see an attack oneself, and has to rely on the mother's story.

*Epidemic mass hysteria* has been described by many authors [40]: it occurs especially in schoolchildren and adolescents. When a woman fainted in church, within 20 min seventy-five children complained of severe headache, vertigo, nausea and abdominal pain, and some had tetany.

For the *Munchausen syndrome by proxy*, including fictitious epilepsy, see p. 35. As always when this syndrome is suspected, it is essential to see the attack oneself, and never to rely on the mother's story.

*Poisons* are important causes of fits. They include boric acid, camphor, carbon tetrachloride, dicophane, lead, mercury, monoamine oxidase inhibitors, plants and insecticides, pyrethrum, rotenone or strychnine.

More than seventy drugs may cause fits [8, 9]. They include acetazolamide, aminophylline, amphetamine, anticonvulsants, antihistamines, chloroquine, diphenoxylate, gamma benzene hexachloride (for scabies), isoniazid, metoclopramide, metronidazole, nose drops, pyrimethamine, theophylline and tranquillizers.

For narcotic withdrawal, see p. 219.

### References

1 Addy P. Nosology of febrile convulsions. *Arch Dis Child* 1986; **61:** 318.
2 Alstatt LB. Transplacental hyponatraemia in the newborn infant. *J Pediatr* 1965; **66:** 985.
3 Annegers JF, Hauser WA, Shirts SB, Kurland LT. Factors prognostic of unprovoked seizures after febrile convulsions. *N Engl J Med* 1987; **316:** 493.
4 Bacon CJ, Bellman MH. Heat stroke as a possible cause of encephalopathy in infants. *Br Med J* 1983; **2:** 328.

5 Bennett HJ, Wagner T, Fields A. Acute hyponatremia and seizures in an infant after swimming lesson. *Pediatrics* 1983; **72:** 125.

6 Bergman I, Painter MJ, Crumbrine PK, *et al.* Neonatal seizures. *Seminars in perinatology* 1982; **6:** 54.

7 Bower BD. Pallid syncope (reflex anoxic seizures). *Arch Dis Child* 1984; **59:** 1118.

8 Chadwick DW. Convulsions associated with drug therapy. *Adverse Drug Reaction Bulletin* 1981; **No. 87:** 316.

9 Davies DM. *Textbook of adverse drug reactions.* Oxford: Oxford University Press, 1981.

10 De Marco P, Ghersini L. Videogames and epilepsy. *Dev Med Child Neurol* 1985; **27:** 514.

11 Derham RJ, Matthews TG, Clarke TA. Early seizures indicate quality of neonatal care. *Arch Dis Child* 1985; **60:** 809.

12 Eriksson M, Zetterstrom R. Neonatal convulsions. *Acta Paediatr Scand* 1979; **68:** 807.

13 Fenichel GM. Neurological complications of immunization. *Ann Neurol* 1982; **12:** 119.

14 Goldberg GN, Lightner ES, Morgan W, Kemberling G. Infantile water intoxication after swimming lessons. *Pediatrics* 1982; **70:** 599.

15 Gordon N. Epilepsy—to treat or not to treat. *Pediatric Reviews and Communications* 1987; **1:** 163.

16 Hellström-Westas L, Rosen I, Swenningsen NW. Silent seizures in sick infants in early life. Diagnosis by continuous cerebral function monitoring. *Acta Paediatr Scand* 1985; **74:** 741.

17 Holmes GL, Russman BS. Shuddering attacks. *Am J Dis Child* 1986; **140:** 72 (leading article p. 19).

18 Illingworth RS. Attacks of unconsciousness in association with fused cervical vertebrae. *Arch Dis Child* 1956; **31:** 8.

19 Lewis HM, Parry JV, Parry RP, *et al.* Role of viruses in febrile convulsions. *Arch Dis Child* 1979; **54:** 869.

20 Levene MI, Trounce JQ. Cause of neonatal convulsions. *Arch Dis Child* 1985; **61:** 78.

21 Livingston S. *Comprehensive management of epilepsy in infancy, childhood and adolescence.* Springfield: Charles Thomas, 1972.

22 Livingston S, Pauli LL. Febrile fits. *Br Med J* 1976; **2:** 1530.

23 Lockman A. Neonatal seizures, diagnosis and treatment. In *Pediatrics Update.* Oxford: Blackwell Scientific Publications, 1980.

24 Lombroso CT, Lerman P. Breath-holding spells (cyanotic and pallid infantile syncope). *Pediatrics* 1967; **39:** 563.

25 Manning D, Rosenbloom L. Non-convulsive status epilepticus. *Arch Dis Child* 1987; **62:** 37.

26 Matsumoto A, Watanabe K, Negoro T, *et al.* Infantile spasms. Etiological factors, clinical aspects and long term prognosis in 200 cases. *Eur J Pediatr* 1981; **135:** 239.

27 Michener RC, Henley WL. Focal convulsions associated with subclinical measles infections. *Clin Pediatr (Phila)* 1983; **22:** 643.

28 Ounsted C, Lindsay J, Norman R. *Biological factors in temporal lobe epilepsy*. Clinics in Dev Med No. 22. London: Heinemann, 1966.

29 Painter MJ, Bergman I, Crumrine P. Neonatal seizures. *Pediatr Clin N Am* 1986; **33**: 91.

30 Rabe EF. Recurrent paroxysmal non-epileptic disorders. *Curr Probl Pediatr* 1974; **4**: 3.

31 Rose AL, Lombroso CT. Neonatal seizure states. *Pediatrics* 1970; **45**: 404.

32 Rükonen R. Infantile spasms: modern practical aspects. *Acta Paediatr Scand* 1984; **73**: 1.

33 Scott O, Macartney FJ, Deverall PB. Sick sinus syndrome. *Arch Dis Child* 1975; **51**: 100.

34 Snyder CH. Conditions that simulate epilepsy in children. *Clin Pediatr (Phila)* 1972; **11**: 487.

35 Stores G. Psychological aspects of nonconvulsive status epilepticus in · children. *J Child Psychol Psychiat* 1986; **27**: 575.

36 Tarby TJ, Volpe JJ. Intraventricular hemorrhage in the premature infant. *Pediatr Clin N Am* 1982; **29**: 1077.

37 Trounce JQ, Fawer CL, Punt J, *et al*. Primary thalamic haemorrhage in first week of life. *Lancet* 1985; **1**: 635.

38 Tsuchiya S, Kagawa K, Fukuyama Y. Critical evaluation of the role of immunization as an etiological factor in infantile spasms. *Brain and Development* 1978; **No. 3**: 17.

39 Warlow CP, Hinton P. Early neurological disturbance following relatively minor burns in children. *Lancet* 1969; **2**: 978.

40 Wason S, Baucher JC. Epidemic mass hysteria. *Lancet* 1983; **2**: 731.

41 Willis J, Rosman NP. The Aicardi syndrome versus congenital infection: diagnostic considerations. *J Pediatr* 1980; **96**: 235.

# Neck Stiffness

Neck stiffness may be a symptom or sign of the utmost importance in childhood, in that it may point to meningitis. On the other hand it may be a trivial matter of no importance. Stiffness in lateral movement of the neck in a newborn baby may be related to a sternomastoid tumour. After the newborn period the commonest causes are the 'rheumatic' stiff neck, cervical adenitis and drugs.

Stein & Trauner [2] listed sixty-six causes of stiff neck. The principal causes are as follows:

Congenital torticollis (sternomastoid tumour)

Meningism, meningitis, poliomyelitis, meningeal leukaemia,
    tetanus
Effects of lumbar puncture
Intracranial haemorrhage, abscess, tumour
'Rheumatic' stiff neck. Epidemic cervical myalgia
Retropharyngeal abscess. Cervical adenitis
Vertebral anomalies or injury
Cervical osteitis, tuberculosis. Discitis
Juvenile chronic arthritis: spondyloarthropathies
Cerebral palsy
Myositis ossificans progressiva
Drugs

For congenital torticollis, see p. 253.

The neck stiffness of *meningism* and meningitis consists of stiffness
in flexing the neck, but not in lateral movement. Ideally the child
should be in the sitting position when the test is carried out. The neck
is fully extended and then flexed. Resistance may be felt throughout
the movement of flexion or only in the terminal part of the movement,
when the chin is almost touching the sternum. It is important to watch
the child's face when testing for meningism, for if there is meningism
there is almost always pain on flexing the neck. A wince of pain in the
last part of the movement may be the only convincing sign of
meningism. The pain is usually felt in the lumbar region, but is
sometimes felt in the muscle at the back of the neck. The child with
meningism may be unable to kiss his knees. When he sits up in bed he
exhibits the tripod sign, placing both arms behind him so that he does
not fall back owing to spasm of the glutei, erector spinae and
hamstrings.

Meningism occurs in a variety of infections in childhood, such as
pneumonia, pyelonephritis, otitis media, tonsillitis, infective
hepatitis, mumps, malaria, Kawasaki syndrome (p. 102),
Legionnaire's disease (p. 151) and typhoid fever. It occurs in many
virus infections of the nervous system, such as poliomyelitis,
encephalitis, the post-infectious encephalomyelitides and pyogenic
meningitis. It also occurs after an intracranial haemorrhage or in the
presence of a cerebral abscess or a tumour.

In a review of 110 cases of *childhood meningitis* [3], the presenting
symptoms were fever (94 per cent), vomiting (70 per cent), drowsiness
(70 per cent), neck stiffness (67 per cent), irritability (41 per cent),

respiratory symptoms (25 per cent), headache (18 per cent), convulsions (15 per cent) and petechiae (13 per cent). As mentioned on p. 250, in neonatal meningitis there is commonly no neck stiffness and no specific sign of meningitis, and there may be no bulging of the fontanelle; the child is just ill, for no obvious reason.

Limitation of movement without pain occurs as a feature of *congenital anomalies of the vertebrae*, including fusion of vertebrae.

The so-called *'rheumatic stiff neck'* is a mysterious entity, at one time ascribed to sitting in a draught. It has nothing to do with rheumatic fever. Tenderness of the muscles distinguishes it from meningism; the pain in the rheumatic stiff neck is mainly on lateral or rotatory movement rather than on flexion. It may be due to a virus infection.

Stiffness of the neck, usually but not always without pain, occurs commonly in *juvenile chronic arthritis* and *spondylo-arthropathies*.

Pain on movement of the neck with stiffness may result from *inflamed cervical lymph nodes* or from *a retropharyngeal abscess*.

*Myositis ossificans progressiva* commonly begins in the neck muscles; there is a deposition of bone between muscle bundles, gradually spreading through the trunk muscles over a period of years. The bone can readily be felt by the examiner's hand [1].

Neck stiffness and opisthotonos may be a side effect of the phenothiazines, metoclopramide, trimethoprim or boric acid poisoning.

### References

1  Illingworth RS. Myositis ossificans progressiva. *Arch Dis Child* 1971; **46**: 264.
2  Stein MT, Trauner D. The child with a stiff neck. *Clin Pediatr (Phila)* 1982; **21**: 559.
3  Valmari P, Peltola H, Korvenranta H, Ruuskanen O. Symptoms, signs and reasons for consulting a physician in cases of bacterial meningitis. *Acta Paediatr Scand* 1985; **Suppl. 322**: 3.

# Torticollis

Apart from the sternomastoid tumour, the 'rheumatic' stiff neck, habit and the effect of drugs, all the causes of torticollis are rare, though several are important for treatment. The causes may be classified as follows:

Muscle

    Sternomastoid tumour (congenital torticollis)

    Myositis ossificans progressiva (rare) (p. 252)

    'Rheumatic' stiff neck

    Poliomyelitis (weakness of muscle)

Cervical vertebrae and joints

    Juvenile chronic arthritis

    Klippel–Feil syndrome, Sprengel's deformity, odontoid anomaly

    Scoliosis (p. 255)

    Osteitis, tumour

    Trauma: subluxation of atlanto-axial joint, strain

Soft tissues—tonsillar abscess, cervical adenitis, retro-pharyngeal abscess

Eye—ocular torticollis

Ear—vestibular disturbance

Intracranial—posterior fossa tumour. AV malformation

Oesophagus—Sandifer's syndrome

Unclassified—paroxysmal torticollis, spasmodic torticollis

    Spasmus nutans

Drugs

Psychological—habit, hysteria, tic

For neck stiffness, see p. 250, and for spasmodic torticollis, see p. 229.

'*Congenital torticollis*' is due to a sternomastoid tumour, itself the result of pressure *in utero* against the sternomastoid muscle—or perhaps rarely the result of damage during delivery. The tumour is felt a few days after birth and torticollis with rotation of the neck develops shortly after. There may be associated cranial and mandibular asymmetry and other indications of the effect of oligohydramnios. A particular risk is a dislocated hip.

The so-called 'rheumatic' stiff neck may be myositis of virus origin. There is local tenderness.

Neck stiffness, occasionally with torticollis, is often a feature of juvenile chronic arthritis.

The *Klippel–Feil syndrome* is diagnosed by the short neck, limitation of neck movement and X-ray, and the *Sprengel deformity* by the high position of the scapula [1].

*Ocular torticollis* is a posture adopted by the child to maintain binocular vision and avoid a squint when there is paresis of an ocular muscle, usually the superior oblique. The head is tilted and rotated. The symptoms often appear at about 2 or 3 years of age.

A *cerebellar tumour* may cause the child to rotate or tilt the occiput towards the shoulder on the affected side.

Torticollis may be the presenting sign in *cervical spine infection* or *tumour* [2].

Some infants, children and adults keep the head tilted to one side for no apparent reason. Bizarre postures may occur in *hysteria*.

### References

1 Hensinger RN. Orthopedic problems of the shoulder and neck. *Pediatr Clin N Am* 1977; **24:** 889.
2 Visudhiphan P, Chiemchanya S, Somburansin P, Dheandhanoo D. Torticollis as the presenting sign in cervical spine infection and tumour. *Clin Pediatr (Phila)* 1982; **21:** 71.

# Opisthotonos

Opisthotonos in the newborn must be distinguished from the posture assumed by a baby delivered by face presentation. Such babies are not hypertonic, unless they have cerebral palsy. Attacks of arching of the back are sometimes an early sign of *athetosis*.

Causes of true opisthotonos include the following:

Severe kernicterus

Airway obstruction—retropharyngeal abscess, tracheal obstruction, vascular ring

Oesophagitis

Sequela of meningitis, encephalitis, cerebral haemorrhage, cardiac arrest

Tetanus, rabies

Gaucher's disease, Tay–Sachs disease, Lesch–Nyhan syndrome

Cerebral tumour

Neck injury

Drugs—especially metoclopramide and phenothiazines, but
also chloroquine and carbamazepine

In a review of 112 cases of boric acid poisoning, Goldbloom &
Goldbloom [1] included amongst the symptoms meningism,
opisthotonos, convulsions, rash, diarrhoea and vomiting.

### Reference

1 Goldbloom RB, Goldbloom A. Boric acid poisoning: report of 4 cases and a
review of 109 cases from the world literature. *J Pediatr* 1953; **43**: 631.

# Scoliosis

The causes of scoliosis can be classified as follows:

Postural—the scoliosis disappearing when the child bends
over [2]

Compensatory—due to unequal length of the legs

Structural—persisting when the child bends over

Unknown causes

Muscular dystrophy, late stage

Poliomyelitis

Rare

Hemivertebra

Congenital asymmetry

Osteogenesis imperfecta

Neurofibromatosis

Marfan's syndrome

Friedreich's ataxia

Prader–Willi syndrome

The clinical diagnosis of most of these conditions is straightforward,
though radiological examination is needed for the diagnosis of hemivertebra and perhaps fragilitas ossium. *Marfan's syndrome* is
diagnosed on the arachnodactyly, tall slender build, subluxation of
the lens of the eye and an aortic valve lesion, often with other
abnormalities. Scoliosis is a common finding in the *Prader–Willi*

*syndrome* (p. 23). It may result from defective leg growth in *juvenile chronic arthritis* involving one knee [1].

### References

1 Holm VA, Laurnen EL. Prader–Willi syndrome and scoliosis. *Dev Med Child Neurol* 1981; **23**: 192.
2 Zorab PA. *Scoliosis*. London: Heinemann, 1969.

# Hypotonia, Muscle Weakness, Polyneuritis

The assessment of muscle tone is part of the routine examination of infants in a welfare clinic or elsewhere. The assessment is made as follows:

**1** Feeling the muscle. The hypotonic muscle, as in Down's syndrome, feels flabby.

**2** Assessing the resistance to passive movement. One tests in particular the elbow, wrist, hip, knee and ankle. In hypertonic children there is increased resistance, and in hypotonic children the resistance is reduced. One has to distinguish voluntary resistance by the child.

**3** Assessing the range of movement. This is increased in the hypotonic child and decreased in the hypertonic child. For instance, in the case of children with Down's syndrome, who are always hypotonic, having flexed the hip to a right angle, abduction is so full that both legs will lie flat extended on the couch. Abduction of the hip is reduced in hypertonia. Dorsiflexion of the ankle is reduced in hypertonia and increased in hypotonia.

**4** One shakes the limb—holding the arm below the elbow and the leg below the knee. The amount of movement of the hand or wrist gives a good idea of the muscle tone.

A severely hypotonic infant lies in the characteristic frog-like posture with the hips abducted and externally rotated, the limbs being in contact with the couch. In ventral suspension the baby cannot hold the head up, and the four limbs hang down lifelessly, with no flexion at hip, knee or elbow. There is complete head lag when he is pulled to the sitting position.

Hypotonia at birth is usually due to severe hypoxia. It can be caused by *drugs* taken by the mother in pregnancy, notably alcohol, barbiturates, chlorpropamide, diazepam, lithium, magnesium sulphate (in labour) and propranolol.

Apart from the hypotonia due to hypoxia, the commonest cause of severe hypotonia with weakness is the Werdnig–Hoffmann syndrome.

Numerous papers have been written about hypotonic or 'floppy' infants, and various classifications have been suggested. The classification below is modified from that of Dubowitz [4].

Hypotonia with weakness
> Motor neurone disease. Werdnig–Hoffmann syndrome
> Duchenne muscular dystrophy. Kugelberg–Wehlander muscular dystrophy
> Congenital muscular dystrophy (rare)
> Myotonic dystrophy (rare) (p. 207)
> Peroneal muscular atrophy (rare)
> Cervical spinal cord injury at birth. Platybasia
> Rare metabolic diseases—glycogenoses, lipoidoses, mucopolysaccharidoses, syndromes of McCardle, Lowe, Leigh, Krabbe, Refsum, Devic
>> Organic acidurias, myoglobinuria, porphyria, abetalipoproteinaemia
>> Hypoparathyroidism, hyperparathyroidism
> Dermatomyositis (p. 45), myasthenia gravis (p. 45)
>> Disseminated lupus (p. 38)
> Acute illness
>> Guillain–Barré syndrome
>> Polyneuropathies
>> Poliomyelitis. Pseudopoliomyelitis. Transverse myelitis
>> Diphtheria
>> Botulism, rabies
>> Potassium deficiency
> Hysteria
> Drugs

Hypotonia without significant weakness
>   Down's syndrome and other severe mental subnormality
>   Benign congenital hypotonia
>   Hypotonic form of cerebral palsy
>   Rare syndromes—Prader–Willi, Marfan, Ehlers–Danlos and
>       congenital laxity of ligaments, Riley's syndrome, Rett
>       syndrome
>   Other metabolic conditions—coeliac disease, hypothyroidism,
>       hypercalcaemia, renal tubular acidosis

## Hypotonia with weakness

*Motor neurone disease* is rare in childhood. There is progressive weakness, wasting and fasciculation of the tongue with loss of reflexes. In the *Werdnig–Hoffmann syndrome* hypotonia is present at birth or develops in the first few weeks. The tendon jerks are usually absent and there may be fasciculation of the tongue. There is indrawing of the chest with inspiration. Contractures develop early. Few survive the first birthday.

The commonest form of *muscular dystrophy* is that of *Duchenne,* affecting boys. Half the affected boys are late in walking (after the age of 18 months), and some mental handicap is common (mean IQ 80), so that they are often somewhat late in other aspects of development. Weakness develops, especially noticeable on climbing stairs. The weakness involves the proximal muscles before the distal ones and the lower limbs before the upper. Toe walking may occur. There is a waddling gait, especially when the boy is tired or running. He cannot perform a standing jump; he cannot rise directly from the supine position—displaying the Gower manoeuvre of rolling over and climbing up the thighs. The prominence of the calf muscles may be obvious.

A benign variant is the Kugelberg–Wehlander syndrome, developing mainly in adolescence, with proximal weakness in the first place.

There may be severe hypotonia in the rare *congenital muscular dystrophy* [12]: the weakness is mainly proximal and it is non-progressive. The creatine phosphokinase is normal or only slightly elevated. For *myotonic dystrophy* as a cause of weakness see p. 207.

In *peroneal muscular atrophy,* which is also rare, weakness develops in the evertors and dorsiflexors of the ankle; reflexes are lost, toe walking may occur, and hammer toes may develop.

*Injury to the cervical spinal cord* may occur, mainly in a breech delivery. There may be considerable hypotonia, with absent tendon jerks. The intercostal musles may be paralysed and there is indrawing of the lower part of the chest on inspiration. The whole picture resembles that of the Werdnig–Hoffmaµn syndrome, but in that condition the child will cry feebly if the foot is pricked, whereas in the child with cervical cord injury there is usually no cry.

There are many metabolic diseases associated with hypotonia and/ or weakness. In *Pombe's type of glycogen storage disease* there is hypotonia from infancy, a large tongue, weakness, mental subnormality and cardiac enlargement. In the *sulphatide lipoidosis* (metachromatic leucodystrophy) weakness and hypotonia begin in the first year, with mental deterioration, optic atrophy and nystagmus: the motor nerve conduction time is prolonged. In *McArdle's syndrome* of phosphorylase deficiency there may be weakness and cramps on exertion. In *paroxysmal myoglobinuria* there are muscle cramps and weakness with myoglobin in the urine. In *familial periodic paralysis* there are attacks of severe weakness in association with potassium deficiency. Episodes of acute weakness occur in *pyruvate carboxylase deficiency* [6]; there is progressive neurological disease with ataxia, weakness of eye movements and peripheral neuritis. In *Leigh's subacute necrotizing encephalomyelopathy* there are hypotonia, ocular palsies, weakness, mental deterioration, dysphagia and failure to thrive. For *Refsum's syndrome* see p. 212. *Neuromyelitis optica* (Devic) may occur at any age; there may be flaccid paralysis, loss of tendon jerks, sensory loss and optic neuritis. *Porphyria* (p. 116) may be manifested by flaccid paralysis, abdominal pain and fits. Hypotonia with sucking and swallowing difficulties may be a feature of *myasthenia gravis,* of the transitory type in the newborn, or of the persistent type.

## *Guillain–Barré syndrome*

This is a condition of varied aetiology, including virus infection and toxic substances. It occurs at any age, including infancy. It commonly begins as a mild upper respiratory tract infection, followed after a period of days or weeks by the rapid onset of symmetrical weakness, often with meningism, hypotonia and loss of reflexes, sometimes with facial palsy and tenderness of muscle or paraesthesiae. The high protein in the CSF with normal cell count is characteristic.

*Other causes of polyneuritis* [7, 10, 15]

These include serum sickness, degenerative polyneuropathies, immunization against mumps, rubella or tetanus, and various infections, including diphtheria, legionnaires' disease, typhus, mumps, Lyme disease (p. 278) and leprosy. There is a rare hypertrophic interstitial polyneuropathy [1] with delayed motor development, hypotonia, weakness and delayed motor nerve conduction.

Numerous *drugs* may cause muscle weakness [3], mostly by causing polyneuritis. They include amphetamine, antibiotics, anticonvulsants, chloroquine, cimetidine, corticosteroids, cytotoxic drugs, indomethacin, isoniazid, metronidazole, nalidixic acid, nitrofurantoin, penicillamine, procainamide, propranolol, salbutamol and tranquillizers.

It may be caused by organophosphate poisoning, solvent sniffing and thallium, gold, arsenic and lead poisoning.

*Hysteria* is an unusual cause of flaccid paralysis with sensory changes.

## Hypotonia without significant weakness

This occurs in Down's syndrome and many other conditions.

*Benign congenital hypotonia* is a non-specific condition which is non-progressive and tends to improve. The usual age at which affected children are able to walk is 5 or 6 years.

There is a rare *hypotonic form of cerebral palsy*, in which there is generalized hypotonia; the exaggerated tendon jerks, the positive stretch reflex, ankle clonus and extensor plantar response establish the diagnosis. These children become spastic as they get older. Many wrongly diagnose hypotonia in the common spastic form of cerebral palsy on account of the excessive head lag when the child is pulled up into the sitting position.

Several rare syndromes are associated with hypotonia without weakness. Hypotonia is an early feature of the *Prader–Willi syndrome* (p. 23). It occurs in *Marfan's syndrome* of arachnodactyly, hyperextensible joints, iridodonesis and congenital heart disease. There may be hypotonia in the *Ehlers–Danlos syndrome* of cutis hyperelastica and in *Riley's syndrome* of familial dysautonomia.

There is a minor degree of hypotonia in many cases of rickets.

**Localized weakness or wasting of mucle**

Weakness of an arm or of the legs without generalized weakness may be due to the following conditions:

>Erb's palsy, Klumpke's palsy
>Pseudoparalysis of scurvy
>Todd's paralysis after an epileptic fit
>Trauma—pulled elbow, nerve damage by injection
>Spinal tumour, abscess, lipoma, sacral agenesis
>Diastematomyelia, syringomelia
>Poliomyelitis: transverse myelitis
>Hysteria

The commonest cause of weakness of an arm from birth is *Erb's palsy*. There is weakness of flexion of the elbow, wrist drop, and the 'chauffeur's tip position' of the hand. The limb is hypotonic—a point of importance, for I have seen it confused with spastic hemiplegia.

The hypertonia of the muscles in mild *spastic hemiplegia* may be so slight that it cannot be detected until the child is older; but in the ipsilateral leg there is likely to be an exaggerated knee jerk and there may be reduced dorsiflexion of the ankle. In cold weather the affected hemiplegic arm and leg are cold as compared with the normal side. In Erb's palsy the biceps jerk is reduced, while in spastic hemiplegia it is increased. After infancy there is no problem, for Erb's palsy almost always disappears within a few days or weeks of birth. For *acute infantile hemiplegia*, see p. 264. *Klumpke's paralysis* is due to damage to the seventh and eighth cervical nerve roots and the first dorsal. There is weakness of the hand and often ipsilateral ptosis and a small pupil if the sympathetic fibres are also involved.

Pseudoparalysis of a limb may be due to *scurvy*, the child not using the limb because it hurts owing to the subperiostal haemorrhage.

After a major epileptic fit there may be weakness of a limb or of an arm and leg, lasting usually for a few hours and occasionally for a few days (*Todd's paralysis*).

Trauma may cause apparent weakness of a limb as does scurvy. Trauma includes fractures, an important cause of which in the early years is child abuse.

A *lipoma* in the region of the cauda equina is an important cause of progressive weakness of the lower limbs, usually with loss of sphincter control [5]. The lipoma can be seen and palpated in the region of the sacrum or buttock.

*Diastematomyelia* is a condition in which the spinal cord is split and tethered by a spicule of bone. It leads to progressive weakness of the legs. It is sometimes revealed by a patch of pigmentation or hair over the spine. For *sacral agenesis*, see p. 312.

Local paralysis may be caused by *poliomyelitis* and other viruses, including the Coxsackie and other viruses of the acute infectious diseases. A few cases of muscle weakness, resembling poliomyelitis, have occurred 4 to 11 days after an *asthmatic attack* [11]. There may be severe flaccid paralysis of a limb or occasionally of several limbs, preceded by muscle pain, as in poliomyelitis. There is no sensory loss. It may be due to a neurotropic virus.

Apparent weakness of an arm may be due to a 'pulled elbow' (p. 277). Apparent paralysis of a limb may be due to hysteria [8].

## Local muscle wasting

Local muscle wasting may be confused with *lipodystrophy*, congenital absence of muscle and congenital asymmetry. In *lipodystrophy* there is loss of fat but not of muscle (p. 27). It usually affects the face first, but may be confined to the lower limbs. *Congenital absence of muscle* such as that of the pectoralis major, sometimes due to the mother taking abortifacients in pregnancy, gives an appearance of unilateral wasting, or of chest asymmetry—and the increased lucency on the affected side in a chest X-ray may be deceptive. In *congenital asymmetry* one side of the body is bigger than the other—hence the old term hemihypertrophy.

*True wasting* may be the result of infection which has damaged the muscle or its innervation [2]. But the commonest cause of local muscle wasting is trauma by an injection—particularly in the arm, buttock or lower limb. No intramuscular injection should be given into the arm; nerve damage has resulted in particular from injection of anti-rheumatic drugs. Local wasting is a well-known result of injecting a depot corticosteroid preparation for hay fever. For a child intramuscular injection should be into the middle of the lateral side of the thigh. Injection into the buttock is not advised [13, 14] because of the risk of injury to the sciatic nerve or the superior gluteal nerve (which would cause muscle atrophy).

A rare result of injections into the thigh (especially repeated ones) is fibrosis and contracture in the quadriceps muscle, causing weakness, and limitation of flexion of the knee and sometimes dislocation of the patella [9, 16].

In spastic hemiplegia, there is some degree of wasting of muscle (and shortening of the limb), but not nearly as much as that caused by poliomyelitis.

Muscle weakness may result from cimetidine, salbutamol or steroids.

*Hypotomia, Muscle Weakness, Polyneuritis*

## References

1 Anderson RM, Hopkin I, Shield LK. Hypertrophic interstitial poly-neuropathy in infancy. *J Pediatr* 1973; **82:** 619.
2 Bergeson PS, Singer SA, Kaplan AM. Intramuscular injections in children. *Pediatrics* 1982; **70:** 944.
3 Blain PG. Adverse effects of drugs on skeletal muscle. *Adverse Drug Reaction Bulletin* 1984; **No. 104:** 384.
4 Dubowitz V. *The floppy infant.* Clinics in Developmental Medicine No. 76. London: Heinemann, 1980.
5 Dubowitz V, Lorber J, Zachary RB. Lipoma of the cauda equina. *Arch Dis Child* 1965; **40:** 207.
6 Evans B. Episodic weakness in pyruvate carboxylase deficiency. *J Pediatr* 1984; **105:** 961.
7 Evans OB. Polyneuropathy in childhood. *Pediatrics* 1979; **64:** 96
8 Goodyer I. Hysterical conversion reactions in children. *J Child Psychol Psychiat* 1981; **22:** 179.
9 Gunn DR. Contracture of the quadriceps muscle. *J Bone Joint Surgery* 1964; **64B:** 492.
10 Hagberg B, Westerberg B. The nosology of genetic peripheral neuropathies in Swedish children. *Dev Med Child Neurol* 1983; **25:** 3.
11 *Lancet.* Post-asthmatic pseudopoliomyelitis in children. Leading article. 1980; **1:** 860.
12 McMenamin JB, Becker LE, Murphy EG. Congenital muscular dystrophy. *J Pediatr* 1982; **100:** 692.
13 Silber DL. Injection technique in infants. *JAMA* 1983; **249:** 1007.
14 *South African Medical Journal.* Complications of intramuscular injection. Leading article. 1985; **68:** 913.
15 Tasker W, Chutorian AM. Chronic polyneuritis of childhood. *J Pediatr* 1969; **74:** 667.
16 Temple AR, Murphy JV, Nerman N. Infantile quadriceps-femoris contracture resulting from intramuscular injection. *N Engl J Med* 1970; **282:** 964.

# Stiffness or Spasticity of Limbs

Many infants in the first days and weeks have greater than usual muscle tone with exaggerated tendon jerks and often with ankle clonus. Unless there are other abnormal signs, such as smallness of the head circumference in relation to the baby's weight or delayed motor development, one pays little attention to it. The signs usually disappear as the child grows older.

The differential diagnosis of *cerebral palsy* depends on the distribution of the spasticity. If a child with spastic quadriplegia has been spastic from birth, the cause would almost certainly be cerebral palsy—but, if he was normal at first and then became spastic, other causes must be considered. If the disease was of acute onset, it could be due to encephalitis (such as post-infectious encephalomyelitis), or to an intracranial vascular accident, such as thrombosis due to dehydration. If the spasticity is of gradual onset, it may be due to one of the numerous degenerative diseases of the nervous system, such as multiple sclerosis (p. 188), AIDS (p. 18), Schilder's disease, which is manifested by the gradual development of blindness, deafness and spasticity beginning in early childhood. There are so many degenerative diseases of the nervous system that it would be impossible to review them all here. The reader should refer to any of the textbooks of paediatric neurology, such as that of Menkes [4] or Drillien & Drummond [1]. Other causes of progressive spasticity involving all four limbs include craniovertebral abnormalities, such as basilar impression and the Klippel–Feil syndrome of fused cervical vertebrae with other anomalies. Neuromyelitis optica and its near relative multiple sclerosis are other causes of spasticity of rapid onset. It should be noted that the spasticity of cerebral palsy may increase as the child grows older, and the development of deformities, such as dislocation of the hip and joint fixation due to muscle contracture may give a false impression that the child has a progressive neurological disorder.

*Acute infantile hemiplegia* is the end result of a variety of conditions, including vascular anomalies, infections, injury, congenital heart disease, disseminated lupus, periarteritis, sickle cell anaemia, homocystinuria, fibromuscular dysplasia [2, 5, 6], epilepsy, polycythaemia, thrombocytopenic purpura and dehydration [3]. The child has a major and often protracted convulsion, followed by coma, and is then found to have a hemiplegia.

Hemiplegia may be a sequel of a major epileptic fit (Todd's paralysis), lasting a few hours, or of migraine (p. 101).

When the spasticity of cerebral palsy is almost entirely confined to the lower limbs, it is easy to diagnose spastic paraplegia, while more careful examination of the upper limbs when the child is building a tower of bricks or performing a timed bead-threading test will show that there is minimal involvement of the upper limbs, so that the true diagnosis is cerebral diplegia. True spastic paraplegia is rare, and should alert one to the possibility that the lesion is spinal and not cerebral. The spinal lesion may be a tumour, cyst or other anomaly, and it should be looked for because it may be treatable.

*Spastic monoplegia* is extremely rare; I saw one possible example in my series of 770 personally observed cases of cerebral palsy. Almost always on full examination one finds an abnormal sign in the ipsilateral limb.

Excessive muscle tone, restricting the range of movement in a joint, may be confused with *deformities of joints,* such as *arthrogryposis* or other congenital abnormalities. Reduced range of movement in a joint such as the hip could be ascribed to increased muscle tone when it is due to *contracture of the muscles,* as a result of the child (usually severely mentally handicapped or hypotonic) always lying in one position.

The *development of excessive muscle tone in a previously normal child* suggests the following possibilities:

Encephalitis or meningitis if acute, and other infections of the
central nervous system, including tetanus
Demyelinating or degenerative disease of the nervous system
Cerebral or spinal abscess or tumour
Brain damage—perhaps decerebrate rigidity—due to anoxia
(e.g. cardiac arrest)
meningo-encephalitis
cerebral tumour or haemorrhage
Drugs

For encephalitis, see p. 224. For toe walking due to spasticity, see p. 270.

*Spasticity of extrapyramidal type* can be caused by diazoxide, phenothiazines, haloperidol, tricyclic antidepressants and metoclopramide.

The number of conditions involved is so considerable, covering a large section of the whole of paediatric neurology, that it would not be profitable to discuss them here. An affected child should be investigated by a paediatrician.

### References

1 Drillien CM, Drummond MB. *Development problems in early childhood.* Oxford: Blackwell Scientific Publications, 1977.
2 Eeg-Olofsson O, Ringheim Y. Stroke in children: clinical characteristics and prognosis. *Acta Paediatr Scand* 1983; **72:** 391.
3 Gold AP, Carter S. Acute hemiplegia of infancy and childhood. *Pediatr Clin N Am* 1976; **23:** 413.
4 Menkes JH. *Textbook of child neurology.* Philadelphia: Lea and Febiger, 1974.
5 Rapola J, Koskimies O, Pesonen E, Jääskeläinen J. Fibromuscular disease in childhood: a generalised arterial disease. *Acta Paediatr Scand* 1980; **69:** 563.
6 Shields WD, Ziter FA, Osborn AG, Allen J. Fibromuscular dysplasia as a cause of stroke in infancy and childhood. *Pediatrics* 1977; **59:** 899

# Inequality of Limb Length

It is said that prenatal maldevelopment of a limb may be caused by the mother taking abortifacients, ergot, cannabis, a contraceptive pill, haloperidol, imipramine, methotrexate, phenytoin or warfarin, or by uterine abnormalities—fibroids, a bicornuate uterus, oligohydramnios—or by hyperthermia in early pregnancy. Irradiation in pregnancy may be a factor. Other drugs are suspected of occasionally causing limb deformities.

The causes of abnormality of limb length may be classified as follows [1, 2, 3, 4]:
1   Congenital bone abnormalities
    Short femur or tibia
    Coxa vara
    Dislocation of hip

2 Soft tissue abnormalities
   Arteriovenous fistula
   Haemangioma (Klippel–Trenaunay syndrome)
   Neurofibromatosis
   Arthrogryposis
   Fixed flexion deformity of knee
3 Abnormality of bone growth
   Achondroplasia
   Fibrous dysplasia
   Pseudoarthrosis of tibia
   Osteoid osteoma
4 Trauma to the epiphysis, causing shortening
   Overgrowth of a limb after fracture [2]
5 Infection—overgrowth due to chronic osteitis
   Tuberculosis
   Osteitis involving the epiphysis
6 Neurological—poliomyelitis
   Cerebral palsy
7 Total growth abnormalities
   Congenital asymmetry

Limb shortening may be a sequel of irradiation damaging the growing end of the bone; and it may follow injection of contrast material into the femoral artery.

The haemangioma involving a lower limb may not be obvious: the limb is enlarged; the slight naevoid markings may be difficult to detect.

A neurofibroma can cause limb enlargement, not necessarily with other signs, such as *café-au-lait* pigmentation.

Cerebral palsy causes shortening of arm or leg, obvious if there is hemiplegia; poiliomyelitis causes more shortening.

In *congenital asymmetry* one side of the body is bigger than the other; hence the old term 'hemihypertrophy'. The difficulty lies in deciding which of the two sides is normal. It may occur in association with the *Beckwith–Wiederman syndrome* of macroglossia, umbilical hernia, hypoglycaemia and gigantism. There may be features of the *Russell–Silver syndrome*—shortness of stature, increased gonad-otrophin output, early sexual development with retarded bone age, *café-au-lait* pigmentation, incurved little finger, turning down of the angles of the mouth and a small triangular face; there is an increased incidence of malignant disease, especially Wilms' tumour, and neurofibromatosis. There may be syndactyly and retinal changes.

## References

1 Bub I, Dekker P, Gericke GS. Asymmetrical limb reduction deformities—aetiological considerations. *South African Med J* 1984; **66:** 338.
2 Klenerman L. Unequal legs. *Br Med J* 1983; **1:** 1302.
3 Pearn J, Viljoen D, Beighton P. Limb overgrowth—clinical observations and nosological considerations. *South African Med J* 1983; **64:** 905.
4 Sharrard WJW. *Paediatric orthopaedics and fractures.* Oxford: Blackwell Scientific Publications, 1979.

# Limitation of Joint Movement

Limitation of joint movement can be a feature of many conditions, including the following:

Cerebral palsy

Joint diseases, e.g. subluxation of hip, juvenile chronic arthritis, arthrogryposis

Muscle contractures, hypertonia

Fetal alcohol syndrome (p. 18)

Diabetes mellitus

Myositis ossificans progressiva (p. 252)

Rare syndromes—Conradi, Hurler (mainly elbow), Cockayne, Morquio (mainly hip), Weaver (p. 20)

Other rare conditions—nail patella syndrome (elbow dysplasia, hypoplasia of patella, dystrophic nails), diastrophic dwarfism, trisomy 8, lipogranulomatosis (p. 48)

Dermatomyositis, fasciitis

Myotonic dystrophy

Joint contractures, often involving only the fifth finger, may occur in *diabetes mellitus*. Brice, Johnston & Noronha [1] found limited joint mobility in 112 diabetic children, especially in older ones and those whose diabetes developed early. It may be an indication of an increased risk of later microvascular disease [2].

*Conradi's syndrome* consists of an achondroplasia-like appearance with cataract; it is commonly related to maternal warfarin ingestion in pregnancy.

*Diffuse fasciitis* [3] resembles dermatomyositis. It is more common in boys. It sometimes follows a febrile episode with myalgia. The skin is firm (sclerema) and swollen, and joint movement is restricted.

### References

1 Brice JEH, Johnston DI, Noronha JL. Limited joint mobility in diabetes. *Arch Dis Child* 1982; **57:** 879.
2 Rosenbloom AL, Silverstein JH, Lezotte DC, Richardson K, McCallum M. Limited joint mobility in childhood diabetes mellitus indicates increased risk for microvascular disease. *N Engl J Med* 1981; **305:** 191.
3 Sills EM. Diffuse fasciitis with eosinophilia in childhood. *Johns Hopkins Med J* 1982; **151:** 203.

# Bow Legs and Knock Knees

Some degree of *bow legs* is normal in late infancy. If the bowing is more marked than usual, so that when the child is lying down there is a gap of over 5 cm between the medial femoral condyles when the internal maleoli are in contact with the legs extended, one should take an X-ray to exclude rickets or *Blount's disease* [2]. Blount's disease is a likely diagnosis if the bowing is unilateral; it is more common in Negroes and in Finland. The X-ray shows irregular ossification on the medial side of the upper tibial epiphysis, leading to beaking on the posteromedial aspect of the metaphysis.

Bow legs are an occasional sequel to *Caffey's disease* (infantile cortical hyperostosis) (p. 37) [1]. Extreme bow legs or knock knees may result from *vitamin D resistant rickets* or *renal osteodystrophy*.

*Knock knees* are normal in toddlers, especially at around the age of 3, except when extreme—there being a gap of over 10 cm between the

internal malleoli when the child is lying down with the legs extended;
in that case an X-ray should be taken.

### References

1  Saul RA, Lee WH, Stevenson RE. Caffey's disease revisited. *Am J Dis Child*
      1982; **136**: 56.
2  Sharrard WJW. Knock knees and bow legs. *Br Med J* 1976; **1**: 826.

# Toe Walking and Toeing In

Many *normal toddlers* walk on their toes by habit. There are no signs of
spasticity or other disease: the tendon jerks are normal, the plantar
responses are flexor, there is a normal range of abduction at the hip
and of dorsiflexion of the ankle. Special investigation is unnecessary.
A child may walk on his toes because of a painful heel.

A *prematurely born baby* on reaching what would have been term is
liable to bear his weight on his toes rather than on the sole of his foot.

By far the commonest cause of toe walking is *cerebral palsy of the
spastic type*. If the toe walking is unilateral, there will be the usual
signs of spastic hemiplegia—the characteristic gait, shortening of the
affected leg and arm, some wasting of the affected limbs, limited
dorsiflexion of the affected ankle, relative coldness of the affected
limbs as compared with the normal ones, limited abduction of the hip,
exaggerated knee jerk and plantar extensor response on the affected
side, and possibly ankle clonus. If both lower limbs are involved,
there will almost certainly be signs of at least slight involvement of the
arms, if the child is old enough to perform fine repetitive movements.

An unusual cause is *congenital shortening of the Achilles tendon*. The
absence of the other signs of cerebral palsy, especially of an exaggerated knee jerk, limited abduction of the hip or an extensor plantar
response, should make a mistaken diagnosis unnecessary. If the
limitation of dorsiflexion of the ankle is due to spasticity, dorsiflexion
will be normal when the knee is flexed. If the limitation is due to
shortening of the Achilles tendon, the dorsiflexion will remain limited
on flexion of the knee.

An early sign of *dystonia musculorum deformans* is often toe walking ('the ballet-dancer's foot) (see p. 230).

Other causes of toe walking are *infantile autism, muscular dystrophy, peroneal muscular atrophy* (p. 258), *unilateral hip dislocation* and *a spinal cord tumour* [2]. Toe walking in Duchenne muscular dystrophy is said to be a postural adjustment to keep the weight-line behind the hip and in front of the knees at the same time in the face of ileotibial band tightness and quadriceps weakness. Toe walking may result from leg shortening or apparent shortening, as in unilateral congenital dislocation of a hip [1].

*Toeing in* is almost always a self-curing condition in the young child [3]; in the commonest form the whole limb is rotated medially, the child walking with the knees partly turned in to face each other. A less common form is metatarsus varus in which there is adduction and varus deformity of the foot, the child walking with the knees forward or turned slightly outwards.

Bilateral talipes in a girl is commonly (in about 40 per cent) associated with congenital hip dislocation. Whenever, in boy or girl, there is significant talipes, one should satisfy oneself that the hip is normal.

### References

1 David T, Parris MR, Poynor MU. Reasons for late detection of hip dislocation in childhood. *Lancet* 1983; **2**: 147.
2 Furrer F, Deonna T. Persistent toe walking in children. A comprehensive clinical study of 28 cases. *Helvetica Paediatrica Acta* 1982; **37**: 301.
3 Sharrard WJW. Intoeing and flat feet. *Br Med J* 1976; **1**: 888.

# Limp, Limb and Joint Pains

When a young child begins to limp, or an older child complains of limb pains, it may be impossible to distinguish bone pain from muscle or joint pain. The young child cannot even say where the pain is; he may be old enough to say that the pain is somewhere in the thigh, but he cannot localize it further; and the younger child just refuses to bear the weight and cannot complain of pain. When a young child begins to limp, there is often a history of minor trauma, but so there is in many other small children, who fall when running, fall off trees or have other knocks and bumps. When there is no history or sign of definite injury, inflammation or arthritis, one often obtains a history of pre- ceding upper respiratory tract infection. That, too, is difficult to assess, because such infections are so common in this age group. *The accurate diagnosis of the cause of a limp (or refusal to bear weight) can be very difficult and often impossible* [17]. It is difficult to say whether the pain has arisen in the soft tissues, muscles, bones, joints or spine.

In a review, Bowyer & Hollister [8] listed sixty-five causes with 120 references. When older children complain of vague limb or back pains, and no abnormal signs can be found, the pain may be due to the normal vigorous pursuits of youth, such as dances, violent games or skateboards. *Traumatic periostitis* may result from a twist or sprain. Recovery occurs in 7 to 10 days. The X-ray may show a periosteal reaction about a week after the injury.

When a previously well child begins to limp, one examines the shoe for a protruding nail, crinkling of the sole or excessive tightness; one then examines the child's lower limbs for a sore place, local heat or bone tenderness (due to fracture), not forgetting to look for enlarged tender inguinal lymph nodes. One then examines the ankle and knee joints for pain on movement and heat on palpation, and the hip joint in order to determine whether the range of movement, particularly in abduction and rotation, is full and painless. One remembers the frequency with which pain in the knee is pain referred from a diseased hip.

Finally one examines the spine for the range of movement, and the abdomen in case the limp is related to psoas spasm due to intra- abdominal inflammation.

I have tried to arrange the causes of limp and limb pains on an anatomical basis, despite overlap. Pain in the lower limbs may be referred from the abdomen (e.g. psoas spasm in appendicitis) or from the spinal cord or vertebrae. *Pain in the knee is commonly pain referred from the hip. When a tibia is fractured (as in a road traffic accident), the pain may be confined to the tibia, when in addition there is injury to the hip.*

For limp due to shortening of a limb, see p. 266.

The following are other causes to consider:

Soft tissue, connective tissue:

Trauma; nail in shoe; ingrowing toe-nail

Inguinal adenitis

Sickle cell disease

Collagen diseases

Muscle:

Growing pains

Trauma. Effect of injection. Strain

Muscular dystrophy. Early poliomyelitis. Weakness of a leg

Cramp—McArdle's syndrome. Dehydration

Trichiniasis, myositis. Other infection

Porphyria

Effect of drugs

Tendons and ligaments:

Sprain, stress. Achilles tendonitis. Tight Achilles tendon. Psoriatic tendonitis

Pes cavus. Flat foot

Bursitis—calcaneal

Periosteum:

Trauma. Non-accidental injury

Scurvy. Rubella syndrome

Caffey's disease. Vitamin A excess. Prostaglandin E

Bone:

Trauma. Non-accidental injury

Stress fracture of heel

Slipped femoral epiphysis

Osteitis. Sickle cell disease

Tumour. Leukaemia. Hodgkin's disease. Osteoid osteoma. Gaucher's disease

Rickets

Osteochondritis:

Perthes' disease of the hip. Scheuermann's disease of the spine

Osgood–Schlatter's disease of the tibia. Kohler's disease of the heel

Freiberg's disease of the metatarsal head

Osteochondritis dissecans. Chondromalacia patellae

Joints:
> Traumas. Pulled elbow. Strain
> Hypermobility
> Transient synovitis
> Infections—pyogenic cocci, dysentery, *Salmonella, Yersinia*
> > Brucellosis, tuberculosis, syphilis
> > Viruses—mumps, rubella, chickenpox, influenza, hepatitis B, glandular fever, arbovirus, adenovirus, cytomegalovirus, parvovirus
> > Miscellaneous—*Mycoplasma, Toxocara,* legionnaires' disease (p. 151), Kawasaki disease (p. 39), toxic shock (p. 92), Lyme disease
> Rheumatic fever. Juvenile chronic arthritis. Psoriasis
> Spondylo-arthropathy. Ankylosing spondilitis
> > Spondylolisthesis
> Gut arthropathy. Reiter's disease. Ulcerative colitis
> > Crohn's disease. Whipple's disease
> Blood diseases—allergic purpura, haemophilia, Christmas disease, leukaemia, sickle cell disease, haemoglobinopathies
> Tumours—haemangioma, histiocytosis
> Miscellaneous—cystic fibrosis, sarcoidosis, gout
> > Haemolytic uraemic syndrome. Allergy to foodstuffs
> > Immunological diseases. Serum sickness
> > Subacute bacterial endocarditis
> > Farber's disease
> > Foreign body in the joint
Drugs
Pain in heel
Psychological

I shall pick out only a few of these for discussion, either because they are common or important or because attention has recently been drawn to them. Before discussing any one of these, one must emphasize the importance of considering *non-accidental injury* as a cause of limp, limb or joint pains. The only objective evidence of a fracture of a bone may be the slight heat on palpation over the break.

One may fail to elicit the history of the particular childhood activity which has cause the limb pain by sprain or strain.

*Inguinal lymphadenitis* as a cause of a limp may be missed if not specifically looked for.

Many children are thought to have rheumatic fever when they have *growing pains*—a misnomer, because the pains occur predominantly before the period of maximum growth. Apley [5] found that one in every twenty-five Bristol school children had such pains. The pains are non-articular, involving mainly the thigh and calf muscles, mainly at night in bed. The cause is unknown. The ESR is normal, an important fact which eliminates rheumatic fever. Øster & Nielsen [28] in a study of 2718 school children aged 6 to 19 years, found that the peak age of growing pains was 11, and at that age approximately 20 per cent of boys and 30 per cent of girls complained of them. The overall incidence in boys was 12·5 per cent and in girls 18·4 per cent. Twenty-eight per cent of those with growing pains also had headaches and 27 per cent had abdominal pain, either simultaneously or at different times. The children were otherwise normal. In a Finnish study [19], the onset of growing pains was mainly age 5 to 7, and the pains largely ceased by 11 years of age. There was a history of headaches in 30 per cent (compared with 12 per cent in controls) and of recurrent abdominal pain in 18 per cent (compared with 6 per cent in controls). There was a strong family history of growing pains.

Some boys with *Duchenne muscular dystrophy* have pain in the legs. *Poliomyelitis* may cause severe limb pain in the preparalytic stage, due to spasm in the muscles about to be paralysed. *Transient myositis* may cause severe pain with fever [37]. Myalgia may be due to *trichiniasis* due to eating uncooked meat: there may be fever, orbital oedema and eosinophilia.

Salbutamol can cause muscle cramps. Cramps may occur in cystic fibrosis owing to sodium depletion.

Periosteal pain may be due to Caffey's disease of infantile cortical hyperosotsis (p. 269), rubella syndrome, scurvy, vitamin A excess, trauma (especially child abuse) or prostaglandin E given for congenital heart disease [29, 30]. Scurvy is rare in Britain, but one has seen it in severely handicapped children.

A *slipped femoral epiphysis* occurs especially between 10 and 15 years, especially in overweight boys. It is bilateral in 20 per cent. The symptom is a limp with little pain, but there may be pain in the knee, groin or anterior aspect of the thigh—possibly suggesting 'growing pains'. The important sign is limitation of hip movement, especially on internal rotation [9]. In the infant and toddler, pain in the hip or a limp may be the result of *congenital dislocation of the hip*.

*Tumours of bone are of great importance and the diagnosis can readily be missed unless specifically looked for. Leukaemia and Hodgkin's disease must be considered when a child complains of persistent limb pain.*

*Osteoid osteoma* occurs at any age, but mainly in children, and more often in boys [27]. It involves especially the tibia and femur, but may affect other bones, including the vertebrae. It causes chronic pain, often severe, especially at night and on exertion. The pains may be of a boring or aching nature, relieved by aspirin. It may be referred from the upper end of the femur to the knee. There is local tenderness and wasting may occur in older children. Below the age of 8 years the affected limb may be longer than the other. The X-rays show no abnormality at first, but later show thickening of the cortex with a lucent area in the bone.

*Transient synovitis of the hip* is common [17, 18]. The age of onset is usually between 18 months and 7 years, and it is rather more common in boys. There may be a history of a preceding cold or minor injury, of doubtful significance. The symptom is refusal to bear weight, or limp, or vague pain in the knee or hip, with limitation of movement. The symptoms usually last a few days, and may be relieved by avoidance of weight bearing. Special investigations are of little help, though an ultrasound study or X-ray is necessary to eliminate Perthes' disease; they may show slight widening of the joint space of the hip [36]. The ESR is raised in about half of all cases. The white cell count is usually normal, but there may be leucopenia or eosinophilia. The condition may be difficult or impossible to distinguish from early Perthes' disease—and some children, thought at first to have transient synovitis of the hip, prove on follow-up examination to have Perthes' disease. The relationship of transient synovitis of the hip to Perthes' disease is still speculative.

Recurrences of transient synotivitis are frequent [18]. The exact frequency of the recurrences is uncertain and depends on the duration of the follow-up study: thirty-six children had a total of eighty recurrences, and recurrences can occur after many years without symptoms. In seventy-two of eighty recurrences there was no evidence of an associated respiratory infection.

The age of onset of *Perthes' disease* is usually 2 to 10 years. It presents with a limp and limitation of hip movement, with pain in the region of the hip or knee, but often no pain at all. It is sometimes found incidentally when an X-ray is taken for another purpose, and the child has had no symptoms to suggest Perthes' disease. It may be bilateral. On examination there is limitation of abduction, external rotation and extension of the hip, but especially of abduction.

*Osteochondritis dissecans* is associated with pain in the knee, especially over the lateral aspect of the medial condyle of the femur. It is due to a fragment of bone underlying the articular cartilage of the knee becoming avascular. *Chondromalacia patellae* occurs in the older child, with pain mainly in the front of the knee, and sometimes with a story of the knee 'giving way' or 'locking'—a similar story to that of the child with a 'clicking knee'—commonly due to a discoid meniscus [35]. In chondromalacia there is tenderness behind the patella and discomfort on rubbing the patella against the end of the femur.

Leg pain may be due to *Achilles tendonitis* [32]; there is warmth and tenderness of the Achilles tendon.

A *pulled elbow* is a common mishap in small children under the age of about five [16]. The child suddenly shows sign of pain in the upper limb or will not move the arm. The pain is usually in the region of the elbow, but in about a quarter of all cases it is localized to the wrist; in others the pain is referred to the forearm or shoulder. The diagnosis is frequently missed, but correct diagnosis is important because it can be cured instantly by appropriate manipulation. It is due to the head of the radius being pulled partially through the annular ligament.

*Hypermobility of joints* may cause limb pains [6, 7, 21]. The hypermobility may be based on features in the muscles, ligaments, capsules or collagen. It may be an advantage in some occupations—for gymnasts, ballet dancers, spin-bowlers, or musicians. It occurs in several syndromes, such as those of Ehrlers–Danlos, Marfan, Cohen (p. 30) and Larsen (general hypermobility, stunted stature, depressed nasal bridge and spatulate digits). Hypermobility is often familial, and symptoms may develop at any age, from 3 onwards. The symptoms may suggest chronic rheumatic disease [21]; in a study of fifty-four cases, 78 per cent were girls, with the mean age of onset of symptoms at 11 years.

In a study of nineteen children with chronic arthritis [12], evidence of old rubella infection was found in seven. Arthritis may follow rubella vaccine, and last for 1 to 6 weeks or more. In older children and adolescents rubella may cause arthritis, as may tetanus toxoid.

*Pyogenic arthritis*, or osteitis near a joint, can readily be confused with rheumatic fever. The diagnosis is made more difficult when two or three joints are involved in osteitis. When there is any doubt (as there often is) a blood culture should be taken before penicillin is given. Arthritis is common in the *mucocutaneous lymph node syndrome* (p. 39).

A wide variety of other infections may cause arthritis or arthralgia. They include pyogenic organisms, tuberculosis, syphilis, viruses, *Mycoplasma*, *Toxocara*, legionnaires' disease, toxic shock, Behçet's disease (p. 15) and Lyme disease. *Lyme disease* [11, 13] has been widely described in many parts of the world, including Britain. It is due to the spirochaete *Borrelia burgdorferi* and is tick-borne. A characteristic rash (erythema chronicum migrans) may be followed several weeks later by arthritis, polyneuritis and cardiac signs. Other features may be periorbital oedema, lymphadenopathy or testicular swelling.

In a study of 2089 children with bacterial meningitis [22], forty-eight had arthritis; the organism was *Haemophilus influenzae* in thirty-eight, *Meningococcus* in nine and *Staphylococcus* in one.

*Rheumatic fever* is now rare in Britain. Its main features are arthritis, lassitude, fever and often carditis, following (in about a third of all cases) a known previous throat infection. The arthritis is typically a 'flitting polyarthritis', involving mainly (and almost entirely) the knee, ankle, wrist and elbow, only occasionally the hip, and rarely other joints. Hip involvement in rheumatic fever is unusual. The arthritis starts in one joint and clears after 2 or 3 days, moving to other joints in rotation, but the arthritis may involve one joint only or at least treatment is given so promptly that other joints are not involved. In my experience all children with arthritis due to rheumatic fever are unwell. If a child complains of pains in the joints and yet feels well and full of energy, rheumatic fever can be almost excluded. Fever may be short-lasting and subside before the child is referred to a doctor. The ESR is invariably high (unless there is heart failure due to carditis, in which case the ESR is normal in about a quarter of all cases). If the ESR was not very high (e.g. if it were merely 15 to 20 mm in an hour, micro-Westergren method), I would almost exclude the diagnosis of rheumatic fever as a cause of the arthritis.

There is almost always a raised sleeping pulse rate in the early stage (e.g. over 100 per min), but there is often a sinus bradycardia (e.g. pulse rate of 60 per min) in the early convalescent stage. If the pulse rate is fast, the sleeping pulse rate alone is of value, because tachycardia due to emotional factors must be excluded. The murmur of an obvious carditis may clinch the diagnosis; but in the early stage of such a murmur it is essential to distinguish it from a functional murmur. The functional murmur is either soft or musical and high-pitched. It is commonly of short duration, tends to be late in systole and louder in the supine position, and is often increased by exertion. Other features include erythema marginatum or rheumatic nodules.

I have seen many children who were thought to have rheumatic fever when in fact they had *febrile aches and pains in the limbs*. These occur in any infection associated with fever and are non-articular.

*Juvenile chronic arthritis.* The peak age of onset of juvenile chronic arthritis is 2 to 4 years, though it may begin long before 2—even in the first year [20]. It is more common in girls than in boys. The presenting symptom is usually pain in a joint. A troublesome presenting symptom or sign, which may last for some months before a joint becomes involved, is unexplained fever. This occurs in some 10 per cent of cases. A single joint may be involved or several joints may be painful at one time. When a single joint is involved, it is most likely to be a knee or ankle. The joint becomes enlarged, movement is painful and becomes restricted, and the joint is hot on palpation. There are signs of effusion into the joint. About half of all cases present with involvement of a single joint, and over a period of months no other joint may be involved. Involvement of the small joints of the fingers (especially the proximal interphalangeal joints) is a common and characteristic feature of other cases. There is commonly wasting of the muscles surrounding an affected joint. Muscle weakness is a common complaint. In about a quarter of all cases there is a characteristic salmon-pink maculopapular slightly raised rash, consisting of lesions 1 to 2 cm in diameter, sometimes oval in shape with a pale centre. The lesions appear mainly in the latter part of the day, especially on the extremities. Pericarditis is a relatively common complication; rare complications include myocarditis and amyloidosis. Secondary scoliosis with gross difference in limb development may occur when a single joint, such as the knee, is affected.

The incidence of splenic and lymph node enlargement in rheumatoid arthritis is often exaggerated. It occurs in not more than one in ten of all affected children. Juvenile chronic arthritis is a seronegative arthropathy, whose true nature may not be obvious for several years [2]: nearly one third of sixty cases turned out to have ankylosing spondylitis or other defined entities.

It may be difficult to distinguish juvenile chronic arthritis from rheumatic fever [34]. Rheumatic nodules may occur in both. The following are the main differentiating points in doubtful cases:

**1**  Stiffness in the mornings strongly favours the diagnosis of juvenile chronic arthritis.

**2**  Duration of joint involvement. Arthritis in one joint does not usually last more than a few days in rheumatic fever, even if no treatment is given.

**3**  Involvement of the neck and proximal interphalangeal joints suggests juvenile chronic arthritis.

**4**  A normal ESR, a negative ASO titre, or the absence of CRP, excludes the diagnosis of rheumatic fever. The ESR is normal in 30 to 40 per cent of children with active juvenile chronic arthritis. A high ESR (over 4 mm in an hour, using the micro-Westergren method) is unusual in juvenile chronic arthritis; an ESR between 10 and 20 mm would almost exclude the diagnosis of rheumatic fever with arthritis unless there were heart failure. The ASO titre is negative in 80 per cent of children with juvenile chronic arthritis, and CRP is absent in 70 per cent. These tests are positive in 99 per cent of children with rheumatic fever and arthritis.

**5**  Iridocyclitis. This occurs in about 15 per cent of children with juvenile chronic arthritis.

**6**  If the child is under 5, he would almost certainly be ill if he had rheumatic fever and would have obvious carditis. I would almost exclude rheumatic fever if a 4-year-old had arthritis without carditis. Under 3, rheumatic fever is exceedingly rare. Unfortunately tests for the rheumatoid factor do not often help in children. The tests are rarely positive in the absence of rheumatic nodules.

Polyarthritis, lasting 1 to 4 months, may follow about 3 weeks after a mild gastrointestinal illness, consisting of abdominal pain, fever and diarrhoea, due to *Yersinia* infections.

*Psoriasis* usually precedes arthritis by several years; it may be preceded by tendonitis. Shore & Ansell [33] described sixty cases in children. In twenty-five the first symptom was psoriasis and in twenty-six the first symptom was arthritis. In nine the onset was with both arthritis and psoriasis. The peak age of onset was 9 to 12 years. In twenty-five there was a family history of psoriasis and it follows that one should always enquire about this. Psoriatic arthritis is indistinguishable from juvenile chronic arthritis except that psoriasis characteristically involves the terminal interphalangeal joints, while juvenile chronic arthritis involves the proximal joints. There is a family history of psoriasis in half. The arthritis commonly begins in the knee, but eventually 87 per cent develop polyarthritis [33]. The polyarthritis is commonly asymmetrical; it frequently affects only a single digit at first. In rare cases there is fever, pericarditis, lymph node enlargement or iridocyclitis.

*Spondylo-arthropathy* usually presents as arthritis of the hip or knee, and less commonly the ankle: later, commonly about 6 years after the onset, there is sacro-illiitis and/or ankylosing spondylitis [2, 3]. It is much more common in boys, most of them 9 or older. A quarter give a history of pain in the heel, due to plantar fasciitis, bursitis or Achilles tendonitis. There may be arthritis in the interphalangeal joints of the toes or the metatarsophalangeal joints. There is sometimes a history of recurrent attacks of transient synovitis of the hip. Six per cent later develop psoriasis, and 8 per cent develop ulcerative colitis or Crohn's disease; other complications include iridocyclitis or aortic incompetence.

The so-called *gut arthropathy* includes arthritis in association with ulcerative colitis, Crohn's disease, Reiter's disease and other bowel infections, such as *Salmonella, Yersinia, Campylobacter* and dysentery. *Reiter's disease* may follow 10 to 20 days after one of these infections—along with conjunctivitis and urethritis. The possibility of one of the above, such as Crohn's disease, should be suspected when in addition to arthritis involving one or two joints, there is loss of weight. Arthritis is sometimes a feature of *cystic fibrosis* [25, 31]. It is usually transient but may recur.

*Sarcoid arthritis* may resemble juvenile chronic arthritis [23, 26]. It is characterized by large, painless, boggy synovial and tendon sheath effusions involving the wrists, ankles, knees and elbows, running a chronic course with uveitis but no hilar lymphadenopathy, and with no abnormal laboratory findings apart from a raised ESR. There is a slowly progressive joint involvement over a 2 to 3 year period. There may be rashes, subcutaneous nodules or uveitis. The arthritis involves mainly wrists and knees. All started before the age of 4 years.

*Juvenile gout* may be secondary to leukaemia or haemolytic anaemia, but may be primary (familial) [10].

A history of recurrent infection, with mild recurrent arthritis, commonly starting at about 3 years of age, may be due to hypogammaglobulinaemia [4].

For Farber's lipogranulomatosis with arthritis, subcutaneous nodules and hepatic enlargement, see p. 48.

Possible causes include a foreign body (such as a thorn), trauma (e.g. by shoes), chilblains, fasciitis or infections of the soft tissues, calcaneal bursitis, bursitis between the Achilles tendon and the calcaneus, periostitis, osteochondritis, ankylosing spondylitis or stress fracture. Food sensitivity (p. 13) has been blamed for joint pains [24]. Confusion is caused by the interval of 4 hrs or a day or two between taking the food and the onset of symptoms.

Many *drugs* may cause arthralgia or joint effusion [1]. Serum sickness may result from diphtheria or tetanus antitoxin. When corticosteroids are discontinued after prolonged administration there may be joint pains, stiffness, paraesthesiae and malaise [15]. Mild arthralgia may accompany almost any drug-induced rash. Barbiturates, methimazole, penicillin and sulphasalazine may cause a joint effusion. Azathioprine, carbamazepine, chlordiazepoxide, cimetidine, ethambutol, heroin, isoniazid and rifampicin may cause joint pains.

Hypervitaminosis A causes angular stomatitis, hepatomegaly and bone pain with periostitis. Cramps may be caused by ergotamine, lincomycin, nalidixic acid, phenothiazines or thiazide diuretics.

Finally a limp or complaint of joint pain my be an *attention-seeking device*, and a limp may be due to *hysteria*.

*Pain in the heel*

The diagnosis of the cause of pain in the heel is commonly difficult, and, although the causes have largely been covered above, I felt that they should be summarized here in spite of the repetition [14].

The main causes are trauma to the soft tissues (e.g. by shoes), infection in the soft tissues, stress fracture, calcaneal bursitis, ankylosing spondylitis, and osteochondritis (Sever, Köhler, Freiberg).

# References

1 *Adverse Drug Reaction Bulletin*. Drug-induced aches and pains. 1971; **No. 30:** 88.
2 Ansell BM. *Rheumatic disorders in childhood*. London: Butterworth, 1980.
3 Ansell BM. Spondyloarthropathy in childhood: a review. *J Roy Soc Med* 1981; **74:** 205.
4 Ansell BM. Arthritis in young children. *Br Med J* 1983; **1:** 1917.
5 Apley J. *The child with abdominal pains*. 2nd edn. Oxford: Blackwell Scientific Publications, 1975.
6 Beighton P, Grahame R, Bird H. *Hypermobility of joints*. Berlin: Springer-Verlag, 1983.
7 Biro F, Gewanter HL, Baum J. The hypermobility syndrome. *Pediatrics* 1983; **72:** 701.
8 Bowyer SL, Hollister JR. Limb pains in children. *Pediatr Clin N Am* 1985; **31:** 1053.
9 Brenkel IJ, Prosser AJ, Pearse M. Slipped capital femoral epiphysis; continuing problem of late diagnosis. *Br Med J* 1986; **2:** 256.
10 *British Medical Journal*. Juvenile gout. Leading article. 1972; **1:** 129.
11 *Canadian Medical Association Journal*. Lyme disease. Leading article. 1986; **134:** 48.
12 Chantler JK, Tingle AJ, Petty RE. Persistent rubella virus infection associated with chronic arthritis in children. *N Engl J Med* 1985; **313:** 1117.
13 *Communicable Disease Report*. Lyme disease. 1986; **No. 19.**
14 Gross RH. Foot pain. *Pediatr Clin North Am* 1977; **24:** 813.
15 Hargreave FE, McCarthy DS, Pepys J, *et al.* Steroid pseudorheumatism in asthma. *Br Med J* 1969; **1:** 443.
16 Illingworth CM. Pulled elbow. *Br Med J* 1975; **2:** 672.
17 Illingworth CM. 128 limping children with no fracture, sprain or obvious cause. *Clin Pediatr (Phila)* 1978; **17:** 139.
18 Illingworth CM. Recurrences of transient synovitis of the hip. *Arch Dis Child* 1983; **58:** 620.
19 Keinänen-Kiukaanniemi S, Hakkinen J, Korhonen J, Kouvalainen K. Growing pains in school children. *Acta Paediatr Scand* 1986; **Suppl 322:** 27.
20 Laaksonen A. A prognostic study of juvenile rheumatoid arthritis. Analysis of 544 cases. *Acta Paediatr Scand* **Suppl 166.** 1966.
21 Lewkonia RM, Ansell BM. Articular hypermobility simulating chronic rheumatic disease. *Arch Dis Child* 1983; **58:** 988.
22 Likitonukul S, McCracken GH, Nelson JD. Arthritis in children with bacterial meningitis. *Am J Dis Child* 1986; **140:** 424.
23 Lindsley CB, Godfrey WA. Juvenile sarcoidosis manifesting as juvenile rheumatoid arthritis. *Pediatrics* 1985; **76:** 765.
24 McCarty EP, Frick OL. Food sensitivity, keys to diagnosis. *J Pediatr* 1983; **102:** 645.
25 Newman AJ, Ansell BM. Episodic arthritis in children with cystic fibrosis. *J Pediatr* 1979; **94:** 594.

26 North AF, Fink CW, Gibson WM, *et al*. Sarcoid arthritis in children. *Am J Med* 1970; **48**: 449.

27 Orlowski JP, Mercer RD. Osteoid osteoma in children and young adults. *Pediatrics* 1977; **59**: 526.

28 Øster J, Nielsen A. Growing pains. *Acta Paediatr Scand* 1972; **61**: 329.

29 Sato Y, Okishima T, Matsuoka Y, *et al*. Periostitis. *Acta Paediatr Japonica* 1982; **24**: 349.

30 Sato Y, Okinshima T, Matsuoka Y, *et al*. Periosteal hypertrophy following administration of prostaglandin E. *Acta Paediatr Japonica* 1982; **24**: 311.

31 Schidlow DV, Goldsmith DP, Palmer J, Huang NN. Arthritis in cystic fibrosis. *Arch Dis Child* 1984; **59**: 377.

32 Shapiro JR, Fallat RW, Tsang RC, Glueck CJ. Achilles tendonitis and tenosynovitis. *Am J Dis Child* 1974; **128**: 486.

33 Shore A, Ansell BM. Juvenile psoriatic arthritis—analysis of 60 cases. *J Pediatr* 1982; **100**: 529.

34 Sills EM. Errors in diagnosis of juvenile rheumatoid arthritis. *Johns Hopkins Med J* 1973; **133**: 88.

35 Snellman O, Stenström RH. Congenital lateral discoid meniscus of the knee joint and its arthrography in children. *Ann Paediatr Fenniae* 1960; **6**: 124.

36 Sprigg A. Modern diagnostic imaging: risks and benefits. In: Meadow R (ed.) *Recent advances in paediatrics*, Vol 8. London: Churchill Livingstone, 1986.

37 Tepperberg J. Transient acute myositis in children. *JAMA* 1977; **238**: 27.

# Back Pains

The commonest cause of back pain in children is ligamentous strain or intervertebral disc lesions in the lumbosacral spine or neck. They are usually due to athletic exercises to which the child is not accustomed or perhaps suited [4]. The pain may be postural, or due to muscle strain. It could be due to spondylolysis—fracture of the pars interarticularis [4]. According to my colleague J. Sharrard FRCS, who has helped me with this section, intervertebral disc lesions in children are not as rare as many think, but are rarely recognized. The so-called fibrositis is probably non-existent; the symptoms are probably due to ligamentous strain or pain referred from the disc region.

Back pain and related symptoms may be due to *discitis* [2, 3, 5]. Symptoms may begin at any age, from 10 months or so, and consist of abdominal pain, refusal to walk, slight fever, irritability, vomiting, malaise, pain in the back, especially on movement, stiff neck, vague pain in the buttocks, knee or thigh, or a limp. On examination there is lumbar lordosis, stiffness of the back and sometimes local tenderness. Straight leg-raising may be restricted. Recovery occurs in 2 to 8 weeks.

*Ankylosing spondylitis* is an important cause of back pain [6] (p. 281).

*Scheuermann's disease of the spine,* mainly thoracic, causes back pain and sometimes adolescent kyphosis.

*Spondylolisthesis* [1] is rare before the age of 5. It consists of a forward slip of one vertebra over the other. The symptoms are low back pain, sometimes sciatic pain, or a crouched posture due to contracted hamstrings.

Pain may radiate from the abdomen (e.g. pancreatitis) to the back.

Other conditions to consider include juvenile chronic arthritis (p. 279) and joint hypermobility (p. 277).

Back pain may be of *psychological origin.* As always, this is a dangerous diagnosis, and I repeat that the diagnosis should only be made on the basis of positive evidence of psychological disturbance after elimination of organic disease on full investigation and follow-up.

## References

1 Bleck EE. Spondylolisthesis. *Dev Med Child Neurol* 1974; **16:** 680.
2 Galil A, Gorodischer R, Bar-Ziv J, *et al.* Intervertebral disc infection (discitis) in childhood. *Europ J Pediatr* 1982; **139:** 66.
3 Hensey OJ, Coad N, Carty HM, Sills JM. Juvenile discitis. *Arch Dis Child* 1983; **58:** 983.
4 King HA. Back pain in children. *Pediatr Clin N Am* 1985; **31:** 1083.
5 *Lancet.* Discitis and the acute abdomen in childhood. Leading article. 1984; **2:** 23.
6 Schaller J, Bitnum S, Wedgewood RJ. Ankylosing spondylitis with chidhood onset. *J Pediatr* 1969; **74:** 505.

# Asymmetry of the Head

It is common to find that a young baby's head is flat on one side, because he has consistently lain on that side, while it bulges out at the other side. The skull becomes more symmetrical as he grows older, and no treatment is necessary.

Many babies are born with some degree of cranial asymmetry, and it is of no importance.

Extreme asymmetry may be due to *craniostenosis*—premature closure of the cranial sutures. As surgical treatment may be possible and necessary, it is important to establish the diagnosis—by palpation of the ridge of fused sutures and by X-ray.

Other causes, both rare, are a *partial Treacher–Collins syndrome* or other anomaly of the first arch, or *congenital asymmetry*.

# A Small Head

The size of the head is closely related to the size of the cranial contents. If the brain does not grow normally, the head is likely to be unusually small. Hence the measurement of the head circumference is an important part of the developmental assessment of an infant, in that it may add confirmatory evidence of defective mental development or of early hydrocephalus. The measurement of the head circumference should be just as much part of the routine examination of a baby in a baby clinic, doctor's surgery or hospital, as is the examination of the hips for congenital subluxation or the back for a congenital dermal sinus, and—after 3 or 4 months—a rough test of hearing.

It is easy to make an erroneous diagnosis of microcephaly and therefore of mental handicap when in fact the child is normal. It is necessary to be aware of the other causes of smallness of the head circumference.

When a child has an unusually small head, one should consider the following conditions:

Normal variation
Small baby
Familial feature
Microcephaly
Craniostenosis

A small baby is likely to have a smaller head than a big baby, and a big baby is likely to have a bigger head than a small baby. *Hence the maximum head circumference must be related to the size of the baby.* This can be done by plotting the head circumference and weight on the relevant centile charts (see Fig. 1). The two normally coincide, though a small or large head may be a familial feature which affects the position on the chart. Hence, when the head is unusual, one must see both parents.

The fact that the head circumference corresponds exactly with the fiftieth centile by no means proves that the head is normal. The child might have microcephaly if he is a particularly big baby, or hydrocephalus if he is a particularly small baby.

When there is true microephaly, the head is not only unusually small, but it is badly shaped, tapering off towards the vertex.

*Craniostenosis* or premature closure of the cranial sutures is a rare cause of undue smallness of the head. The fused sutures may be palpated by the experienced finger, but the diagnosis is established by X-ray. The anterior fontanelle would be closed; but early closure is frequently a normal variant.

If brain damage occurs in the early months (especially in the first year), serial head measurements are likely to show a deceleration in the growth of head size. Brain damage after the first year or two does not have this effect, because most of the normal brain growth has already occurred before the damage.

# A Large Head

Erroneous diagnosis or unnecessary suspicion of the presence of hydrocephalus is common. The usual error is to fail to relate the size of the head to the size of the baby. The best (and the easiest) measurement to which to relate the head size is the weight [1, 2]. A big baby is likely to have a bigger head than a small baby. Serial measurements are more important than single ones: serial measurements enable one to determine whether a child's measurement is deviating from his position on the centile charts (see Fig. 1). It is commonly forgotten that if there is an unusually fast rate of increase of head size, as shown on the head chart, the most common cause is a correspondingly rapid increase in the size of the baby; hence the position on the centile head chart must be compared with the position on the centile weight chart.

Another common source of error is the genetic or familial one. There may be a familial tendency to have an unusually large (or small) head. The child's head size is correlated with home socio-economic conditions.

Two other sources of error are common. The *preterm baby* has a relatively large head; and an older infant (e.g. 9 to 12 months of age) with 'failure to thrive' has a relatively large head because the brain suffers less from malnutrition than the rest of the body.

A widely open fontanelle, which is not bulging, may be merely a normal variant, often familial.

Significant causes of head enlargement are as follows:

Hydrocephalus
Subdural effusion
Cerebral tumour or cyst
Megalencephaly (rare) [4]
Hydraencephaly (rare)
Other rare diseases—cerebral gigantism, Canavan's disease, agenesis of the corpus callosum, neurofibromatosis, Russell–Silver syndrome, myotonic dystrophy (p. 207), Osler–Rendu–Weber syndrome (p. 364)

Certain storage diseases, e.g. sulphatide lipoidosis and gangliosidosis, incontinentia pigmenti achromians of Ito

Fragile X syndrome

The diagnosis of *hydrocephalus* would be confirmed by the finding of a bulging fontanelle, widely separated sutures, and serial measurements plotted on the centile chart which indicate that the head size in relation to the weight of the child is enlarging excessively.

The child with *achondroplasia* has a large head, partly because of a slight ventricular enlargement and partly because of *megalencephaly*, a large brain, usually of poor quality. (For discussion of 109 cases of megalencephaly, see Lorber & Priestly [4].

*Hydranencephaly* is a rare condition in which the head seems to be full of cerebrospinal fluid with compression of brain tissue. The diagnosis is made in part by transillumination in a darkened room.

In *cerebral gigantism* [5], there is a prominent forehead, acromegalic features, excessive growth in height, large hands and feet, clumsiness and mental subnormality. There is excessive growth in the first 3 or 4 years.

*Canavan's disease* is an autosomal recessive condition, showing itself in early infancy with poor head control, spasticity, optic atrophy and progressive macrocephaly. Lacey [3] described forty children with *agenesis of the corpus callosum*. There were mental retardation, convulsions, congenital anomalies, learning disorders, and macrocephaly or microcephaly. In the *Russell–Silver syndrome* there is dwarfism with a large head.

For incontinentia pigmenti, see p. 359.

### References

1 Illingworth RS, Eid E. Head circumference in relation to weight, chest circumference, supine length and crown rump length in the first six months of life. *Acta Paediatr Scand* 1971; **60**: 333.

2 Illingworth RS, Lutz W. The measurement of the infant's head circumference and its significance. *Arch Dis Child* 1965; **40**: 672.

3 Lacey DJ. Agenesis of the corpus callosum. *Am J Dis Child* 1985; **139**: 953.

4 Lorber J, Priestley BL. Children with large heads. *Dev Med Child Neurol* 1981; **23**: 494.

5 Sotos JF, Cutler EA. Cerebral gigantism. *Am J Dis Child* 1977; **131**: 625.

*A Large Head*

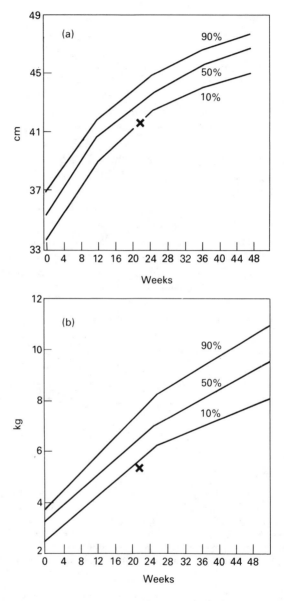

**Fig. 1.** (a) Head and (b) weight charts with head circumference and weight corresponding.

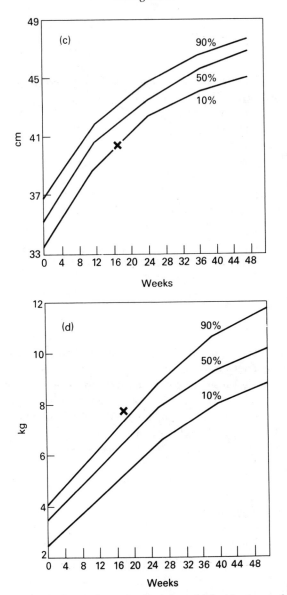

**Fig. 1 cont.** (c) Head and (d) weight charts for a child with microcephaly showing a small head in relation to weight.

# Asymmetry of the Chest

When the chest is notably asymmetrical the following conditions should be considered:

> Congenital deformity
> Congenital absence of the pectoralis major
> Scoliosis
> Intrathoracic disease—atelectasis, pleural effusion, air-containing cyst, etc.
> Congenital asymmetry (hemihypertrophy, hemiatrophy)

For congenital absence of the sternal head of the pectoralis major, see p. 262.

# Crying

All babies cry long before they laugh, and the causes of crying (or laughing) are not always clear [1].

Many of the causes of crying are obvious. The usual ones are hunger, wind or other discomfort. Some babies cry when the light is put out; others cry when the light is put on; all are likely to cry if the limbs or head are tightly held by one's hand.

One may summarize the causes of crying as follows:

## A. Infants

1  *Crying without disease*
> Hunger, sometimes due to fear of over-feeding. Thirst
> Discomfort—wind, cold, heat, itching, evening colic, wet napkin, loud noises, teething
> Cow's milk allergy
> Irritability on the breast
> Personality
> Crying on passing urine

Habit
Loneliness: desire to see surroundings, or to be picked up
Fatigue
Food forcing
Child abuse
Drug withdrawal (newborn). Use of drugs
Unexplained
2  *Crying with disease*
Infection
Headache, earache
Strangulated hernia. Torsion of testis
Intestinal obstruction and intussusception
Pink disease
Phenylketonuria
Coeliac disease
Autism

**B. Older children** (excessive crying only)

Personality, insecurity, habit
Hunger
Fatigue
Puberty
Early chorea
Illness
Child abuse
Autism
Drugs

The obvious cause of crying by an infant is hunger. A sensible mother feeds her young baby when he wants it, whether in the day or night. Rigid ideas about the feeding schedule, due to fears of causing 'bad habits', lead to a great deal of crying. Another rigid idea which leads to much crying from hunger is the fear of over-feeding. Many babies cry from hunger because someone is so obsessed by the fear of over-feeding them that they are half-starved. A baby's cry may be due to thirst caused by hypernatraemia as a result of making the feeds with dried milk too strong (for instance, a heaped measure of milk powder in 30 ml of water), or by over-clothing and excessive sweating.

*Discomfort* from any cause may lead to crying. Causes include excessive cold or excessive heat, pruritus (as from eczema), a wet napkin or a sudden loud noise. For 'evening colic' see p. 109.

Allergy to cow's milk (p. 13) is a possible but unlikely cause of excessive crying. It is a difficult diagnosis to establish with certainty, and, apart from laboratory investigation, trials with and without cow's milk are likely to be needed.

*Teething* is a convenient condition to blame when a baby, 6 months or more of age, cries excessively, especially in the evening. It is reasonable to suggest that the eruption of a tooth through the periosteum may cause pain; but *much of the crying which is ascribed to teething is in fact related to habit formation in connection with sleep, due to parental mismanagement.* The usual age at which this sleep problem arises is 9 to 12 months. The baby discovers that if he cries when put to bed he will be picked out of his cot and taken downstairs—and so he cries every time when put to bed. He may also discover that if he cries as soon as he awakens he will be picked up and taken either downstairs or into his parents' bed—and so he cries out every night. This crying is commonly ascribed by parents to 'indigestion' or 'awful wind', when in fact it is purely a habit which they have themselves caused.

A unique study of the effect of teething was carried out in Finland [2], studying the effect of teething in 126 normal babies in a home for illegitimate infants. The eruption of a tooth was *not* associated with bronchitis, diarrhoea, rashes, convulsions or fever. There was only a marginal increase of restlessness by day, with no significant increase of crying.

*Irritability and screaming in the newborn period when the baby is put to the breast* is an annoying symptom, which leads to some babies being put to the bottle. It may be due to the baby's nose becoming obstructed by his upper lip when feeding, or being blocked by the mother's breast tissue. It may be partly due to the mother trying to force the baby to suck, or fearing that the baby will bite her, so that she withdraws as soon as he begins to suck. The problem settles down within about 10 days if patience is shown.

However wise the management, some babies cry excessively, and one can only ascribe it to the *personality*—which is largely inherited. Some babies seem to sense their mother's anxiety and tenseness and cry as a result. The amount of crying by a baby commonly represents an interaction between his personality and developing mind and the personality of his parents, especially the mother.

Babies commonly cry, often with a shriek, when *passing urine*. It is a normal feature, especially around the age of 6 months.

Many babies cry when left alone and are quiet when picked up. Many intelligent babies, from the age of 6 weeks or so, are not content to be left lying down with nothing to see. They are quiet when propped up so that they can see the fascinating activities of the kitchen.

In the weaning stage much crying is due to *efforts to force the child to take food*, especially food which he does not like, or not allowing him to feed himself when he wants to. Rarely such crying may be due to food allergy.

It must be admitted that much crying by infants occurs without discoverable cause. If the crying continues when the child is picked up and fed, it must be assumed that it is due to some discomfort— perhaps *abdominal pain* or *headache*. Crying is usual when the baby feels tired.

Crying when the baby is unwell may be due to *infection*, such as otitis media or pyelonephritis, or to intestinal obstruction (if there is also vomiting). One must examine the *hernial orifices* for a strangulated hernia and look for torsion of the testis. The acute onset of screaming attacks should suggest the possibility of *intussusception*.

*Pink disease* should no longer occur, because mercury is no longer a constituent of teething powders, but one must remember the possibility of the mother having obtained a teething powder from an old stock, or having applied an ointment containing mercury (p. 221).

Crying is a feature of *phenylketonuria* until by proper treatment the serum phenylalanine level is reduced to normal. Crying is a common feature of coeliac disease, until gluten is excluded.

*In older children* excessive crying may be a feature of the *personality*. It may be due to insecurity, and one must investigate the home and school background.

Crying at night is usually due to *habit formation*, the habit having continued from infancy. The child repeatedly cries out at night because he knows that his mother will come to him, perhaps read to him, play with him, give him a warm drink or take him into her own bed (p. 298).

A child may cry because he is *hungry or tired*. Children at *puberty* commonly burst into tears with little or no provocation.

When an older child is excessively lachrymose one must eliminate organic disease, such as *anaemia* or *pyelonephritis* or a persistent *streptococcal throat infection.*

When a child who previously behaved normally becomes unusually tearful, one should consider early *chorea,* in which emotional behaviour is a common early symptom, or other serious disease such as cerebral tumour. The symptom could also be due to drug abuse, particularly amphetamines, bromides, barbiturates, heroin and methylphenidate.

An occasional cause of persistent inconsolable crying is *autism.*

Despite the most careful history-taking and investigation, it may be impossible to determine the exact cause of excessive crying; but the more carefully the history is taken, the fewer are these cases. Some of them may be related to the mother's fatigue, or to domestic friction. Some complaints of a baby's constant crying represent a mother's urgent call for help, in a 'pre-battering' situation. It is often difficult to decide whether a mother's complaint that the baby cries excessively is an index of her fatigue or personality problems, or represents an unrealistic idea of the amount of crying by normal babies.

**References**

1 Illingworth RS. *The normal child.* London: Churchill Livingstone, 9th edn, 1987.
2 Tasanen A. General and local effects of the eruption of deciduous teeth. *Ann Paediatr Fenniae* 1968; **14:** suppl. 29.

# Types of Cry

There is an increasing interest in the nature of the cry of infants. Analysis of the cry by spectographic methods has yielded interesting and useful information [3]: the cries of the asphyxiated, hypothyroid, Down's syndrome and other abnormal babies all have their special characteristics when studied by these methods. Fisichelli & Karelitz [1] showed that normal infants cry more rapidly after a stimulus than do children with brain abnormalities. Babies with cerebral irritability, meningitis, hydrocephalus and kernicterus have a shrill, high-pitched cry.

The hoarseness of *laryngitis* is characteristic. More important is the presence of hoarseness in a child with stridor dating from birth.

A hoarse gruff cry is characteristic of *hypothyroidism*.

The cat-like cry of the *'cri-du-chat'* syndrome is characteristic. This occurs in microcephalic infants. There is often some degree of hypertelorism, an antimongoloid slant of the eyes and low-set ears. It is associated with deletion of the distal portion of the short arm of one of the 4 to 5 chromosomes. The crying of the child with the *Cornelia de Lange syndrome* is said to resemble a bleating lamb [2].

Other characteristic cries are the weak cry of the child with *Werdnig–Hoffmann disease* (or similar muscle weakness) or the child with *myasthenia gravis,* and the whimper of a *seriously ill* child.

The child with *pneumonia* may have a grunting type of cry.

### References

1 Fisichelli VR, Karelitz S. The cry latencies of normal infants and those with brain damage. *J Pediatr* 1963; **62:** 724.
2 McArthur RG. Edwards JH. De Lange syndrome. Report of 20 cases. *Can Med Ass J* 1967; **96:** 1185.
3 Michelsson K, Wasz-Hockert O. The value of cry analysis in neonatology and early infancy. In Murry T, Murry J (eds) *Infant communication: cry and early speech.* Houston: College–Hill Press: 1980, p. 124.

# Insomnia and Sleep Disturbance

Refusal or failure to sleep, or awakening and crying, is almost always a behaviour problem, and an extremely common one; as with most behaviour problems, it represents a clash between the child's personality and developing mind, and the personality and attitudes of the parents, especially the mother. I have discussed the problem in detail elsewhere [3].

The following are the main causes of defective sleep:
  Mismanagement, including hunger
  Evening colic (p. 109)
  Mental subnormality
  Vomiting, diarrhoea, polyuria, frequency of micturition
  Pruritus
  In the older child—insecurity, fears, anxieties, depression
  Drugs

*Mismanagement* may consist of leaving the infant crying from hunger because of the fear that night feeds cause bad habit formation. Usually, however, sleep disturbance arising from mismanagement begins later in infancy, especially at about 9 to 15 months, when the child is allowed to discover that, as soon as he cries (e.g. when put to bed, or on wakening), his mother will pick him up, take him downstairs, play with him, give him a warm drink or take him into her own bed.

Some *mentally subnormal children* have an inverted sleep rhythm, sleeping by day and being wakeful at night.

Anything causing *vomiting, diarrhoea, polyuria* or *frequency of micturition* will cause sleep disturbance.

*Pruritus,* as from infantile eczema or scabies, may cause troublesome insomnia.

In the older child, *bad habit formation* beginning in infancy is the cause of insomnia.

Other causes of sleep disturbance in the older child are *worries and anxieties about home or school, fear of the dark or of shadows on the wall.* Depression may cause sleep disturbance, in the form of insomnia or excessive somnolence.

Certain *drugs* may cause insomnia. They include amphetamine, carbamazepine, diazepam, diphenoxylate, ephedrine, griseofulvin, imipramine, methylphenidate, niclosamide, theophylline and vincristine. Fenfluramine may cause nightmares. Barbiturates or antihistamines may have a paradoxical effect and cause sleeplessness.

*Sleep-walking* is a common problem of normal children, mainly after the age of 4 or 5 years, occurring mainly in deep stage 4 sleep early in the night. It is often a familial feature. According to Klackenberg [4], the peak age for somnambulism in children is 11 to 12 years. It is usually unassociated with other sleep disturbances or behaviour problems, except that it seems to be more common after a large meal shortly before going to bed. It has been said to be occasionally associated with the Tourette syndrome [1]. For a review of the symptoms of sleep-walking, nightmares, bruxism and head-banging in sleep, see the paper by Parkes [5] entitled *The parasomnias*.

*Nightmares* (night terrors) are more common than sleep-walking: most children have occasional episodes. They tend to occur particularly at the onset of an infection, or when there is a sudden loud noise [2]. If they are excessively frequent, they may be due to insecurity at home or school. *Beta blockers* may cause nightmares. Nasal decongestants have also been blamed (p. 172).

*Excessive somnolence* may be a feature of depression. It may occur with narcolepsy; it is a feature of diabetic coma, uraemia and other serious illnesses. It is a feature of the *Pickwickian syndrome* of obesity, hypoventilation and hypercapnia. For hypersomnia in the *Kleine–Levin syndrome*, see p. 226.

Excessive sleeping may be due to the Munchausen by proxy syndrome, the mother deliberately giving drugs to get the child into hospital (or to kill him).

*Narcolepsy*, in which the child suddenly falls asleep (especially when bored or doing nothing), is unrelated to epilepsy, but may be associated with cataplexy in which there is sudden loss of muscle tone with laughter or strong emotion [6].

## References

1 Barabas G, Matthews WS, Ferrari M. Somnambulism in children with Tourette syndrome. *Dev Med Child Neurol* 1984; **28:** 457.
2 Fisher C, Kahn E, Edwards E, Davis DM, Fine J. A psychological study of nightmares and night terrors. *J Nerv Ment Dis* 1974; **158:** 174.
3 Illingworth RS. *The normal child*. London: Churchill Livingstone, 9th edn, 1987.
4 Klackenberg G. Somnambulism in childhood—prevalence, control and behavioral correlations. *Acta Paediatr Scand* 1982; **71:** 495.
5 Parkes JD. The Parasomnias. Lancet 1986; **2:** 1021.
6 Wittig R, Zorick F, Roehrs T, Sicklester J, Roth T. Narcolepsy in a 7 year old child. *J Pediatr* 1983; **102:** 725.

# Mental Subnormality

When one considers the obvious fact that approximately half the population has an IQ of less than 100, it is clear that backwardness is a common problem. Not all backwardness is due to a low level of intelligence, and many other conditions have to be kept in mind when one is considering the problem of a backward child.

The most common cause of backwardness in childhood is mental subnormality, and that condition will be considered first. I have discussed developmental diagnosis and the diagnosis of mental subnormality in detail elsewhere [1]. Below is a summary of the main points in the diagnosis.

The first essential to the diagnosis of mental subnormality is a thorough knowledge of the normal, the variations from the normal, and the reasons for those variations—for one has to try to distinguish backwardness due to a low innate endowment from backwardness due to factors such as unsatisfactory postnatal environment, illness or handicap, especially sensory handicap, affecting vision or hearing, which are potentially remediable, and which have only an indirect bearing on developmental potential. One needs to know the normal in order to determine how far the infant has developed as compared with an average baby of the same age.

It is also useful to know about conditions which somewhat increase the likelihood that a child will be retarded—the factors which place him 'at risk' of mental subnormality. One may summarize these factors as follows:

> Prenatal—familial or genetic factors, infections in pregnancy, intra-uterine growth retardation, placental insufficiency or hypoxia *in utero*, multiple pregnancy, maternal drug addiction, preterm labour; fetal congenital abnormalities
>
> Perinatal—hypoxia, other perinatal problems

One must not exaggerate the importance of those factors. For instance, a mentally subnormal woman, even one with Down's syndrome, may give birth to a normal infant. Maternal rubella in the first 3 months is hazardous to the fetus. Innumerable low-birth-weight infants are mentally normal or superior. Maternal toxaemia only slightly increases the risk of fetal abnormality. Any major congenital deformity, such as a cleft palate or congenital heart disease, slightly increases the risk of mental handicap. Many children who suffered severe hypoxia at birth are mentally and physically normal. Cerebral palsy, neonatal convulsions other than those due to hypocalcaemia and hyperbilirubinaemia significantly increase the risk of a mental handicap.

It follows that one must take the history of the factors above, but that one must not pay too much attention to them. One bears them in mind and is alerted to the increased risk, but does not exaggerate their importance. The next step (after the newborn period) is to obtain a history of milestones of development, so that one can assess the rate of development from birth until the present time. One needs to determine whether the rate of development is accelerating, average or falling off (as in serious illness or harmful environment).

The physical examination must include neurological examination for signs of cerebral palsy and other conditions. The diagnosis of Down's syndrome and hypothyroidism should be obvious. The examination must include in particular a measurement of the maximum circumference of the head, because the size of the head is governed largely by the growth of the cranial contents. If the brain does not grow normally, the head is usually small. The head circumference of mentally subnormal infants is nearly always small in relation to their weight, unless they have hydrocephalus, megalencephaly or hydranencephaly.

With regard to the developmental examination, it is essential to remember the all-important principle that the mentally subnormal child is backward in all aspects of development, except occasionally in the motor field (sitting and walking). Hence the full-term mentally subnormal baby at birth resembles a preterm baby, in that he tends to sleep a large part of the day and night, he may have difficulty in sucking and swallowing, regurgitate and fail to demand feeds. He is then late in passing the milestones of development. He is late in beginning to smile at his mother (average in normal full-term infants—4 to 6 weeks); he is late in followng with his eyes and turning his head to sound (average 3 to 4 months), he is late in reaching out and grasping objects without their being placed in his hand (average 5 months), in chewing (average 6 or 7 months), in helping his mother to dress him by holding his arm out for a sleeve, in imitating byebye and playing pat-a-cake (all average 10 months), and later in speech. (The average child begins to combine words spontaneously at 21 to 24 months.) He is likely to be late in feeding himself with a cup without help (average 15 months) and in acquiring sphincter control (average 18 months for the first signs). Above all he shows less interest in his surroundings and concentrates badly, being easily distracted. He is late in ceasing to take objects to the mouth, and in ceasing to cast objects to the ground, one after the other (average in both about 15 months).

The diagnosis of mental subnormality is a most serious one to make, and it can only be made after careful consideration of the history, the child's development to date, the findings on examination, and an interpretation of the significance of each. It is wrong even to breathe a suspicion that the child is mentally handicapped until one is certain of one's ground, for it will cause the gravest distress and anxiety to the parents. I would strongly advise the family doctor to seek the opinion of an expert before imparting his diagnosis to the parents.

**Reference**

1 Illingworth RS. *Development of the infant and young child, normal and abnormal.* Edinburgh: Churchill Livingstone, 9th edn, 1987.

# General Backwardness

There are many causes of general backwardness other than mental subnormality; they are relevant to the subject of under-achievement at school—performance below the level which should correspond with the child's tested intelligence. I have discussed these in detail elsewhere [5, 6]. The factors are outlined in this and subsequent sections.

Many conditions other than mental subnormality may cause generalized backwardness in infancy and especially in later childhood. For convenience I have listed them in three groups—factors in the child, in the home, in the teaching—though realizing that there is some overlapping between these groups. They may be summarized

as follows:
a   Factors in the child
    Delayed maturation
    Major physical problems, such as cerebral palsy
    Major sensory problems, such as blindness or deafness
    Personality problems—laziness, day-dreaming, insecurity,
        emotional block, effect of failure
    Psychoses—autism, schizophrenia
    Drug addiction
b   Factors in the home or environment
    Emotional deprivation. Child abuse
    Malnutrition, adverse socio-economic factors, poverty, low
        expectations, poor example, one-parent family
c   Factors in the school
    Poor teaching, lack of motivation
    Absence from school
    Changes from school to school
    Special school instead of ordinary school
    Effects of friends, gangs
    Drugs

## Factors in the child

Though *delayed maturation* is not as common as some parents imagine, it is a real entity. An infant may be retarded in all aspects of development and yet prove to be normal later. This could not be expected if there were microcephaly—and this fact alone indicates the importance of including a measurement of the maximum head circumference in the examination of a baby. The diagnosis of mental subnormality in infancy, unless it is severe, is difficult: the diagnosis of mental subnormality in an infant with a head of normal size in relation to weight is more than difficult—it is dangerous.

Delayed maturation causes trouble at school—the child doing badly in the subjects of the curriculum, and yet doing well later.

*Physical problems,* such as cerebral palsy or muscular dystrophy may cause serious retardation apart from the commonly associated mental subnormality. Amongst other things these conditions reduce the child's opportunity for learning.

*Defective vision and hearing.* When a child has poor eyesight or hearing from birth, he cannot know that he does not see or hear properly. It is the responsibility of others to make the diagnosis.

## The personality

The personality of the child has an important effect on his progress at school. Laziness is partly a personality problem, partly the effect of the bad influence of others, and partly lack of interest in the work—which may be a matter of the child's lack of aptitude for a particular subject or the way in which the subject is taught. Day-dreaming may interfere with school work. Sensitive children may develop emotional blocks to learning when they are afraid of the teacher or are being unduly hurried.

*Insecurity* is a most important cause of backwardness in intelligent children. The insecurity may be due to difficulties at home, bullying at school or fear of a teacher. It has a powerful effect in lowering the standard of a child's work. Failure in work has a bad effect on a child's progress. Success leads to success, and failure to a further lowering in the standard achieved. For depression, see p. 226.

## Poor concentration

The most common cause of defective concentration is low intelligence—or an intelligence quotient below that of other members of the class. But it may also be due to the child being gifted, finding the work too easy, or to his having interests and aptitudes outside the school curriculum.

Poor concentration may be due to day-dreaming, insecurity, or finding the work too easy. It may be due to boredom, dislike of the work, lack of motivation in the teaching, or dislike of the teacher. It may be due to a defect of the eyesight or of hearing. *Drugs* are an important cause of defective concentration. They include anti-convulsant drugs, antihistamines, fenfluramine, theophylline and tranquillizers. Barbiturates are particularly important offenders—either by causing drowsiness or irritability, or by a direct action on the brain, interfering with learning and memory. Anti-convulsant drugs may also interfere with folate metabolism, which can affect performance.

Frequent petit mal attacks may result in defective concentration.

The so-called 'petit mal status' consists of a rapid succession of attacks; these attacks may interfere with school work.

## Infantile autism

Infantile autism is regarded as a basic cognitive deficit, involving language and behaviour [7, 9]. There is a genetic factor [3, 9]. In 40 per cent of cases there is an elevated blood serotonin level [1], and in 25 per cent chromosome studies show a fragile X [4]; it is said that a similar chromosome variant is seen in Rett's syndrome (p. 213). Fenfluramine has been said to be helpful in some cases [8], but this is disputed. Various prenatal and perinatal factors, such as rubella in pregnancy and hypoxia at birth, have been implicated [2, 9].

An autistic child, from the earliest infancy, shows no affection, preferring toys to persons. He has no desire to be picked up and cuddled when he is a baby. He may be poor at sucking, late in smiling, surprisingly undemanding if left alone and annoyed on being disturbed. He may cry unusually rarely—or cry excessively. He may fail to respond to the human voice while he responds to other sounds. His speech is seriously retarded. He may use words and intonate them well, but they bear no relation to the person listening to them and no relation to the existing situation. His head is of normal size and shape and he looks intelligent; yet he functions as a mentally subnormal child. He disregards his parents and tends to avert his gaze when spoken to. He is really an extreme introvert and isolates himself from the world. He may play with one toy in an obsessional way for hours, and is often especially fond of spinning toys; and he hates to change his occupation, having an intense desire for 'sameness'. He likes one particular routine, one particular toy or furniture arrangement and may develop a panic reaction if change occurs. He may adopt bizarre attitudes and postures, flicking his fingers in front of his eyes and walking on his toes.

The prognosis is serious, though some improvement may occur. One in four develops epilepsy in adolescence.

Similar symptoms are often seen in severe mental subnormality, and the original description of infantile autism by Leo Kanner at Baltimore has been expanded by some to include 'autistic behaviour' in severe mental subnormality. I think that this is unwise.

*Schizophrenia*

The symptoms of schizophrenia [11] are severe impairment of emotional relationships, solitariness, remoteness, lack of feeling for people, abnormal postures, striking immobility (katatonia) or aimless over-activity, ritualistic mannerisms (e.g. rocking and spinning), pathological preoccupation with particular objects, resistance to change, excessive or abnormal response to sensory stimuli—for example insensitivity to pain or other discomfort—illogical anxieties, hallucinations (rare in autism), and irrelevance of speech. The parents cannot understand the child; a book by professional parents [10] gave a vivid description of their own schizophrenic son. Schizophrenia is rare before school age while autism manifests itself in early infancy; there is a stronger genetic factor in schizophrenia than in autism.

*Other factors in the child*

Sometimes psychoses are superimposed on mental handicap and this increases the difficulty of assessment.

Unsatisfactory performance at school may be a relic of the fetal alcohol syndrome (p. 18) or of other maternal drug addiction in pregnancy.

**Factors in the home**

Factors in the home have a profound effect on the child's progress from infancy onwards [5, 6]. They include the home interests and example, the opportunities for the child to learn outside the home and school, praise for good work, expectation of success, and the right attitude to homework (implying that it is an understood thing that the homework will be done after the meal on returning from school). Other important factors include love and security, the amount of conversation between child and parent and its quality, the provision of suitable play material, the chance to develop independence, loving discipline, a good example, good nutrition and the prevention of disease, the encouragement of special interests, the encouragment of questions and argument, ambition but not over-ambition, regular school attendance and the expectation of success. A poor home causes a considerable degree of retardation. Emotional deprivation is likely to cause delay in speech and cognitive processes rather than in motor development. Some parents actively discourage the child from doing his homework—or provide no place in which he can work away from the family and the television set.

## Poor teaching and other school problems

Backwardness may be due to poor teaching. Unless the teacher likes the child and the child the teacher, there are likely to be learning difficulties [5]. Some teachers use the methods of threats, punishment, ridicule, sarcasm, instead of encouragement and praise, and then blame the child for not doing well. Lack of motivation is an important cause of backwardness: when a subject is badly taught and made uninteresting, the children are not likely to do well in it.

*Prolonged absences from school* are usually due to faulty management at home, parental disinterestedness in education, illness, or care of a sibling. Children are kept off school far too readily—and miss a great deal of education as a result. They are kept away from school for the most trivial cough or wheeze—and yet are taken shopping and attend the child health clinic with the baby brother. Frequent moves from school to school cause an emotional upheaval, and the child may find that work is being taught differently, or that he has missed much that has been taught. It has been shown that frequent short spells of absence from school cause more deterioration in performance than one long period of absence.

Some children are retarded by being sent to a special school instead of an ordinary school. The standard of education cannot be as high in a special school, where there is a wider scatter of age groups and intellectual levels in a class than in an ordinary school, and where less time is devoted to lessons.

## References

1 Ciaranello RD. Hyperserotonemia and early infantile autism. *N Engl J Med* 1982; **307**: 181.
2 Finegan J, Quarrington B. Pre-, peri- and neonatal factors and infantile autism. *J Child Psychol Psychiat* 1979; **20**: 119.
3 Folstein S, Rutter M. Genetic influences and infantile autism. *Nature* 1977; **265**: 726.

4  Gillberg C, Wahlström J. Chromosome abnormalities in infantile autism. *Dev Med Child Neurol* 1985; **27**: 293.
5  Illingworth RS. *The child at school: a paediatrician's manual for teachers.* Oxford: Blackwell Scientific Publications, 1974.
6  Illingworth RS. *The normal child.* London: Churchill Livingstone. 9th edn, 1987.
7  Ornitz EM, Ritvo ER. The syndrome of autism: a critical review. *Am J Psychiat* 1976; **133**: 609.
8  Ritvo ER, Freeman BJ, Yuwiler A. Study of fenfluramine in outpatients with the syndrome of autism. *J Pediatr* 1984; **105**: 823.
9  Rutter M. The treatment of autistic children. *J Child Psychol Psychiatr* 1985; **26**: 193.
10  Wilson L. *This stranger my son.* London: John Murray, 1968.
11  Wolff S, Barlow A. Schizoid personality in childhood: a comparative study of schizoid, autistic and normal children. *J Child Psychol Psychiat* 1979; **20**: 29.

# Backwardness in Individual Fields of Development

In considering individual fields of development one must make due allowance for preterm delivery; e.g. if a baby were born 2 months prematurely, the average age for beginning to smile would be 4 to 6 weeks plus 2 months.

## Smiling

All mentally subnormal and most autistic children are late in beginning to smile at the mother. A blind child will probably be late in beginning to smile.

## Sitting and walking

The common causes of lateness in sitting and walking are:

        Mental subnormality
        Delayed motor maturation, usually familial
        Hypertonia—cerebral palsy

Hypotonia
Muscular dystrophy
Emotional deprivation: institutional care
Lack of opportunity to sit and walk: illness
Excessive caution and timidity: dislike of bumps

By no means all mentally subnormal children are late in learning to sit and walk, but most are. A few children with Down's syndrome learn to sit at the usual age, but almost all are late in learning to walk.

When a child is late in sitting or walking, and no other abnormality can be found, it is common to find that the mother, father or sibling behaved in the same way. We presume that this is a matter of delayed maturation.

Cerebral palsy, particularly of the spastic and athetoid types, delays walking and in severe cases may make it impossible. The hypotonias delay sitting and walking. A child with the Werdnig–Hoffmann syndrome may never walk. Children with a more benign hypotonia may walk at 5 or 6 years of age. Children with *muscular dystrophy* of the Duchenne type are late in learning to walk. About half the boys with Duchenne muscular dystrophy have not started to walk alone by 18 months; but a confusing feature of these boys is the frequently associated mild mental retardation, which in itself delays walking.

Children brought up in an institution are late in sitting and walking, partly because of emotional deprivation and partly because of lack of practice. If a child is kept on his back for prolonged periods, the age of sitting and walking is delayed.

*Obesity* rarely delays walking [5].

Many children refuse to walk without a hand held, long after they have become sufficiently mature to walk unaided.

Congenital subluxation of the hip rarely delays walking. Many children are referred to orthopaedic surgeons on account of lateness in walking. This is irrational, and such children should be referred to the paediatrician.

*Delayed sphincter control and enuresis*

The following are the main causes of delayed control of the bladder:

Delayed maturation, usually a familial feature (primary enuresis)
Mismanagement of toilet training

Severe constipation
Emotional deprivation
Organic causes
    Mental subnormality
    Urinary tract infection
    Bladder-neck or urethral obstruction
    Ectopic ureter entering the vagina. Ureterocele
       Diverticulum of the anterior urethra
    Meningomyelocele
    Sacral agenesis, diastematomyelia, lipoma of the cauda
       equina
    Epispadias. Ectopia vesicae
    Absent abdominal muscles
    Trauma
    Epilepsy

A full review is that of Kolvin, MacKeith & Meadow [7].

Many psychiatrists maintain that enuresis is entirely a psychological problem, while many paediatricians hold that there are two types of enuresis, primary and secondary, the primary kind being that in which the child has never been dry at night, and the secondary variety in which the child is dry for a period of months or years and then begins to wet the bed. They feel that the primary type usually has an organic basis, there being delay in maturation of the relevant part of the nervous system, some children being late in acquiring control of the bladder, just as others are late in learning to sit, walk or talk. In this variety there is usually a family history of the same complaint. If one of identical twins wets the bed, the other usually does; but if one of non-identical twins does, the likelihood of the other doing so is much less. No one would deny that psychological difficulties can be added to the problem of the child with primary enuresis. For instance, the mother is likely to smack the child for wetting his bed, may ridicule him or try to shame him for it—and so make him worse. If she shows excessive anxiety about his toilet training, she is likely to cause emotional disturbance and add to his problem.

There is an overlap between so-called primary and secondary enuresis and it is uncertain whether the distinction is worth while. Daytime wetting without night wetting is more likely to be psychological than organic. It is commonly associated with urgency of micturition [1].

*Mismanagement of toilet training* may cause delay in control of the bladder or relapse once control has been achieved. It may add psychological factors to the problem of delayed maturation. Mismanagement consists usually of excessively enthusiastic 'potting', compelling the child to sit on the potty when he wants to get off and smacking him for not using it. Occasionally a parent does not give the child a chance to use the potty when he wants it, and delays the acquisition of control. It is the usual thing for a mother to smack her child for wetting the bed—until she finds that it does not help, and then she merely scolds him. MacKeith [10] wrote that the sensitive or critical period is important; when the child has reached that degree of maturation which enables him to learn to control the bladder, mismanagement of toilet training is particularly liable to delay the acquisition of control. Unkindness or strict methods are especially important. Parents can delay the acquisition of control, but they can do little to accelerate it until the nervous system is ready.

A child brought up in an institution, or otherwise exposed to *emotional deprivation,* is likely to be late in acquiring control of the bladder.

There are many possible *organic causes* of urinary incontinence. The mentally subnormal child, being late in almost all aspects of development, is likely to be late in acquiring sphincter control.

The role of *urinary tract infection* is difficult to interpret. It is common in girls, but by no means all girls are cured of enuresis when the infection has been treated. It is uncertain whether the infection is the cause or the result of the problem.

Other organic causes of urinary incontinence were fully reviewed in the article by Smith [14]. When a child has constant dribbling incontinence, day and night, urethral valves may be the cause in the boy, or an ectopic ureter or ureterocele in a girl. The older boy may dribble only after micturition, because some urine remains in the posterior urethra until the voluntary squeeze of the external urethral musculature relaxes, thus allowing the urine to dribble through. A diverticulum of the anterior urethra acts in the same way. The ectopic ureter in the girl may open into the urethra, or between the urethral and vaginal orifice, or near the hymen. In boy or girl, the diagnosis should immediately be suspected if there is dribbling incontinence. When the mother's story is equivocal, one should see that the child has a dry nappy on (if he still has one), and then observe when it becomes wet, by examining it every 10 min or so.

The other organic causes, such as meningomyelocele, ectopia vesicae, absent abdominal muscles or lipoma involving the cauda equina, are obvious if looked for. The 'neurogenic bladder' is diagnosed by the dribbling of urine, the patulous anus, perineal anaesthesia, and the fact that urine can be expressed by firm suprapubic pressure. It is easy to miss the diagnosis of *epispadias* by failing to examine the penis. *Diastematomyelia* is less easy to diagnose. It may be associated with a meningomyelocele, or there may be a tuft of hair in the middle of the back which draws attention to the possibility of an underlying bone deformity. In addition to the incontinence there may be progressive weakness of the legs. The diagnosis is established by X-ray studies. *Sacral agenesis* may be impossible to diagnose without X-ray studies. If only one or two segments are missing, a gap may be felt on palpation. When there is complete sacral agenesis, the buttocks are flat, the intergluteal cleft is small, and there may be lower limb deformity. There may be other orthopaedic abnormalities, a lipoma, hypospadias or an imperforate anus [4]. The symptom is usually urinary incontinence of the dribbling variety, often with recurrent urinary tract infection. One should examine for a patulous anus [15]. The condition is sometimes related to maternal diabetes.

Incontinence following circumcision may be the result of putting a stitch through the urethra.

Bed-wetting in the case of an epileptic child may be the result of a fit.

*Secondary enuresis* is usually due to psychological stress or insecurity. The cause may lie in worry at home or school, a move from house to house, a move to a new school or a spell in hospital. It is important to realize that, when a child has recently acquired control of the bladder, anything causing frequency or polyuria is liable to cause enuresis, especially when this develops at the sensitive or critical period [10]. Hence in all cases one should examine the urine for sugar (i.e. for diabetes mellitus) and for the specific gravity (for renal failure and other causes of polyuria). One must also examine a clean specimen under the microscope for excess of white cells and for organisms and culture it in order to eliminate a urinary tract infection (see p. 320). Berg, Fielding & Meadow [2] studying forty children with day and night incontinence and forty-six with incontinence only at night, found that day and night incontinence in boys is commonly associated with soiling and that one in two girls with it has bacteriuria. In another study [1], it was found that in day wetting there was a strong association with urgency, but little evidence of psychological causes. It is probable that in many, if not most, cases there is an interaction of many causes; delayed maturation, conditioning, faulty training methods, the sensitive period, the personality of mother and child, psychological stress, the mother's ignorance of normal development and its variations, social factors, bladder capacity and sometimes organic disease [7].

Gross constipation is an occasional cause of wetting.

*Giggle incontinence* is more common in girls; it begins before puberty, and usually disappears in a few years [8].

## Delayed speech

The following are the usual causes of delayed speech:

Mental subnormality
Delayed maturation, usually a familial trait
Emotional deprivation
Deafness
Multiple pregnancy (twins)
Psychological factors
Psychoses—autism and schizophrenia
Aphasia
Unknown causes

The most common cause of delayed speech is *mental subnormality*. Probably all mentally subnormal children are late in learning to speak. Otherwise, the usual cause is delayed maturation: one nearly always finds that the mother, father or sibling was late in learning to speak.

Children with infantile autism are late in speaking, and deafness is commonly suspected. Children with schizophrenia may be late in learning to speak.

A child brought up in an institution or otherwise subjected to *emotional deprivation* is likely to be late in learning to speak. Delayed speech is an almost universal finding on follow-up examination of children who have suffered child abuse [9].

An important cause of delayed speech is *deafness*, which may be only for high tones. One must not be put off by the story that the child hears footsteps and many other noises. Suitable high tones for testing the child's hearing are the sounds PS, PHTH, and the crumpling of tissue paper, assuming that he cannot see the source of sound and that the source of sound is on a level with the ear and reasonably near (e.g. within 30–60 cm).

*Twins* are often late in speech—perhaps because the mother has less time to talk to twins than to singletons. The delay is unlikely to be due to the twins understanding each other without speaking properly.

Delayed speech is *not* due to laziness, it is *not* due to 'everything being done for him', it is *not* due to tongue-tie, and it is most unlikely to be due to jealousy. There is some association between delayed speech and delay in the establishment of handedness. Whatever the causes, parents and doctors should realize that a child fails to speak because he cannot speak. Adults tend to talk less to him, so that he hears less and is still further retarded. Emotional causes include emotional deprivation, such as that due to institutional care, insecurity and worries. Poor teaching may be a cause.

Aphasia or 'elective mutism' is rare. After a period of normal speech the child limits his speech to familiar situations or a small group of intimates [6]. There are commonly other behaviour problems and often domestic friction.

We cannot always determine the cause of delayed speech. We do know that many children who are late in learning to speak are subsequently late in learning to read or write. When a child of 3 or 4 years of age is not saying any words and his hearing is known to be normal, and he is not autistic or mentally handicapped (i.e. has aphasia), the outlook is uncertain. All children with delayed speech development should be referred to an expert for diagnosis.

*Indistinct speech*

Indistinctness of speech, now termed a 'phonological disorder', is usually due to substitution of letters, of which the commonest is the substitution of 'th' for 's'—the central lisp, due to protrusion of the tongue between the teeth when pronouncing the 's'. It is readily treated by the speech therapist, though milder ones cure themselves. The speech therapist may treat other substitutions, but it is uncertain how much of the improvement to be expected is due to therapy and how much to maturation, for most of these substitutions are self-limiting.

*Nasal speech* is due to a cleft palate, a submucous cleft, or adenoids. A submucous cleft may be suspected because of a history of nasal regurgitation in infancy, and the finding of a bifid uvula, decreased palatal movement on phonation and a palpable notch on the posterior edge of the hard palate. It may follow adenoidectomy.

It may be due to certain *drugs*, namely diazepam, imipramine, metoclopramide, phenytoin, primidone or sulthiame.

When a child has never spoken normally, *dysarthria* may be due to cerebral palsy, in which there is spasticity or incoordination of the muscles of speech, to a cleft palate (or submucous cleft), or to structural abnormalities of the jaw, including malocclusion and macroglossia. Malpronunciation of the sounds m, n and ng may be due to nasal obstruction.

*Loss of speech* may be a premonitory sign of migraine (p. 101). In convalescence after *Reye's syndrome* [11] speech may be lost or difficult. Early loss of speech is a common feature of many degenerative diseases of the nervous system, or a result of a cerebral tumour.

In the *Landau–Kleffner syndrome* [3] a child's previously normal speech regresses with the onset of convulsions. Deafness may be suspected; some, especially older children, make a complete recovery.


## *Learning disorders, attention-deficit disorders*

There is a vast literature on the subject of learning disorders; these disorders include difficulties in reading, spelling, speaking, writing, languages, mathematics and spatial appreciation. They may form part of the group of conditions termed 'attention-deficit disorders'—over-activity, poor concentration, clumsiness and aggresiveness. Useful reviews include those of Rutter [12] and Shaywitz and colleagues [13].

This group of conditions is multifactorial in origin. An obvious cause of many of them is mental subnormality; but the IQ score of many children with these complaints is average or superior. The help of an experienced psychologist is needed for the diagnosis.

Causative factors include adverse prenatal conditions (p. 18), perinatal conditions such as hypoxia, hyperbilirubinaemia or hypo-glycaemia, or postnatal factors such as child abuse, sexual abuse, and the effect of handicaps such as sensory defects, diabetes, juvenile chronic arthritis, Duchenne muscular dystrophy or haemophilia. *Drugs* taken by the child may be relevant: they include anti-convulsant drugs, smoking and passive smoking, cannabis and other drugs of addiction, and food additives. There is some connection between these disorders and the establishment of handedness. Some of the conditions represent delayed maturation in specific fields of development.

Chromosomal disorders may be relevant. The XO karyotype may be relevant to non-verbal performance in tests and visuospatial, directional and constructive abilities [16], and the XXY karyotype to verbal development, especially speech, spelling and reading. The fragile X syndrome has been found in some cases.

So-called *specific dyslexia* is a genetic condition which is more common in boys, and is often accompanied by clumsiness and over-activity. These children tend to leave too large a space between letters, to reverse letters, such as h and y, d and b. They commonly read from right to left, and interpret, for instance BUT as TUB, WAS as SAW. I saw a page of an intelligent boy's exercise book with sums calculated like

$$16+1 = 71$$
$$13+1 = 41$$

Some of the children do mirror-writing. They may have inadequate auditory discrimination of speech and sound, interpreting, for instance, BUD as BUT, though their hearing is normal. They may show an inability to synthesize into correct words letters which have individually been sounded correctly—interpreting, for instance, CLOCK as COCK. They may be able to spell a word correctly but be unable to write it: they cannot correlate sound with the written word. They are commonly ambidextrous or left-handed. They tend to write slowly and hesitantly, wriggling and distorting the face as they read. As they mature most of the symptoms disappear, leaving only some reading difficulty. The problem may lead to behaviour disorders and truancy.

### References

1  Berg I. Day wetting in children. *J Child Psychol Psychiatr* 1979; **20**: 167.
2  Berg I, Fielding D, Meadow R. Psychiatric disturbance, urgency and bacteriuria with day and night wetting. *Arch Dis Child* 1977; **52**: 651.
3  Bishop DVM. Age of onset and outcome in acquired aphasia with convulsive disorder (Landau–Kleffner syndrome). *Dev Med Child Neurol* 1985; **27**: 705.
4  Fourie I van H. Sacral agenesis and neuromuscular bladder dysfunction. *South African Med J* 1984; **65**: 55.

5 Jaffe M. The motor development of fat babies. *Clin Pediatr (Phila)* 1982; **21:** 619.

6 Kolvin I, Fundudis T. Elective mute children. Psychological development and background factors. *J Child Psychol Psychiatr* 1981; **22:** 219.

7 Kolvin I, MacKeith RC, Meadow SR. *Bladder control and enuresis.* Clinics in Developmental Medicine Nos. 48 and 49. London: Heinemann, 1973.

8 *Lancet.* Giggle incontinence. Leading article. 1982; **1:** 1000.

9 Lynch MA. The prognosis of child abuse. *J Child Psychol Psychiat* 1978; **19:** 175.

10 MacKeith RC. Is maturation delay a frequent factor in the origins of primary nocturnal enuresis? *Dev Med Child Neurol* 1972; **14:** 217.

11 Reitman MA, Casper J, Coplan J, *et al.* Motor disorders of speech and voice in Reye's syndrome survivors. *Am J Dis Child* 1984; **138:** 1129.

12 Rutter M (ed.) *Developmental neuropsychiatry. Symposium on learning disorders.* London: Churchill Livingstone, 1984.

13 Shaywitz S, Shaywitz B, Grossman HJ. Learning disorders (symposium), *Pediatr Clin N Am* 1984; **31:** 277.

14 Smith ED. Diagnosis and management of the child with wetting. *Aust Paediatr J* 1967; **3:** 193.

15 Thompson IM, Kirk RM, Dale M. Sacral agenesis. *Pediatrics* 1974; **57:** 236.

16 Walzer S. Chromosome abnormalities and cognitive development. Implications for understanding normal human development. *J Child Psychol Psychiat* 1985; **26:** 177.

# Mental Deterioration

The main causes of mental deterioration include the following:

> Psychological causes. Insecurity. Emotional deprivation. Domestic problems. Bereavement
>
> Socio-economic causes. Adverse home conditions
> Malnutrition
>
> Education factors. Poor teaching. Boredom
> School absences. Moves from school to school
> Bullying. Influence of friends and gangs
>
> Development of handicaps. Duchenne muscular dystrophy.
> Ill health
>
> Head injury
>
> Cerebral tumour, abscess, or vascular accident
> Meningitis. Encephalitis

Epilepsy
Metabolic diseases. Thyroid deficiency. Hypoglycaemia
Other degenerative diseases of the nervous system
AIDS
Late effect of cerebral irradiation
Psychoses
Drugs and poisons. Drugs of addiction

Many factors other than organic disease may cause deterioration in school work. They include insecurity and worries for any reason, teasing for obesity, dislike of a teacher, domestic friction, school problems, boredom, socio-economic factors and poor teaching.

The development of *handicaps*, such as visual or auditory defects, or serious chronic illnesses, such as juvenile chronic arthritis or Duchenne muscular dystrophy, may be relevant—partly because of their psychological effect, partly because they may interfere with the teaching. But it is easy to ascribe deterioration in work to psychological factors when the true cause is a cerebral tumour or other serious disease.

*Epilepsy* does not in itself cause serious mental deterioration, though epileptic fits may themselves be caused by a cerebral lesion which also causes mental deterioration. Petit mal is not usually a factor, though frequent attacks, particularly a rapid succession of attacks (petit mal status), may cause a child to lose the thread of a lesson. Subictal epilepsy consists of a series of electrical discharges which may cause confusion (without convulsive movements) and mental deterioration if untreated (p. 234). Temporal lobe epilepsy is more likely than other forms of epilepsy to interfere with school work. Any prolonged epileptic fit may damage the brain by hypoxia. Psychological problems associated with epilepsy may cause significant deterioration in school work. Drugs given for the treatment, especially barbiturates, or other drug in an overdose, may cause drowsiness, defective concentration, bad behaviour and learning difficulties.

A wide variety of *metabolic and other degenerative diseases* of the nervous system are major causes of mental deterioration. Severe hypoglycaemia, or repeated attacks of less severe hypoglycaemia, may cause brain damage. The development of thyroid deficiency may pass unnoticed for some months, and cause deterioration in work.

Metabolic and degenerative diseases include particularly abnormalities of amino acid and carbohydrate metabolism. There are so many of these diseases that it is not useful to attempt to relate particular symptoms to particular diseases. The classification by Lagos [2] is useful, because it is based on the age of onset of symptoms. Unfortunately there is some overlapping between the groups; but the classification does help one to refer to any of the larger textbooks of paediatrics for further information. All are rare. The classification (modified) is as follows:

1  *Deterioration starting at birth*
    Phenylketonuria
    Pyridoxine dependency
    Maple syrup urine disease (fits, vomiting, hypotonia)
    Homocystinuria (resembling Marfan's syndrome, with
        dislocation of the lens, long fingers, but with fits
        and thromboses)

2  *Starting in the first two years*
    Amaurotic family idiocy
    Hyperuricaemia (Lesch–Nyhan disease: p. 231)
    Subacute necrotizing encephalopathy (feeding dif-
        ficulties, vomiting, hypotonia, weakness,
        respiratory problems)
    Leucodystrophies
      Sulphatide lipoidosis (starting at 12 to 18 months,
        with motor weakness, ichthyosis and hepato-
        splenomegaly [1]
      Krabbe's disease (normal till 4 to 6 months: fits)
      Pelizaeus–Merzbacher disease (starting in the first
        year: nystagmus, choreo-athetosis)
      Hypersarcosinaemia, carnosinaemia, hyperlysinaemia
      Canavan's disease. Leigh's disease (p. 16)
      Gaucher's disease (hypertonia, splenomegaly)
      Niemann–Pick disease (especially Jews)
    Generalized gangliosidosis
    Mucopolysacharidoses
    Glycogen storage disease

3  *Starting after 2 years*
    Amaurotic family idiocy (late forms)
    Myoclonic epilepsy
    Schilder's disease (blindness, deafness, spasticity)

Subacute sclerosing panencephalitis (commonly related
to measles virus)

Heller's infantile dementia (no neurological signs)

Mental deterioration, sometimes with spasticity, may be the result
of *AIDS* infection. Deterioration may be a late result of cerebral
irradiation for leukaemia.

For schizophrenia, see p. 306.

*Drugs and poisons* are important causes of deterioration. Lead
poisoning may cause severe brian damage. Mentally subnormal
children are more likely than others to eat dirt or take objects to the
mouth, and so are at risk of developing lead poisoning.

*Drugs of addiction* (p. 217) should be considered as possible causes of
a child's deterioration in school work.

### References

1  Burk RD, Valle D, Thomas GH. Early manifestations of multiple sulfatase
   deficiency. *J Pediatr* 1984; **104:** 574.
2  Lagos JC. *Differential diagnosis in pediatric neurology.* Boston: Little Brown,
   1971.

# Symptoms Related to the
# Genito-urinary Tract

## URINARY TRACT INFECTION

A urinary tract infection is difficult to diagnose with certainty in
general practice (and there are often difficulties in making the
diagnosis in hospital). Mistakes are commonly made in two
directions: the diagnosis is made when there is in fact no urinary
infection, and it is missed when there is an infection. The reasons for
the mistakes are varied. Many regard scalding on micturition or frequency as definitely indicating an infection, and regard these
symptoms as necessary before making the diagnosis. Both of these
beliefs are incorrect. Discomfort on micturition may be due to meatal

ulcer or balanitis in the boy, or soreness of the vulval region, as in a nappy rash, in the girl. There are many other causes of frequency (p. 324). Symptoms of urinary tract infection vary with the age of the child. Normand & Smellie [1] analysed this in 336 children as follows:

| | Age Total | 0–2 years 120 Percentage | 2–5 years 91 Percentage | 5–12 years 125 Percentage |
|---|---|---|---|---|
| Failure to thrive | | 33 | 3 | — |
| Diarrhoea | | 13 | 0 | — |
| Vomiting | | 20 | 8 | 2 |
| Fever | | 18 | 29 | 26 |
| Convulsions | | 3 | 4 | 2 |
| Haematuria | | 3 | 8 | 3 |
| Frequency, dysuria | | 2 | 16 | 22 |
| Enuresis | | 0 | 13 | 15 |
| Abdominal pain | | 0 | 13 | 30 |

These symptoms are the exception rather than the rule in a urinary tract infection. In an acute infection the common symptoms are fever, vomiting, rigors, meningism and a febrile convulsion (under the age of 5). There may be abdominal discomfort and sometimes diarrhoea. There is unlikely to be tenderness in the loin. Another common misbelief is the idea that there must be albumin in the urine or that the presence of albumin confirms the diagnosis. In fact albumin is present in less than half of all cases. Frank haematuria is definitely unusual. In a chronic urinary tract infection the only symptoms are commonly lack of energy, poor appetite and other vague symptoms which do not point to the urinary tract.

Outside the hospital the only satisfactory method of obtaining a culture of urine is the dipslide or one of its modifications, in which the child passes urine on to a dipslide or the dipslide is inserted into the clean urine container, put into the sterile bottle provided and sent to the laboratory.

### Reference

1 Normand IC, Smellie J. The child with urinary tract infection. *Medicine UK* 1975; **No. 29,** 1588.

## DELAYED MICTURITION IN THE NEWBORN

Delayed micturition in the newborn baby was discussed by Moore & Galvez [2] and by Johnston [1]. Johnston found that 67 per cent pass urine in the first 12 hrs, 25 per cent in the next 12 hrs, and 7 per cent only after 24 hrs. He suggested that sometimes there is no discoverable cause for transient urinary retention. Absence of micturition with an empty bladder and without ascites (which would suggest rupture of the urinary tract with urethral obstruction) indicates severe bilateral renal agenesis. Causes to consider include:

> Restriction of fluid
> Tubular or cortical necrosis
> Renal agenesis
> Bilateral renal vein thrombosis
> Congenital nephrotic syndrome
> Nephritis
> Neurogenic bladder
> Urethral diverticulum
> Ureterocele

### References

1 Johnston JH. Abnormalities of micturition in the neonate. *Br J Hosp Med* 1976; **16:** 462.
2 Moore ES, Galvez MB. Delayed micturition in newborn period. *J Pediatr* 1972; **80:** 867.

## SUPPRESSION OR RETENTION OF URINE

For convenience these will be discussed together.

The causes of suppression or retention of urine can be listed as follows:

> Normal—newborn
> Behaviour problem

Urethral obstruction
 Valves in posterior urethra
 Congenital contracture of vesical outlet
 Hypertrophy of the verumontanum
 Labial adhesions
 Hydrocolpos
 Congenital stricture
Anterior sacral meningocele, sacral teratoma, retrovesical cyst
Neuromuscular disease—spina bifida, myelitis, tumour of the
    cord, sacral agenesis, poliomyelitis, transverse myelitis,
    Guillain–Barré syndrome
Diverticulum at the base of the bladder
Faecal impaction
Meatal ulcer
Foreign body
Stone
Transient instrumentation
Trauma
Acute nephritis
Drugs—phenothiazine group

Retention of urine is a rare behaviour problem, an unusual attention-seeking device.

Dribbling of urine with a poor stream in the case of a baby suggests urethral obstruction. Sacral agenesis (p. 312) may cause the same symptoms. Labial adhesions or hydrocolpos are readily diagnosed by inspection of the vulva.

Faecal impaction is diagnosed by rectal examination.

*Imipramine and sulphasalazine* may cause difficulty in micturition.


## Oliguria

Oliguria may be due to:
        Fever, dehydration, shock
        Acute nephritis, haemolytic uraemic syndrome
          Acute tubular necrosis
        Renal vein thrombosis
        Incompatible transfusion
        Drug—carbamazepine

## FREQUENCY, POLYURIA OR SCALDING
## ON MICTURITION

It is normal for a baby in the first few months to scream on micturition. Some scalding on micturition may be due merely to the urine being concentrated as the result of a raised temperature in an infection.

A toddler may develop what appears to be frequency of micturition, when it is in reality an attention-seeking device. The child discovers that, as soon as he indicates that he wants to pass urine, his mother drops everything and rushes him to his potty; he then wants to pass urine every few minutes, and his mother, in her anxiety to train him, does not realize the true nature of the frequency. When she consults a doctor, he may wrongly prescribe treatment without establishing the diagnosis by culture.

A toddler who is learning to control the bladder always has urgency and cannot wait once he feels the desire to pass urine. Children with enuresis of primary type, especially if they have daytime wetting, may retain this urgency for years.

When a child seems to have discomfort on micturition, a local examination of the genital area must be carried out. A common cause is a nappy rash, meatal ulcer or soreness of the vulva. One has seen many children treated as urinary tract infection when the cause of the dysuria is nothing more than local soreness. In adolescent girls, dysuria may be due to vaginitis (e.g. caused by candida, herpes or trichomonas) [1].

Frequency or scalding are not usually prominent symptoms of urinary tract infection unless there is cystitis. Normand & Smellie (p. 321) showed that in the first two years dysuria or frequency was a feature of urinary tract infection in only 2 per cent; in the 2 to 5 year age group the figure was 16 per cent and in the 5 to 12 year group it was 22 per cent.

Dysuria or frequency may occur in acute nephritis or pelvic appendicitis (in which the diagnosis is further confused by the finding of an excess of white cells in the urine).

The causes of *polydipsia* and *polyuria* are mainly the following:

Habit polydipsia (probably the commonest cause)
Diabetes mellitus, diabetes insipidus
Renal failure: chronic nephritis, etc.
Renal tubular acidosis, hypercalcaemia

Rare syndromes—salt-losing type of adrenocortical hyper-
plasia, Conn's syndrome, Bartter's syndrome, De Toni–
Fanconi syndrome, cystinosis
Catecholamine-secreting tumour (e.g. phaeochromocytoma
(p. 46) rare)
Carbohydrate malnutrition (p. 13)
Drugs

Polydipsia and polyuria are usually (but not always) merely a habit;
this has to be distinguished from organic causes by laboratory means
[2].

Polyuria is sometimes a symptom in acute pancreatitis (p. 114),
sickle cell crises or Kawasaki disease (p. 39). For Conn's and Bartter's
syndromes, see p. 16.

*Drugs* which cause dysuria include acetazolamide, tranquillizers
and isoniazid. Sulphonamide crystalluria may cause dysuria.

Drugs which cause frequency and polyuria include antihistamines,
carbamazepine, clonazepam, fenfluramine, tetracycline and vitamin
D excess.

Habit polydipsia in child or adult has to be distinguished by
complex laboratory procedures from polydipsia of organic origin,
such as diabetes insipidus [2].

## References

1 Demetriou E, Emans SJ, Masland RP. Dysuria in adolescent girls: urinary
    tract infection or vaginitis? *Pediatrics* 1982; **70**: 299.
2 Kohn B, Norman ME, Feldman H, Thier SA, Singer I. Hysterical polydipsia
    in children. *Am J Dis Child* 1976; **130**: 210.

## HAEMATURIA

The commonest causes of haematuria are acute nephritis, infection,
obstruction and tumours. The causes may be summarized as follows:
Blood diseases, especially anaphylactoid purpura, leukaemia
Scurvy. Haemolytic uraemic syndrome
Connective tissue or collagen diseases
Kidney—nephritis, focal nephritis, pyelonephritis, tuber-
culosis. Glandular fever (rare cause)
Tumours. Wilms' tumour. Polycystic kidney. Angioma

Hydronephrosis
Calculi. Crystalluria
Renal vein thrombosis, infarction. Varices, angioma, telangiectasia
Tropical infections—schistosomiasis, malaria
Ureter—stone
Bladder—foreign body, tumour, haemorrhage, cystitis
Urethra—foreign body, trauma
Effect of exertion or cold (p. 65)
Factitious haematuria
Drugs, poisons
Unexplained

*Blood diseases* which cause haematuria include haemophilia, haemorrhagic disease of the newborn, sickle-cell anaemia, thrombocytopenic purpura and leukaemia. Haematuria commonly follows Henoch–Schönlein purpura (p. 63) as a result of complicating nephritis. This can occur without a rash, so that the diagnosis may be difficult. Scurvy, glandular fever and the collagen diseases are occasionally accompanied by haematuria.

Acute nephritis is now a rare cause of haematuria in Britain, but in tropical countries it is common, especially in association with infections of the skin. The symptoms may be acute, with headache, vomiting, fits or puffiness of the eyes, but there may be no visible oedema.

Recurrent haematuria is commonly due to focal nephritis [6]. Haematuria is an unusual symptom in acute urinary tract infection; in the analysis by Normand & Smellie (p. 321) it occurred in 4 per cent of 336 children.

*Tuberculosis* of the kidney is now rare in Britain. The tuberculin test will be positive. The diagnosis is confirmed by the finding of sterile pyuria, detection of tubercle bacilli in the centrifuged deposit, and isolation of the tubercle bacillus on culture or guinea-pig inoculation.

*Tumours and cysts* of the kidney include the nephroblastoma (Wilms' tumour), polycystic disease and angioma of the renal pelvis. Wilms' tumour occurs particularly in the first 4 years. It may be associated with aniridia, Beckwith's syndrome, Bloom's syndrome congenital asymmetry, the von Hippel–Landau syndrome (p. 210), cerebral gigantism, bilateral retinoblastoma, neurofibromatosis, multiple pregnancy or anomalies of the urinary tract. The symptoms or signs are principally abdominal swelling, haematuria, dysuria, abdominal pain and sometimes fever.

*Renal calculi* are rare in children, except in tropical countries, unless they are confined to bed for prolonged periods with orthopaedic conditions.

*Renal vein thrombosis* occurs mainly in the first few months of life, commonly following an infection elsewhere [3]. The diagnosis is suspected when a child suddenly develops haematuria, a renal mass and perhaps oedema. The kidney is palpable in half the cases. There may be a thrombocytopenia, uraemia, albuminuria and acidosis. *Infarction of the kidney* may occur in subacute bacterial endocarditis.

*Conditions in the bladder* include polypi, diverticula and foreign bodies. The latter are important in girls. I have seen a child admitted to hospital on ten occasions on account of haematuria, before a safety pin was found in the bladder. Polypi and diverticula are diagnosed by cystograms and cystoscopy. *Haemorrhagic cystitis* may result from an adenovirus infection of the bladder, cyclophosphamide, or *Bacillus proteus* cystitis and urethritis (blood appearing especially at the end of micturition) [4].

Bleeding may arise from a *urethral caruncle* in a girl or a *meatal ulcer* in a boy. The blood in such a case would be seen at the end of micturition. Urethral obstruction may cause haematuria.

In an occasional child haematuria follows *exertion* [1].

*Drugs* which cause haematuria include anticoagulants, acetazolamide, aminophylline, bacitracin, cephalosporins, cyclophosphamide, kanamycin, methicillin, PAS, phensuximide, phenytoin, salicylates, sulphonamides and troxidone.

*Factitious haematuria* has to be considered when there are no other obvious causes [5]: it may be a feature of the 'Munchausen by proxy' syndrome, in which the mother adds blood to the child's urine.

After the most complete investigation, including renal biopsy, it may be impossible to determine the cause of haematuria [7]. Symptomless haematuria is said sometimes to be an unexplained familial condition [2].

For conditions causing a colour change in the urine suggestive of haematuria, see p. 328.

## References

1 Illingworth RS, Holt KS. Transient rash and haematuria on exercise and emotion. *Arch Dis Child* 1957; **32:** 254.

2 *Lancet*. Benign familial haematuria. Leading article. 1984; **1:** 1450.

3 McFarland JB. Renal vein thrombosis. *Q J Med* 1965; **34:** 269.

4 Mufson MA, Belshe RB, Horrigan TJ, Zollar LM. Cause of acute haemorrhagic cystitis in children. *Am J Dis Child* 1973; **126:** 605.

5 Outwater KM, Lipnick RN, Luban NLC, Ravenscroft K, Ruley EJ. Factitious hematuria. *J Pediatr* 1981; **98:** 95.

6 Roy LP, Fish AJ, Vernier RL, Michael AF. Recurrent macroscopic hematuria, focal nephritis and mesangial deposition of immunoglobulin and complement. *J Pediatr* 1973; **82:** 767.

7 West CD. Asymptomatic hematuria and proteinuria in children. *J Pediatr* 1976; **89:** 173.

## CHANGES IN THE COLOUR OF URINE

The following conditions are associated with unusual coloration of the urine:

Dark colour
  Concentration, as in fever
Yellow
  Bile (dark yellow)
  Carotene-containing foods
  Riboflavin, rifampicin, phenazopyridine (pyridium)
Red or red brown
  Urates
  Beeturia
  Blackcurrant juice, blackberries, rose hip syrup
  Eosins or rhodamine B in foodstuffs
  Haemoglobinuria, myoglobinuria
  Porphyria
  *Serratia marcescens* infection
  Favism
  Danthron ('Dorbanex' for constipation), senna
  Phenothiazines, phenolphthalein, phensuccimide, nitrofurantoin
Dark brown or black
  Nitrofurantoin, metronidazole, quinine, cascara, senna
  Alkaptonuria, tyrosinosis, melanosis
Blue
  Hypercalcaemia
  Copper clasp on nappy holder

Green
  Prochlorperazine, amitriptyline
  *Pseudomonas* infection
Haemoglobinuria occurs when there is rapid haemolysis.

The red colour of the urine in *beeturia* is due to the pigment betanin in the beet. The red colour changes to yellow when alkali is added, and returns to red on acidification [2].

*Urates* disappear on boiling.

In *porphyria*, the urine may be normal in colour when passed, but changes to Burgundy red on exposure to light. There may be haemolytic anaemia, photosensitivity and hypertrichosis.

The urine in *myoglobinuria* is red brown and gives a positive benzidine or guaiac test. It follows crush injuries, electric shocks, severe exercise or other causes. There may be muscle pains, chills and vomiting.

In *alcaptonuria* the urine becomes dark on standing. The nappy may show a black stain. The urine gives a colour change with Benedict's reagent and ferric chloride gives a fleeting blue colour.

A blue colour in the nappy may be due to a *Pseudomonas* or *Serratia marcescens* infection [1].

**References**

1  Thearle MJ, Wise R, Allen JT. Blue nappies. *Lancet* 1973; **2**: 499.
2  Tunnessen WW, Smith C, Oski FA. Beeturia. *Am J Dis Child* 1969; **17**: 424.

## PAIN IN THE PENIS

This is an unusual symptom, apart from pain on passing urine. Pain in the penis may be due to irritation at the bladder neck, as by a stone.

## PAIN OR SWELLING IN THE SCROTUM

The obvious causes are:
  Hernia or hydrocele (they may be both present)
  Torsion of the testis, spermatic cord or appendages
  Blood diseases—allergic purpura, leukaemia

Trauma. Insect bite
Scrotal oedema
Tumour of testis. Cyst. Angioma
Epididymo-orchitis or orchitis alone
Filariasis (in the tropics). Lyme disease (p. 278)

Unless there has been definite injury, pain in the scrotum should be regarded as being due to torsion of the testis until proved otherwise. The torsion may be that of the spermatic cord or the testicular appendages [2]: in the latter case there may be a localized spot of tenderness at the upper pole of the testis.

Indications of torsion of the spermatic cord include [9] high-lying ipsilateral testis, change in the normal posterolateral location of the epididymis, and tenderness throughout the testis and epididymis. Epididymis in children may be associated with urinary tract anomalies and various organisms, including the *Staphylococcus* [6].

Unilateral acute scrotal pain has been described as an initial finding in acute appendicitis [8].

*Torsion* can occur at any time in childhood, from the first day onwards [7, 10]. It is more common in the first year. The pain often starts in sleep or during exercise; it commonly begins in the inguinal region of the abdomen just above the internal inguinal ring and may be referred to the abdomen. The testis may untwist and retwist, with recurrence of pain. About a third of all cases had had one or more preceding attacks of pain [4]. There is often vomiting and shock. *The correct diagnosis is urgent,* so that surgical treatment can be given immediately. The peak age incidence is in the perinatal or peripubertal period [3]. Of eighty-five cases described by Chapman and Walton [2], six were in the first year. Fourteen cases were torsion of the hydatid of Morgani. In a study of 150 boys [1] with acute scrotal swelling, in thirty-eight the diagnosis was testicular torsion, in thirty-nine hydatid of Morgagni, in thirty-five epididymitis, in twelve hydrocele or hernia, trauma in nine, and in others, blood diseases, tumour, oedema, insect bite or varicocele.

Torsion of the testis can be confused with epididymitis but that is exceedingly rare in the absence of a urinary tract infection or other gross urological abnormality; but it has been described with *haemophilus influenzae* infection [3]. In one series, thirty of sixty-seven acute cases of torsion had been wrongly diagnosed as epididymitis. It .has to be distinguished also from the orchitis of mumps and tuberculosis, testicular neoplasm or injury, or haemorrhage in purpura. Orchitis apart from mumps is rare; and orchitis in mumps hardly ever occurs prior to puberty. Orchitis could be confused with a strangulated hernia.

A *large testis* may be a feature in the fragile X syndrome, and a *small testis* may be a feature of Klinefelter's syndrome. (See also pp. 340, 346).

### References

1 Caldamone AA, Valvo JR, Altebarmakian VK, Rabinowitz R. Acute scrotal swelling in children. *J Pediatr Surg* 1984; **19:** 581.
2 Chapman RH, Walton AJ. Torsion of the testis and its appendages. *Br Med J* 1972; **1:** 164.
3 Chesney PJ, Saarti T, Mueller G. Acute epididymo-orchitis due to *Hemophilus influenzae* Type B. *J Pediatr* 1978; **92:** 685.
4 Haynes BE, Bessen HA, Haynes VE. The diagnosis of torsion of the testis. *JAMA* 1983; **249:** 2522.
5 Kelalis PP, Stickler GB. The painful scrotum: torsion vs epididymo-orchitis. *Clin Pediatr (Phila)* 1976; **15:** 220.
6 Likitnukul S, McCracken GH, Nelson J, Votteler T. Epididymitis in children and adolescents. *Am J Dis Child* 1987; **141:** 41.
7 Perera WSN. The red-hot scrotum: a 10 year review. *Records of the Adelaide Children's Hospital* 1979; **2:** 185.
8 Simmons WP, Jennings W. Unilateral acute scrotal pain as initial finding in acute appendicitis. *Clin Pediatr (Phila)* 1986; **25:** 352.
9 Stoller ML, Kogan BA, Hricak H. Spermatic cord torsion: diagnostic limitations. *Pediatrics* 1985; **76:** 929.
10 Williamson RCN. Death in the scrotum. Testicular torsion. *N Engl J Med* 1977; **297:** 338.

# Oedema

### General oedema

Arrangement of causes below is not entirely satisfactory, because of overlapping of the basic causes.
In the newborn
> Immaturity of the kidney
> Hydrops
> Hypoxia

Severe infection. Syphilis
Vitamin E deficiency
General causes
    Increased capillary permeability. Cold injury (p. 65), anaemia,
        allergic purpura
    Hypoproteinaemia. Defective protein intake
        Kwashiorkor.    Beriberi.    Protein    loss—burns,    eczema,
            suppuration. Protein-losing enteropathy
    Sodium retention. Excess sodium of fluid infusion
        Feeding errors
    Congestive heart failure
        Constrictive pericarditis
    Steatorrhoea
    Diabetes mellitus
    Kidney disease. Nephritis, nephrotic syndrome, renal vein
        thrombosis, haemolytic uraemic syndrome (p. 57)
    Liver disease. Galactosaemia
Rare
    Collagen diseases
    Intestinal lymphangiectasia
    Dystrophia myotonica [12] Yellow nail syndrome (p. 366)
    Obstruction of the inferior vena cava
    Angioneurotic oedema
    Drugs
    Unknown causes [4]

*Hydrops fetalis* was in the past ascribed to haemolytic disease; but
now other causes are more important—and in some the cause is
uncertain [1, 7, 8]. Known causes include the twin transfusion
syndrome, congenital heart disease, congenital nephrotic syndrome,
Gaucher's disease, Turner's syndrome, Down's syndrome, hepatic
insufficiency and infections in pregnancy (toxoplasmosis, herpes,
cytomegalovirus, rubella).

*Excessive sodium or fluid intake* is usually due to excessive
intravenous infusion. An over-concentrated formula, especially for a
preterm baby, may cause oedema.

Generalized oedema due to *heart failure* is rare in children. It could
be due to heart block; this is usually congenital, but may occur in
disseminated lupus (p. 38) or Sjögren's syndrome (p. 51). Heart
failure may be due to other forms of congenital heart disease. Heart

failure without a murmur may be due to paroxysmal tachycardia, coarctation of the aorta, Fallot's tetralogy (in early infancy), transposition of the vessels, or anomalous venous drainage. When heart failure develops, the murmur of a patent ductus or of a septal defect may disappear. Heart failure without a murmur may be due to fibroelastosis, viral myocarditis, or severe anaemia.

Slight oedema in the newborn may be due to maternal *diabetes*. In around 10 per cent of children slight oedema occurs for a few days after starting treatment for diabetes [10].

Oedema without albuminuria may be a presenting symptom in *cystic fibrosis*, and occurs in other types of steatorrhea.

The *nephrotic syndrome* is the end result of many conditions. It may be congenital, or caused by disseminated lupus, renal vein thrombosis (p. 327), syphilis, amyloid disease, diabetes or quartan malaria. It may be caused by heavy metals, ampicillin, daunorubicin, penicillamine, phenindione, potassium perchlorate, rifampicin, sulphonamides, thioridazine, troxidone or old stocks of tetracycline.

The oedema of nephritis or nephrotic syndrome may be asymmetrical in distribution—especially on the face, when the child has been lying on one side in sleep.

Oedema of the upper part of the body may be due to obstruction of the superior vena cava, and oedema of the lower part of the body to obstruction of the inferior vena cava (or ascites).

Oedema may be due to aspirin sensitivity or corticosteroids. For face, eyelids and conjunctiva, and *angioneurotic oedema,* see p. 49.

## Hands and feet

Oedema of the hands and feet, without evidence of oedema elsewhere, may be due to the effect of cold, especially in the chilblain type of circulation. It may be an early sign of dermatomyositis or periarteritis. It occurs in the Kawasaki syndrome (p. 39). It may be a socio-economic problem and has been given the name 'deprivation hands and feet' [6]; in the inner city area of Nottingham thirteen examples were seen with this condition in socially disadvantaged homes. Physical growth was defective. *Lymphoedema praecox* is a term applied [11] to oedema of the legs developing in adolescent girls. It is thought to be due to an imbalance between lymph formation and transport.

**Arms**

Oedema of the arm of a newborn baby may be due to an arm presentation.

A mother may be greatly alarmed when she picks up a baby from his bed in the morning and finds that one arm is swollen, cold and blue. There is pitting oedema. This is due not to the child lying on the affected arm, but to the arm having become uncovered when the temperature of the room is low. In a few hours the oedema disappears and the arm becomes normal in colour and appearance.

**Abdominal wall**

Shaul [13] noted oedema of the abdominal wall in neonatal appendicitis (p. 111), and in necrotizing enterocolitis of the newborn. It may occur in peritonitis.

**Legs**

*Congenital asymmetry* may be confused at first with oedema. In this condition one half of the body is larger than the other, but there is no oedema. Oedema of the limbs is often a feature of *cold injury* in the newborn period.

Unilateral limb enlargement from birth may be due to a *lymphangioma* or *arteriovenous abnormality* (Klippel–Trenaunay syndrome) but there is not usually oedema. If the oedema is unilateral, and dates from birth, *Milroy's oedema* should be considered. This is largely lymphatic and there is little pitting.

Oedema of both legs in a girl, or in a boy in whom the testes cannot be palpated, suggests *Turner's syndrome*. In a boy or girl there may be oedema of the feet in Noonan's syndrome; in that case the chromosomes will usually be normal.

Oedema of both legs may result from *ascites*.

*Sickle-cell anaemia* may cause oedema of the limbs.

Oedema may be due to *compression stenosis of the left common iliac vein* by an overriding right common iliac artery ('iliac compression syndrome') [3].

## Genitalia

Oedema of the genitalia is common in normal newborn infants.

Oedema of the scrotum may be caused by an insect bite or sensitivity to detergents used for washing the nappies or pants [2]. The cause of oedema of the scrotum is not always clear [9]. The onset is often rapid, with little pain, sometimes slight fever, clearing up in 12 to 48 hrs. It might be allergic in origin, or due to bites or superficial cellulitis in association with an abrasion or pustule.

Oedema of the scrotum has to be distinguished from epididymitis, in which there would be marked tenderness, and from torsion of the testis, which may present as oedema with local tenderness. It could also be confused with *rupture of the urethra* with extravasation of urine.

Oedema of the scrotum can be an early manifestation of *anaphylactoid purpura.*

## Lower part of body

This may be due to an adherent pericardium or obstruction of the inferior vena cava.

## Sternum

This occurs at the onset of mumps [5]. Oedema over the sternum occurs in almost 6 per cent of cases of mumps, usually developing 5 to 8 days after the commencement of the glandular swelling, and lasting about 5 days.

## References

1 Andersen HM, Drew JH, Beischer NA, *et al.* Non-immune hydrops fetalis, changing contribution to perinatal mortality. *Br J Obst Gynaecol* 1983; **90**: 636.
2 Cochran W. Severe dermatitis and biological detergents. *Br Med J* 1970; **2**: 362.
3 Cockett FB, Thomas ML, Negus D. Iliac vein compression—its relation to ileofemoral thrombosis and the post-thrombotic syndrome. *Br Med J* 1967; **2**: 14.
4 Fisher DA. Obscure and unusual edema. *Pediatrics* 1966; **47**: 506.

5  Gellis SS, Feingold M. Mumps and presternal edema. *Am J Dis Child* 1976; **130**: 417.
6  Glover S, Nicoll A, Pullan C. Deprivation hands and feet. *Arch Dis Child* 1985; **60**: 976.
7  Hutchison AA. Non-immunologic hydrops: a review of 61 cases. *Obstet Gynecol* 1982; **59**: 347.
8  Im SS, Rizos N, Joutsi P, Shime J, Benzie RJ. Non-immune hydrops fetalis. *Am J Obst Gynecol* 1984; **148**: 566.
9  Kaplan GW. Acute idiopathic scrotal edema. *J Pediatr Surg* 1977; **12**: 647.
10 Klein R, Marks JF, Roldan E, Sherman FE, Fetterman GH. The occurrence of peripheral edema and subcutaneous glycogen deposition following the initial treatment of diabetes mellitus in children. *J Pediatr* 1962; **60**: 807.
11 Lewis JM, Wald ER. Lymphedema praecox. *J Pediatr* 1984; **104**: 64.
12 Pearse RG, Höweler CJ. Neonatal form of dystrophia myotonica. *Arch Dis Child* 1979; **54**: 331.
13 Shaul WL. Clues to the early diagnosis of neonatal appendicitis. *J Pediatr* 1981; **98**: 473.

# Delayed Puberty in the Girl and Amenorrhoea

By the term delayed puberty I mean absence of menstruation by the age of 16. By primary amenorrhoea I mean the absence of menstruation; by secondary amenorrhoea I mean amenorrhoea after one or more menstrual periods.

Much the commonest finding in delayed puberty is merely that it is a normal variation, frequently familial. Puberty is delayed by severe malnutrition or severe general disease. Girls of small build are likely to reach puberty later than those of big build; so, for obscure reasons, are those in large families. Rare cases include the following:

Turner's syndrome and other forms of gonadal dysgenesis
Pituitary disease, especially craniopharyngioma and gonado-
    trophin deficiency
Testicular feminization syndrome: ovarian insufficiency

For *Turner's syndrome*, see pp. 340, 344. Most children with this syndrome are small in height. *Pituitary dwarfism* may be unexplained, or due to a tumour; the child is dwarfed but with normal proportions, and usually with no secondary sexual characteristics. Pituitary disease is unlikely if physical growth is normal. *Gonadotrophin deficiency* may be congenital. Affected children may be tall, and there will be no secondary sexual characteristics.

The *testicular feminization syndrome* is characterized by a normal female appearance with normal or increased height and normal breast development with pale areolae. There is little or no body hair, pubic or axillary. There is often a family history of amenorrhoea.

If there is no sign of puberty by the age of 16, and there is no relevant family history, full investigation is required.

When there are normal secondary sex changes, but no menstruation, disease is unlikely to be found. About 10 per cent of girls do not menstruate until there is full breast development or a bone age of 13 or 14. Much the commonest cause of delayed menarche in the presence of normal secondary sexual characteristics is malnutrition, deliberate or otherwise. Frisch, Wyshak & Vincent [1] noted the high incidence of primary or secondary amenorrhoea in eighty-nine young ballet dancers; there was a strong correlation between the occurrence of amenorrhoea and excessive thinness. Menstruation does not occur, or ceases to occur, when the weight drops below a critical level.

It is usual for menstruation to be irregular or scanty for several months after the first period has occurred. It is normal for a year or more to elapse between periods in the second year. Approximately forty periods occur before the regular adult pattern is established.

Amenorrhoea commonly occurs during the summer, or when there is emotional stress, as on starting school, especially when weight reduction occurs.

Amenorrhoea may result from anatomical causes, including in particular *hydrocolpos* or *haematocolpos*, readily found on physical examination. Another cause is the *adrenogenital syndrome*, in which there is enlargement of the clitoris with small stature. *Hyperthyroidism* or *hypothyroidism* are rare causes of amenorrhoea.

*Drugs* which may cause amenorrhoea include those causing hyperprolactinaemia. It may follow the use of the contraceptive pill. Relevant drugs are haloperidol, methyldopa, metoclopramide, phenothiazines or tranquillizers.

*Pregnancy* may be the cause of the amenorrhoea.

## Reference

1 Frisch RE, Wyshak G, Vincent L. Delayed menarche and amenorrhoea in ballet dancers. *N Engl J Med* 1980; **303**: 17.

# Some Other Gynaecological Problems

## Vaginal bleeding

A small amount of vaginal bleeding in the girl between the age of 5 and 10 days is normal. It is due to maternal oestrogens and is not related to haemorrhagic disease of the newborn.

Vaginal bleeding at any subsequent age, without associated signs of puberty, should raise the possibility of trauma, child abuse, foreign body or possibly a tumour. It may also occur as a result of blood disease. The blood may arise from the vulva, vagina or uterus. The blood may have come from the urethra.

Vaginal bleeding is rarely the first indication of sexual precocity.

It is said that ethosuximide can cause vaginal bleeding.

It is essential that vaginal bleeding before the age of puberty should be investigated because of the importance of possible causes.

## Vaginal discharge

It is normal for the newborn girl in the first few days to have a thin vaginal discharge, and between the fifth and the tenth day some bleeding may occur.

After infancy a clear mucoid discharge is common and of no significance. Unless it is offensive or purulent it should be ignored. It may be due to lack of cleanliness, eczema, nappy rash or mild itching leading to rubbing. A small girl playing in a sandpit may readily introduce some sand into the vagina by direct contact with the sand or by the hands. Soreness may be associated with masturbation.

At puberty some leucorrhoea is physiological, resulting from oestrogen stimulation.

Vaginitis may be due to threadworms, *Candida* infection, *E. coli, staphylococci, streptococci, gonococci* or *virus infections* such as herpes

[2], Lichen sclerosus and diabetes. A blood-stained discharge may be due to *Shigella* or group A streptococci. *Trichomonas* infection is rare before puberty. Infection is liable to occur because of proximity of the vagina to the anus, the lack of labial fat pads, the lack of pubic hair, the wrong wiping direction and dirty fingers.

The possibility of sexual abuse has to be remembered.

A *foreign body* is an important cause of purulent blood-stained vaginal discharge. An X-ray may demonstrate it, but a Kelly cystoscope may be needed to establish the diagnosis. Foreign bodies responsible for vaginal discharge [1] include toilet paper, safety pins, hairpins, folded paper, crayons, twigs, splinters of wood, cherries, paper-clips, beads, bits of toys, pencil erasers, sand, stones, marbles, cotton, shells, nuts, corks and insects.

A rare cause of vaginal discharge is a tumour.

## Dysmenorrhoea

This is rare for 2 or 3 years after the onset of menstruation, because the menstrual cycles are usually anovular. It can be suggested by the mother or older girls, and the commonest cause of dysmenorrhoea in the young adolescent is psychological.

## Menorrhagia

The commonest cause of abnormal uterine bleeding in an adolescent is hyperplasia of the endometrium—a self-limiting condition which does not require treatment.

Other important causes of excessive blood loss are anaemia, blood disease and an incomplete abortion.

## Reference

1 Henderson PA, Scott RB. Vaginitis caused by toilet tissue. *Am J Dis Child* 1966; **111:** 529.
2 Singleton AF. Vaginal discharge in children and adolescents. *Clin Pediatr (Phila)* 1980; **19:** 799.
*For general references see*
 Beynon CL. Menstrual problems in adolescence. *Practitioner* 1975; **214:** 192.
 Dewhurst CJ. *Gynaecological disorders of infants and children.* London: Cassell, 1974.
Root AW. Endocrinology of puberty. *J Pediatr* 1973; **83:** 187.

# Delayed Puberty in the Boy

By delayed puberty I mean the absence of signs of puberty by the age of 17.

The causes of delayed puberty include the following:

Normal variation, often familial

Malnutrition: severe chronic illness. Cystic fibrosis. Asthma

Pituitary disease: isolated gonadotrophin deficiency; Fröhlich's syndrome

Delayed treatment of cryptorchidism or torsion of testis; postoperative complications

Rudimentary (autosomal or X-linked) or absent testes

Mumps

Male intersex

Myotonic dystrophy

Neurofibromatosis

Rare syndromes—Klinefelter, Turner (male), Noonan, Kallman, Laurence–Moon–Biedl, Carpenter, Del Castillo, Prader–Willi, Fanconi, Rud

Drugs—cannabis. Cyclophosphamide

There are considerable *normal variations* in the age of onset of puberty, often familial [1]. It tends to be later in large families. Boys of small build are likely to reach puberty later than those of big build. As in the case of the girl, malnutrition or severe illness may delay the onset of puberty, but obesity does not.

*Pituitary disease* includes in particular the craniopharyngioma and the chromophobe adenoma. There is severe growth failure. Optic atrophy, particularly unilateral, may point to the diagnosis. Fröhlich's syndrome is so rare that it can be virtually ignored; in order to make the diagnosis there must be evidence of disease of the hypothalamus, with polyuria, polydipsia and glycosuria, obesity and dwarfism.

In Klinefelter's syndrome the penis is of normal size, but the testes are small. There is commonly gynaecomastia.

In the male Turner's syndrome there may be genital underdevelopment, short stature, webbing of the neck, low posterior hair line, coarctation of the aorta, cubitus valgus and mental subnormality. Noonan's syndrome is similar, but with a normal karyotype.

Isolated deficiency of gonadotrophins may be associated with anosmia (*Kallman's syndrome*). It is also found in the *Laurence–Moon– Biedl* syndrome of polydactyly, retinitis pigmentosa and dwarfism, and occurs in association with neurofibromatosis.

In Carpenter's syndrome there is hypogonadism, acrocephaly, polydactyly or syndactyly, obesity and mental subnormality.

In the Del Castillo syndrome there is germinal cell aplasia, with normal sexual maturation but small testes.

For the Prader–Willi syndrome, see p. 22; for the Fanconi syndrome, see p. 60; for the syndrome of Rud, see p. 356.

Cannabis (p. 218) and cyclophosphamide may delay the onset of secondary sexual characteristics.

The causes of delayed puberty should be sought if there are no signs of puberty by the age of 17 [1].

## Reference

1  Root AW. Endocrinology of puberty. *J Pediatr* 1973; **83:** 187.

# Early Normal Breast Enlargement

It is normal and usual for male and female full-term infants to have breast enlargement; it is rare in preterm infants under 32 weeks gestation. The enlargement usually begins 2 to 3 days after birth, reaching a peak in the second week [1]. Most infants secrete milk by 7 days, seventeen of nineteen are still secreting by the second week, but none after the eighth week. There is no difference in the breast size in boys and girls until after the age of 6 months, when the breasts of girls tend to be larger.

The enlargement may occur after the newborn period, and persist for 5 years or more, without other indications of puberty [2, 3], or may regress after birth and then recur—regressing again after that. When breasts enlargement occurs before 2 years of age, it usually regresses completely. The enlargement may be asymmetrical.

## References

1  McKiernan JF, Hull D. Breast development in the newborn. *Arch Dis Child* 1981; **56**: 525.
2  Mills JL, Stolley PD, Davies J, Moshang T. Premature thelarche: natural history and etiologic investigations. *Am J Dis Child* 1981; **135**: 743.
3  Pasquino AM, Tebaldi L, Cioschi L, *et al*. Premature thelarche: a follow-up study of 40 girls. *Arch Dis Child* 1985; **60**: 1180.

# Sexual Precocity

## The girl

Sexual precocity in a girl may be either isosexual or heterosexual. The former implies the early appearance of pubertal features appropriate to the sex of the patient, while the latter implies the development of secondary sexual characteristics such as enlargement of the clitoris.

The causes of precocity are as follows:

> Constitutional sexual precocity
> Rare
>> Intracranial tumours
>> Hydrocephalus
>> Hypothyroidism
>> Polyostotic fibrous dysplasia
>> Adrenocortical tumour. Hepatoma
> Heterosexual
>> Congenital adrenal hyperplasia
>> Ovarian tumour or cyst [4]
>> Drugs

Sexual precocity before the age of 9 years is the so-called 'constitutional' type, i.e. without any disease, in 90 per cent of cases. It can occur at a few months of age. The sequence of changes may be the same as that of an older child; but the first sign of sexual precocity may be vaginal bleeding alone, pubic hair alone or breast changes, or any combination of these. The child is usually tall for her age at first, but, owing to premature closure of the epiphyses, smallness of stature is the end result. It is important that endocrinological investigations should be carried out in order to eliminate the other causes. The 17-oxosteroid output is higher than in ordinary children of the age but normal for puberty. At puberty a vaginal smear shows oestrogenization.

It should be noted that breast enlargement may occur without other signs of puberty in normal children, and pubic hair can occur without breast enlargement or other signs of puberty [1]. In these cases the stature is average, and the urinary 17-oxosteroids are normal for the age. Gonadotrophins are either not found in the urine or at a low level, normal for the age. The vulva has a normal atrophic appearance and vaginal and urethral cells are not oestrogenized. The skeletal maturation, the urine and plasma oestrogens are normal for the age. When there is breast enlargement without any other signs of puberty (premature thelarche) the areola is usually pale and unpigmented.

Sometimes vaginal bleeding without pubic hair may occur in a young child, and not recur for some years until normal adolescence occurs. The stature would be average for the age, and there would be no oestrogenization in the vaginal smear.

*Intracranial conditions* should be revealed in the ordinary physical examination of the child, including ophthalmoscopy for papilloedema.

*Polyostotic fibrous dysplasia* (Albright's syndrome) consists of sexual precocity, pigmentation of one side of the body (perhaps only a patch on the buttocks or thigh), with X-ray evidence of fibrous dysplasia in the femur or other bones on the same side as the pigmentation. The exact mechanism of the sexual precocity is uncertain. Vaginal bleeding commonly precedes other signs of precocity.

*Adrenocortical tumours* usually make themselves obvious by the rapid onset of puberty, often with the full appearance of Cushing's syndrome, obesity of the buffalo type, with little fat in the extremities, a plethoric facies, hypertension, commonly stunting of growth and hypertrichosis. There is an excess of 17-oxogenic steroids in the urine. The common cause is carcinoma.

Sexual precocity also occurs in association with *adrenocortical hyperplasia*, which is normally associated with pseudohermaphroditism. There is enlargement of the clitoris from birth, usually with advanced skeletal maturation and increased 17-oxosteroids in the urine.

When the cause of sexual precocity is an *ovarian tumour,* the vaginal bleeding tends to be marked, with minimal breast changes and pubic hair. The diagnosis should be suspected if vaginal bleeding precedes the development of pubic hair or of breast changes. The tumour is usually felt on bimanual examination. If there is a granulosa cell tumour, there is a great excess of oestrogens in the urine, and in the case of a teratoma there is an excessive output of gonadotrophins from the tumour. Premature puberty has followed treatment of leukaemia [3].

Transient breast enlargement has been ascribed to ovarian cysts [4], the enlargement being temporary only. Breast enlargement has occurred in cystic fibrosis [6].

Breast enlargement has resulted from contamination of food, tablets or cosmetics by oestrogens. It occurred in Puerto Rico and Italy because of contamination of meat by oestrogenic substances [5] and contamination of meat or poultry by anabolic steroids.

## The boy

Whereas in 90 per cent of cases of sexual precocity in girls the cause is 'constitutional' and not related to disease, the majority of cases in boys are due to serious disease.

As a rule, if the penis is fully developed as at puberty, and the testes are normal in size for puberty, the cause is likely to be intracranial. If the penis is large but the testes are small and undeveloped the cause is likely to be adrenal.

The causes of sexual precocity are as follows:

    Isosexual
        Constitutional
        Hypothalamic tumour, hydrocephalus, postencephalitis
        Hypothyroidism [2]
        Congenital adrenal hyperplasia
        Hepatoma
        Tumour of testis
        Exogenous androgens
    Heterosexual
        Feminizing tumour of adrenal cortex
        Exogenous oestrogens

As in the girl, breast enlargement may be due to drugs.

## References

1 Altchek A. Premature thelarche. *Pediatr Clin North Am* 1972; **19**: 543.
2 Hemady ZS, Siler-Khodr TM, Najjar S. Precocious puberty in juvenile hyothyroidism. *J Pediatr* 1978; **92**: 55.
3 Leiper A, Stanhope R, Kitchin P, Chessells J. Precocious and premature puberty associated with treatment of acute lymphoblastic leukaemia. *Arch Dis Child* 1987; **62**: 1107.
4 Lyon AJ, De Bruyn R, Grant DB. Transient sexual precocity and ovarian cysts. *Arch Dis Child* 1985; **60**: 819.
5 Rodriguez C, Bongiovanni A, Borrego L. An epidemic of precocious development in Puerto Rican children. *J Pediatr* 1985; **107**: 393.
6 Russi EW. Gynaecomastia in cystic fibrosis. *Br Med J* 1984; **1**: 1160.

# Gynaecomastia in Boys

When a boy has enlargement of the breast, the following conditions have to be considered:

> Normal newborn breast enlargement
> Normal gynaecomastia of adolescence
> Disease involving the skin, pituitary, thyroid, lung, adrenal, liver, kidney, testis. Malnutrition. Paraplegia
> Klinefelter's syndrome after puberty
> Effect of drugs

Enlargement of the breast is normal in newborn full-term male babies, but rare in prematurely born ones. An obese boy may appear to have breast enlargement, but the appearance is due to nothing more than fatty tissue.

Gynaecomastia is common in *adolescence*. In a study of 1855 non-obese adolescent boys, it was found in 38·7 per cent. The figure for the 14–14½ year old group was 64·6 per cent. In 23·3 per cent the enlargement was unilateral. It persisted for up to 2 years in 27·1 per cent and up to 3 years in 7·7 per cent. It may be unilateral [3].

Gynaecomastia is occasionally seen in various diseases in adults, including generalized skin conditions, severe malnutrition, acromegaly, thyrotoxicosis, carcinoma of the lung, feminizing adreno-cortical tumour, cirrhosis of the liver, renal failure, or tumour of the testis. It may occur in paraplegic patients. It is not clear how many of these conditions cause gynaecomastia in children [1].

Gynaecomastia may be a feature of *Klinefelter's syndrome*. Some 25 per cent of such children are mentally subnormal. The testes are small for the age. The diagnosis is established by the buccal smear and chromosome analysis.

The following *drugs* may cause gynaecomastia: amphetamine, anabolic steroids, cannabis, cimetidine, cytotoxic drugs, digitalis, gonadotrophins, griseofulvin, isoniazid, metronidazole, oestrogens, PAS, progesterone, reserpine, spironolactone, testosterone and tranquillizers. It has resulted from digoxin poisoning. It has been ascribed to oestrogen-containing haircream [2].

### References

1  Carlson HE. Gynecomastia. *N Eng J Med* 1980; **303:** 795.
2  Edidin DV, Levitsky LL. Prepubertal gynecomastia associated with estrogen-containing hair cream. *Am J Dis Child* 1982; **136:** 587.
3  Nydick M, Bustos J, Dale JH, Rawson RW. Gynecomastia in adolescent boys. *JAMA* 1961; **178**: 449.

# Lactorrhoea

Lactorrhoea occurs in a variety of conditions, mainly associated with increased circulating prolactin levels. The secretion of prolactin is inhibited by dopamine, and hyperprolactinaemia is therefore caused by several drugs, including metoclopramide, reserpine, sulpiride and tranquillizers. It may be caused by cimetidine, which increases the serum prolactin.

*Blood-stained nipple discharge in infants.* This may be a benign condition, resolving spontaneously [1]. It could be due to a small duct papilloma; there may be an elevated blood progesterone level [2].

**References**

1 Berkowitz C, Inkelis SH. Bloody nipple discharge in infancy. *J Pediatr* 1983; **103**: 755.
2 Sigalas J, Roilides E, Tsanakas J, Karpouzas J. Bloody nipple discharge in infants. *J Pediatr* 1985; **107**: 484.

# Recurrent Infections

Most children suffer recurrent infections, and in most cases the cause is unknown. Malnutrition is a factor, probably because of its effect on complement, phagocytes and secretory IgA antibody responses. Concomitant and interrelated factors include poverty, poor housing and dirt. Infants in developing countries, when not fully breast-fed, suffer greatly from recurrent gastroenteritis. Common respiratory infections, colds and tonsillitis reach their peak when the child starts at school, attends a nursery, or when an older sibling starts school and brings the infection home. After 2 or 3 years at school the incidence of these infections falls off steeply. The infections are largely viral, but some are streptococcal infections of the throat. Repeated virus infections do not usually denote a recognized immunological deficiency.

Knowledge of relevant immunological factors is rapidly increasing [8]. A whole volume of *Pediatric Clinics of North America* (May 1977, pp. 275–425) was devoted to this subject. There are more than forty immunological deficiency syndromes.

A simple grouping of causes, modified from the review by Johnston [9], is as follows:

Non-immunological
    Obstruction—Eustachian tube, bronchi, urinary tract
    Vascular obstruction
    Alteration of bacterial flora by antibiotics
Phagocyte function
    Defect of neutrophil migration, opsonin deficiency, leucopenia, splenectomy or absence of spleen
    Chronic granulomatous disease

Humoral system
  Cell-mediated immunity—T cell defect
  Hypogammaglobulinaemia, IgA deficiency, complement
    deficiency
Malnutrition
Immunosuppression by drugs or severe infection
  Kawasaki disease
  AIDS
Abnormal communication in the cerebrospinal fluid pathways
Domestic or other reservoir of infection
Unknown

Obstruction of secretions commonly causes infection. Examples are incompletely opened nasolacrymal duct in infancy, the pre-auricular sinus, congenital dermal sinus, adenoidal hypertrophy and narrow postnasal space obstructing the Eustachian tube, cystic fibrosis obstructing the airway by thick secretions, and Riley's syndrome causing bronchial hypersecretion and obstruction. Recurrent urinary tract infections may be related to an underlying structural defect.

*Foreign bodies* in the ear, nose, bronchus and vagina, or an in-dwelling urethral catheter, cause persistent or recurrent infection.

*Granulopenia* is commonly due to infection, drugs, especially chloramphenicol, and blood diseases.

*Chronic granulomatous disease* is a fatal genetic condition with phagocytic dysfunction [1, 6]. Onset is usually in the first year, with lymphadenitis, pneumonia, fever and perirectal abscess, diarrhoea, sometimes with liver abscess, osteitis, skin infection and otitis media. It is more common in boys. There is commonly hepatosplenomegaly.

*Cyclic neutropenia* is a rare condition in which every few weeks there are mouth ulcers and other infections, with fever and arthralgia. In *exocrine pancreatic insufficiency* there are neutropenia, dwarfism and infections.

The *Chediak–Higashi syndrome* is an autosomal recessive, with undue susceptibility to infection, pyoderma, hypopigmentation and neutropenia.

*Splenectomy*, especially in the first five years, and especially in the first two postoperative years, carries a risk of overwhelming infection, especially pneumococcal [2]. This also occurs in adults [4]. The reason for the splenectomy is probably irrelevant. There is a similar susceptibility in hereditary splenic hypoplasia and in asplenia with or without congenital heart disease [7].

In *T cell deficiency syndromes* there is a special tendency to virus or *Candida* infection. There is normal primary immune function, phagocytosis and inflammatory response, but there are deficiencies in tests of cell-mediated functions. They include *Di George's syndrome* of congenital aplasia of the thymus, hypoparathyroidism, tetany, abnormal susceptibility to viral and fungal infections, failure to thrive and anomalies of the great vessels. The increased susceptibility to infection in *ataxia telangiectasia* (see p. 212), the *Wiskott–Aldrich syndrome*, purpura and eczema (p. 64) are largely thymic dependent. The development of serious failure of resistance to infection in early infancy may be related to prenatal cytomegalovirus, rubella or Epstein–Barr infection, or to maternal drug addiction before or after the child's birth.

*Impaired inflammatory response* results from a lack of inhibition of certain complement components; there is a special susceptibility to staphylococcal infections. A familial deficiency has been described.

The *gamma-globulin deficiencies* include agammaglobulinaemia, hypogammaglobulinaemia and dysgammaglobulinaemia. *Burton's disease* is an example of hypogammaglobulinaemia; it usually develops in the second year, with recurrent staphylococcal or *Haemophilus influenzae* infections, and often with arthritis (especially boys). Buckley, Wray & Belmaker [3] described undue susceptibility to infection in association with hyperimmunoglobulinaemia E.

Immunosuppression by drugs, such as corticosteroids, or by severe infections are an important factor. Infections include the Kawasaki disease (p. 39) and acquired immune deficiency syndrome (AIDS) [11, 12] (p. 18). In association with malnutrition in developing countries, infections may cause serious immunosuppression.

It is said that severe psychological stress may depress cell-mediated immunity [10] and lead to recurrent infections.

*Recurrent meningitis* is usually due to a communication between the subarachnoid space and the air sinuses, mastoid, ear or skin (by a congenital dermal sinus). Cerebrospinal fluid rhinorrhoea may be due to a congenital defect in the cribriform plate or elsewhere, or result from injury [13]. Other causes of recurrent meningitis [9, 13] include Behçet's disease, familial Mediterranean fever, disseminated lupus and immunological deficiencies, including asplenia. It has been ascribed to trimethoprim with sulphamethoxazole [5], to isoniazid and to non-steroidal anti-inflammatory drugs.

350    *Recurrent Infections*

*Recurrent antrum or skin infections* may result from frequent reinfection from a reservoir or infection in the home (or school). When a child has a chronic or recurrent antrum infection, it is important to ensure that neither of the parents or any other person in the home has a similar infection. Domestic animals may be a reservoir of infection, streptococcal or otherwise. Threadworm and roundworm infections are difficult to eradicate because of the presence of infection in other members of the family, school mates and dust. Recurrent herpes infections may arise from a reservoir in the family.

## References

1 Ament ME, Ochs HD. Gastrointestinal manifestations of chronic granulomatous disease. *N Engl J Med* 1973; **288:** 382.
2 Bisno AL. Hyposplenism and overwhelming pneumococcal infection: a reappraisal. *Am J Med Sci* 1971; **262:** 101.
3 Buckley RH, Wray BB, Belmaker EZ. Extreme hyperimmunoglobulinemia E and undue susceptibility to infection. *Pediatrics* 1972; **49:** 59.
4 Desser RK, Ultmann JE. Risk of severe infection in particular with Hodgkin's disease or lymphoma after diagnostic laparotomy and splenectomy. *Ann Int Med* 1972; **77:** 143.
5 Haas EJ. Trimethoprim–sulphamethoxazole: another cause of recurrent meningitis. *JAMA* 1984; **252:** 346.
6 Hayakawa H, Kobayashi N, Yata J. Chronic granulomatous disease in Japan: a summary of the clinical features of 84 registered patients. *Acta Pediatr Japonica* 1985; **27:** 501.
7 Hjelt L, Hakosalo J. Congenital asplenia. *Annales Paediatr Fenniae* 1959; **5:** Suppl 12.
8 Janeway CA. Recurrent infections. In: Green M, Haggerty RJ (eds) *Ambulatory pediatrics.* Philadelphia: Saunders, 1977.
9 Johnston RB. Recurrent bacterial infections in children *New Engl J Med* 1984; **310:** 1237.
10 *Lancet.* Emotion and immunity. Leading article. 1985; **2:** 133.
11 Oleske J, Minnefor A, Cooper R, *et al.* Immune deficiency syndrome in children. *JAMA* 1983; **249:** 2345.
12 Rubenstein A. Acquired immunodeficiency syndrome in infants. *Am J Dis Child* 1983; **137:** 825.
13 Symposium. Recurrent meningitis. *Proc Roy Soc Med* 1974; **67:** 1141.

# Symptoms Related to the Skin

## PRURITIS

Pruritus, or the itch, is a common symptom in childhood. Perhaps the commonest causes are infantile eczema or urticaria, irritation by contact with wool or a sweat rash. The following are the main causes to consider:

> Moderate or severe pruritus
> > Eczema and dermatitis: dermatitis herpetiformis
> > Scabies
> > Urticaria, bites, stings
> > Lichen planus
> > Mycosis fungoides
> > Chilblains
> > Prickly heat
> Slight pruritus
> > Sweat rash. Irritation by wool next to skin
> > Psoriasis, pityriasis rosea and pityriasis rubra pilaris
> > Pyogenic skin infections. Pemphigus
> > Pediculosis. Ringworm. Chickenpox
> > Jaundice, uraemia, diabetes mellitus
> > Leukaemia. Reticuloses
> Psychological
> Drugs

There are other conditions which cause pruritus, but the above are the principal ones. The list is such a long one that it would not be profitable to discuss the differential diagnosis.

Severe *psychological stress* may cause urticaria. It may have an immunological basis.

*Scabies* is diagnosed by the burrows, found especially on the sides of the fingers, wrists, anterior axillary folds and buttocks. In infants scabies may affect the scalp and the soles of the feet. The intense itching, and the common history of itching in other members of the family, suggests the diagnosis. But the diagnosis is commonly confused by superadded infection, by unwise topical applications, or by urticarial wheals, vesicles, bullae, eczema, impetigo or pustules.

Innumerable *drugs* may cause urticaria or pruritus. They include aminophylline, antibiotics, anticonvulsants, antihistamines, antisera, aspirin, chloral, chloroquine, codeine, clonidine, corticosteroid ointment, diphenoxylate, gold, griseofulvin, nalidixic acid, non-steroidal anti-inflammatory drugs, opiates, piperazine, quinine, salicylates, tetanus toxoid, tranquillizers, vitamin A excess and vitamin $B_3$ (nicotinamide) excess.

## URTICARIA

Acute urticaria may be caused by allergy to foods and to food additives, notably tartrazine and other azo dyes, sodium benzoate and 4-hydroxybenzoic acid used as preservatives in pickles, sauces, instant coffee and other foods [2]. Tartrazine is used as a yellow dye in orange squash, many foods, and scores of drugs. *Penicillin, aspirin* and *cotrimoxazole* are common offenders; a possible cause is the presence of penicillin in cow's milk. Urticaria may be due to sensitivity to topical applications—to the antibiotic or to the base or vehicle used.

Urticaria may result from bites, stings, inhalants, vigorous exercise, emotional stress or exposure to extreme cold or light.

Other causes of urticaria include fungi, virus infections and reticuloses. It may have an immunological basis.

Chronic *papular urticaria* is usually due to sensitivity to insect bites, such as fleas from a dog or cat or other household pets [1]. It is commonly aggravated by aspirin. It may be a reaction to scabies.

Papular urticaria may be associated with bullae on the legs.

### References

1 *British Medical Journal*. Chronic urticaria. Leading article 1976; **3**: 68.
2 Delayney JC. Response of patients with asthma and aspirin sensitivity to tartrazine. *Practitioner* 1976; **217**: 285.

## ECZEMA

Eczematous skin lesions occur in a variety of diseases other than infantile eczema. They include:

Contact dermatitis
Nappy rash

Rare

    Mycoses

    Histiocytosis

    Wiskott–Aldrich syndrome (purpura and eczema)

    Agammaglobulinaemia

    Phenylketonuria, Hartnup disease

    Ataxia telangiectasia

    Ahistidinaemia

    Acrodermatitis enteropathica

    Coeliac disease

    Mucopolysaccharidoses

    AIDS

Drugs—aminoglycosides, amitriptyline, antihistamines, iodides, meprobamate, penicillin, phenothiazines, quinine, salicylates, sulphonamides, thiazide diuretics.

## HAIR LOSS AND HYPERTRICHOSIS

Hair loss in the newborn is frequent and normal.

### Hair loss

Loss of hair may be due to the following conditions:

    Head rolling

    Trichotillomania

    Alopecia areata. Down's syndrome

    Ringworm and other infections

    Pituitary, thyroid, parathyroid or adrenal insufficiency

    Abnormalities of hair structure—trichorrhexis, pili torti, monilethrix

    Any severe chronic illness or acute weight loss

    Vitiligo

    AIDS

    Rare syndromes

      Ectodermal dysplasia

      Progeria

      Dystrophia myotonica

      Argininosuccinicaciduria

      Hallerman–Streiff

Acrodermatitis enteropathica
Disseminated lupus
Incontinentia pigmenti
Drugs

Infants often denude their heads in a patch or patches by *head rolling*. Toddlers and other children sometimes acquire the habit of pulling their hair out; it is usually a manifestation of insecurity.

*Alopecia areata* may be due to several causes. The hair tends to break off 2 or 3 mm from the root. The broken hair is the shape of an exclamation mark, being thicker at the top than the base. It may be associated with agammaglobulinaemia. There is an association between *Down's syndrome,* diabetes, Addison's disease and alopecia areata, probably dependent on an auto-immune mechanism [3]. Alopecia in the case of older children sometimes follows psychological stress, as in adults.

*Ringworm* is diagnosed by fluorescence under Wood's light or by detection of the fungi in potassium hydroxide on a slide.

*Trichorrhexis nodosa* is a condition in which there are nodular swellings on the hair with fractures of the hair shaft. *Pili tori* consist of twisted hair. The condition is hereditary and is sometimes associated with deafness. Affected infants are commonly born without hair. After some growth of hair, the eyelashes, hair of scalp and hair of eyebrows fall out. *Monilethrix* is a developomental anomaly of the hair shaft. The diagnosis is made by microscopy.

Hair loss may be the sequel of any *chronic illness* or acute weight loss.

Numerous *rare syndromes* are associated with hair loss [6, 7, 8, 9]. *Menke's kinky hair syndrome* [2] consists of pili torti, loss of hair, slow growth, mental deterioration and convulsions; hypothermia is an important symptom. It is an X-linked recessive due to a defect of copper metabolism. For *acrodermatitis enteropathica* see p. 362.

*Drugs* which cause hair loss include amphetamine, antibiotics, anticoagulants, anticonvulsants, antithyroid drugs, arsenic, bismuth, chloroquine, cytotoxic drugs, dextran, ethionamide, etretinate, fenfluramine, gold, heparin, lead, lithium, mepacrine, thallium, tranquillizers and vitamin A or $B_3$ excess. Hair loss may follow several weeks after anticoagulant therapy.

## Hypertrichosis [4]

Generalized hypertrichosis is often racial. Other causes, except those related to drugs, are rare. They included the following:

> Endocrine—Cushing's syndrome (p. 343), adrenocortical hyperplasia, adrenal insufficiency, polycystic ovary
>
> Other metabolic conditions—porphyria (p. 116), mucopolysaccharidoses
>
> Severe weight loss or malnutrition. Degenerative diseases of the nervous system. Lipodystrophy
>
> Chromosomal—Turner's syndrome, trisomy E
>
> Cornelia de Lange syndrome
>
> Leprechaunism
>
> Congenital asymmetry
>
> Epidermolysis bullosa
>
> Dermatomyositis
>
> Syndrome of hereditary gingival hyperplasia with hypertrichosis [10]
>
> Drugs

Hirsutism may result in the female from administration of *androgens*. It may occur in ovarian and adrenal diseases and in Turner's syndrome. A hairy face may occur in the *fetal alcohol syndrome*.

Local hypertrichosis or patches of excessive hair occur in the *hairy naevus, linear naevus sebaceous syndrome* [5] and on the back in relation to *diastematomyelia* or *congenital dermal sinus*.

Of the several mucopolysaccharidoses, *Hurler's syndrome* is the most likely to be associated with hirsutism; there is progressive hepatosplenomegaly, cataract and mental deterioration.

The *Cornelia de Lange syndrome* presents with a characteristic facies in which the eyebrows are continuous with each other. There is hirsutism, malformation of the hands with a proximally placed thumb, and mental subnormality.

Various *drugs* cause hypertrichosis [1, 4, 10]. They include anabolic steroids, androgenic hormones, chlorpromazine, corticosteroids, diazoxide, minoxidil, penicillamine, phenytoin, psoralens and streptomycin.

## References

1 Bruinsma W. *A guide to drug eruptions.* Oosthuizen, Holland: De Zwaluw, 1977.
2 Danks DM, Campbell PE, Stevens BJ, *et al.* Menke's kinky hair syndrome. *Pediatrics* 1972; **50**: 188.
3 Du Vivier A, Munro DD. Mongolism and alopecia areata. *Proc Roy Soc Med* 1974; **67**: 596.
4 Forbes A. Hypertrichosis. *N Engl J Med* 1965; **273**: 602.
5 Gellis SS, Feingold M. Linear nevus sebaceous syndrome. *Am J Dis Child* 1970; **120**: 138.
6 Price VH. Disorders of the hair in children. *Pediatr Clin N Am* 1978; **25**: 305.
7 Rook A, Wilkinson DS, Ebling FJG. *Textbook of dermatology.* Oxford: Blackwell, 4th edn, 1979.
8 Verbov J. *Modern topics in paediatric dermatology.* London: Heinemann, 1979.
9 Verbov J, Morely N. *Colour atlas of paediatric dermatology.* MTP Press, 1983.
10 Winter GB, Simpkiss MJ. Hypertrichosis and hereditary gingival hyperplasia. *Arch Dis Child* 1974; **49**: 394.

# ICHTHYOSIS

Ichthyosis simplex (xeroderma) is a dominant inherited condition. Rare causes include [2, 3]:

Ichthyosiform erythroderma (lamellar ichthyosis of the newborn), ichthyosis following the collodion skin syndrome (harlequin fetus)

Refsum's syndrome (p. 212)

Sjögren–Larsson syndrome—ichthyosis, spasticity, mental subnormality

Rud's syndrome—dwarfism, fits, mental subnormality, hypogonadism

Netherton's syndrome in girls [4]. Abnormal hair shafts, allergic manifestations, renal disease, deafness and dwarfism

Ichthyosis nigricans—sex-linked recessive, males: early infancy—large scattered brown-black scales; often mental subnormality

Ichthyosis and osteopetrosis [1]

Sulfatide lipoidosis (p. 259)

Various chromosome abnormalities

**References**

1 Dowd PM, Munro DD. Ichthyosis and osteopetrosis. *Proc Roy Soc Med* 1983; **76**: 423.
2 Frost P, Van Scott EJ. Ichthyosiform dermatoses: classification based on anatomic and biometric observations. *Arch Dermatol* 1966; **94**: 113.
3 *Lancet*. Scaly skin. Leading article. 1978; **2**: 615.
4 Rayner A, Lampert RP, Rennert OM. Familial ichthyosis, dwarfism, mental retardation, renal disease and deafness. *J Pediatr* 1978; **92**: 766.

## DESQUAMATION

General desquamation occurs in scarlet fever, sometimes in measles, the toxic shock syndrome (p. 92), ichthyosis, disseminated lupus, pityriasis alba, pityriasis rosea (herald spot on trunk, followed 10 to 14 days later by oval pinprick scaly patches on trunk, neck, arms above elbows, legs above knees).

*Exfoliative dermatitis* may result from drugs—anticonvulsants, chloroquine, etretinate, gold, griseofulvin, isoniazid, nitrofurantoin, penicillin, phenothiazines, salicylates, streptomycin, sulphonamides or thiouracil.

*Desquamation of hands and feet* occurs in dermatitis, lichen planus, psoriasis and the Kawasaki syndrome.

## PIGMENTATION

Below is a brief summary.

*Normal pigmentation*

This includes racial factors; sunburn; freckles; mongolian pigmentation.

Mongolian pigmentation (naevus of ITO or OTA) is almost universal in coloured races [2], and is said to be almost universal in Eskimos. It has been found in up to 9 per cent of white children in whom it has a blue-grey colour, resembling an old bruise [5, 8]. In a study of 3230 Chinese children in Hong Kong [6], mongolian pigmentation was found in 75 per cent of those under 2 years, 25 per cent of those at 6 years and 2 per cent of those at 12 years of age. The pigmentation occasionally persists into adult life. The pigmentation is predominantly in the lumbosacral area, often in front of the ankle and occasionally on the arms.

*Café-au-lait lesions* are normal unless multiple and large. Single lesions—1 to 3 cm long occur in 20 per cent of normal children. If they are more than six in number, and are more than 4 to 6 cm long, they should be regarded as *neurofibromatosis* until proved otherwise. Crawford [3] suggested that the diagnosis of neurofibromatosis in a child should be made on the basis of two or more of the following— five or more café-au-lait spots, biopsy, family history and a characteristic bone lesion.

Causes:
(i) Neurofibromatosis (Von Recklinghausen's disease)
(ii) Tuberous sclerosis (epiloia). A quarter of all cases of epiloia have café-au-lait spots with mountain ash leaf-shaped white macules and hypopigmented areas
(iii) Silver's syndrome
(iv) Association with pulmonary stenosis and mental sub-normality [11]
(v) Gaucher's syndrome
(vi) De Toni–Fanconi syndrome (p. 00)
(vii) Phaeochromocytoma

Vitiligo [1, 7, 10] occurs in diabetes mellitus, collagen vascular disease, auto-immune disease and hypogammaglobulinaemia.

*Other patchy pigmentation*

Albright's syndrome (polyostotic fibrous displasia) p. 343.
*Multiple lentiginoses* [4]—a dominant condition with multiple pigmented skin lesions, ECG conduction defects, hypertelorism, pulmonary stenosis, abnormal genitalia, retarded growth, deafness and mental subnormality.
Peutz–Jeghers syndrome—pigmentation around the nose, mouth, nails, hands; pigmentation in the oral mucosa; intestinal polyposis.

*Incontinentia pigmenti*

There are two forms [1], the incontinentia pigmenti achromicans of
Ito, with streaks of hypopigmentation and hyperpigmentation, and
a variety of congenital anomalies including megalencephaly,
mental subnormality, optic atrophy, hypotonia, alopecia and fits,
but without previous vesicular lesions, and the more common
Bloch–Salzberger type, especially in girls, beginning as a vesicular
rash and followed by linear and patchy pigmentation on the trunk
and limbs, with mental subnormality.

*Diffuse pigmentation*

Yellow—jaundice: mepacrine skin staining; carotenaemia: excessive
intake of carrots (p. 127)
Blue or blue black—chlorpromazine, chloroquine, acanthosis
nigricans, heavy metals
Brown or grey-brown—heavy metals, phenothiazines, repeated
transfusions
Addison's disease, Gaucher's disease
Niemann–Pick disease, xeroderma pigmentosum
Bronze—phototherapy (neonate)
Other rare conditions causing diffuse or extensive patchy
pigmentation include:
Xeroderma pigmentosa—pigmented area related to ataxia,
athetosis, deafness, keratoses, large freckles, delayed
sexual, mental and physical development, photosensi-
tivity and telangiectasia
Cushing's syndrome
Thyrotoxicosis
Pellagra and sprue
Hartnup disease (error of tryptophane metabolism, ataxia,
pellagra-like lesions)
Porphyria. Violaceous skin
Syndrome of spastic paraplegia with mental subnormality and
pigmentation [9]
Effect of drugs—antimalarial drugs, arsenic, bismuth,
busulphan, clonazepam, corticosteroids, cytotoxic

drugs, gold, griseofulvin, mercury, nitrofurantoin, phenothiazines, phenytoin, silver, vitamin A excess. Mepacrine causes a yellow pigmentation. Rifampicin in a large dose may cause red pigmentation

## Hypopigmentation

Patchy hypopigmentation and hyperpigmentation occurs in vitiligo, epiloia (tuberous sclerosis), and the Rothmund–Thomson syndrome (p. 364).

A white forelock is a feature of the Waardenburg syndrome (p. 202).

Striking hypopigmented areas follow eczema, nappy rashes and other skin conditions in coloured children [2].

Patches of hypopigmentation, in the young child perhaps only seen under Wood's light, are characteristic in *epiloia* (tuberous sclerosis). Depigmented areas occur in pityriasis alba, naevus depigmentosus and lichen sclerosus. For streaks of pigmentation, see p. 359.

Generalized hypopigmentation may occur in albinism, phenyl-ketonuria, hypopituitarism and the Chediak–Higashi syndrome, a recessive, consisting of hypopigmentation of the skin, hair and eyes, with a predisposition to infection and later to lymphoma.

## References

1 Bleehan S. Disorders of melanin pigmentation. *Br J Hosp Med* 1975; **13**: 590.
2 Brauner GJ. Cutaneous disease in black children. *Am J Dis Child* 1983; **137**: 488.
3 Crawford AH. Neurofibromatosis in the pediatric patient. *Orthop Clin North Am* 1978; **9**: 11.
4 Gorlin RJ, Anderson RC, Blaw M. Multiple lentigines syndrome. *Am J Dis Child* 1969; **117**: 652.
5 Jacobs A, Walton R. Mongolian pigmentation. *Pediatrics* 1976; **58**: 218.
6 Lau JTK, Ching RML. Mongolian spots in Chinese children. *Am J Dis Child* 1982; **136**: 863.
7 Lerner AB, Nordlung JJ. Vitiligo. What is it? Is it important? *JAMA* 1978; **239**: 1183.
8 Levin S. Mongolian spot: Afro-Asian stain; sacral stain. *S African Med J* 1981; **60**: 123, 450.
9 Mukamel M, Weitz R, Metzker A, Varsano I. Spastic paraparesis, mental retardation and cutaneous pigmentation disorder. A new syndrome. *Am J Dis Child* 1985; **139**: 1090.
10 Wall LM. Disorders of pigmentation. *Medicine (UK)* 1980; p. 1582.
11 Watson GH. Café-au-lait spots, pulmonary stenosis and dull intelligence. *Arch Dis Child* 1967; **42**: 303.

## PHOTOSENSITIVITY

Photosensitivity may be caused by the following conditions:

> Drugs—amitriptyline, antidepressants, anti-emetics, antihistamines, barbiturates, carbamazepine, chloroquine, cotrimoxazole, cytotoxic drugs, demeclocycline (ledermycin), diphenoxylate, frusemide, gold, griseofulvin, nalidixic acid, phenothiazines, sulphonamides, tetracyclines, thiazide diuretics, viprynium

> Topical—cosmetics

> Pellagra

> Rare
>> Porphyria
>> Cockayne's syndrome (p. 364)
>> Hartnup disease
>> Bloom's syndrome (p. 364)
>> Xeroderma pigmentosum (p. 359)
>> Ultraviolet light causes a rash in pellagra and disseminated lupus

## BULLOUS OR VESICULAR SKIN LESIONS

Bullous skin lesions occur in a wide variety of conditions [4, 6, 7], including the following:

> Scalds, burns, sunburn, frostbite, bites, stings

> Impetigo. Herpes

> Scabies. Urticaria: urticaria pigmentosa (mast-cell disease, blisters, urticarial wheals, pigmented maculopapular eruptions)

> Pemphigus neonatorum

> Rare
>> Erythema multiforme
>> Epidermolysis bullosa. Lesions usually present at birth: blisters on pressure areas—may be only on hands and feet
>> Bullous disease of childhood—a persistent or recurrent disease, involving especially the pubis, scalp and trunk [6]. It usually starts in the first 10 years, with remission in a few months to 3 years

Incontinentia pigmenti

Toxic epidermal necrolysis: resembles scalded skin. Usually staphylococcal; also caused by barbiturates, phenytoin, penicillin, sulphonamides

Acrodermatitis enteropathica—a chronic, probably recessive, disease, usually starting in the first 18 months—vesicular or bullous warts on extremities or around mouth and anus; loss of hair; diarrhoea. May be due to zinc deficiency [5].

Porphyria; vesicles or bullae on exposure to sun

Syphilis

Cockayne's syndrome—dominant, recurrent bullous eruption of hands and feet

Dermatitis herpetiformis

Kaposi's varicelliform eruption—herpes infection super-imposed on eczema or other chronic skin disease

Stevens–Johnson syndrome (p. 145)

Orf—usually single pustule on finger or hand, infected by sheep: it clears spontaneously in a few weeks. It can occur on the mouth, as a result of a child kissing lambs

Self-inflicted, dermatitis medicamentosa

Drugs—acetazolamide, antibiotics, clonidine, cytotoxic drugs, frusemide, iodides, nalidixic acid, penicillamine, quinine, salicylates, thiazides, tranquillizers and sedatives [2]. Cetrimide sensitivity can cause a bullous reaction on the scalp [1].

*Vesicular eruptions* may be due to any of the causes of photosensitivity.

Vesicular eruptions in the newborn have resulted from infection by *Haemophilus influenzae* [3], *Staphylococcus aureus*, the cytomegalovirus and herpes. After the newborn period the commonest cause is chickenpox; it can also be caused by herpes simplex or zoster, or the Coxsackie virus (hand, foot and mouth disease—causing vesicles on the tongue, hands and feet, and sometimes on the knees). *Dermatitis herpetiformis* is a relapsing condition, bullous or vesicular, affecting the limb and trunk. The first symptom is often pruritus, and later vesicles appear. The onset is especially around 6 to 11 years. It is associated with a coeliac-like enteropathy. *Pityriasis lichenoides varioliformis* resembles chickenpox, but lasts several weeks. Other infections causing a vesicular eruption include the enterovirus and mycoplasma pneumoniae.

For scabies, see p. 357.

## References

1 Ahmed AR, May R. Chronic bullous dermatosis of childhood. *Am J Dis Child* 1982; **136:** 214.
2 *British Medical Journal.* Drug induced bullous eruptions. Leading article. 1981; **1:** 421.
3 Halal F, Delorme L, Brazeau M, Ahronheim G. Congenital vesicular eruption caused by *Haemophilus influenzae* Type B. *Pediatrics* 1978; **62:** 494.
4 Katz SJ. Blistering skin diseases. *N Engl J Med* 1985; **313:** 1657.
5 Moynahan EJ. Acrodermatitis enteropathica: a lethal inherited zinc deficiency syndrome. *Lancet* 1974; **2:** 399.
6 Ramsdell W, Jarratt M, Fuerst J, Stern J. Bullous disease of childhood. *Am J Dis Child* 1979; **133:** 791.
7 Schachner L, Press L. Vesicular, bullous and pustular disorders in infancy and childhood. *Pediatr Clinics N Am* 1983; **30:** 609.

## ERYTHEMA NODOSUM

Erythema nodosum is a non-specific response to:

Bacteria—streptococci, tuberculosis, BCG, *Leptospira, Pasteurella, Yersinia*

Viruses—e.g. cat scratch fever

Psittacosis

Malaria

Fungal infections

Sarcoid, ulcerative colitis, Crohn's disease, Hodgkin's disease, disseminated lupus, Behçet syndrome (p. 175)

Drugs—barbiturates, bromides, iodides, penicillin, salicylates, sulphonamides, thiouracil; and may follow the discontinuation of corticosteroids

## TELANGIECTASIA

Some degree of telangiectasia on the back of the neck in infancy, and on the interscapular area in older children, is normal. Much the commonest cause of telangiectasia otherwise is prolonged use of topical corticosteroids. Other causes are rare; they include:

Osler–Rendu–Weber syndrome. This is a dominant genetic condition, the most common manifestations of which are telangiectasia on the face and in the nasal mucous membrane (causing epistaxis, not often before puberty). There may be similar lesions in the retina, larynx, bone and gastrointestinal tract. There may be a large head, due to megalencephaly, multiple angiomata and cirrhosis of the liver

Louis–Bar syndrome of ataxia telangiectasia

Bloom's syndrome—facial telangiectasia with a butterfly distribution, with dwarfism and photosensitivity

Cockayne's syndrome—facial telangiectasia with a butterfly distribution, loss of facial subcutaneous fat, characteristic facies, retinitis pigmentosa, cataract, deafness and kyphosis, photosensitivity, dwarfism and mental subnormality

Rothmund–Thomson syndrome—telangiectasia, cataract, sparse hair and dwarfism

Blue bleb syndrome—blue nodular naevi on the skin with intestinal telangiectasia

Turner's syndrome—with intestinal telangiectasia

Wyburn–Mason syndrome—facial telangiectasia with cerebral arteriovenous aneurysm

Bonnet–Dechaume–Blanc syndrome of facial telangiectasia with involvement of the retina and brain

# NAEVI

The common naevi are:

The 'stork-bite' naevi on the inner end of the upper eyelid of the newborn baby, disappearing after a few months

The wedge-shaped naevus on the forehead of the newborn baby. There is always a coexistent naevus on the back of the neck [2]. These naevi disappear in a few months

The strawberry naevus, which is capillary or cavernous,

appearing a few days after birth, growing for up to 6
months and disappearing within 5 to 10 years

The cavernous haemangioma—a markedly elevated naevoid
mass

Facial port-wine stain. When the stain is above the eye, there is
usually an angioma in the pia, calcifying after a few
months, with hemiplegia, mental subnormality and fits
(Sturge–Weber syndrome)

Pigmented naevi and melanomata

Rare[1]

Fabry's syndrome (angiokeratoma corporis diffusum), with
purplish black naevi, and naevi in the skin, cardio-
vascular, pulmonary and renal systems

Kasabach–Merritt syndrome—cavernous haemangioma with
thrombocytopenia

von Hippel–Landau syndrome—naevi involving the retina,
skin and cerebellum, sometimes with polycystic kidney,
haemangioma of liver and Wilms' tumour

Klippel–Trenaunay syndrome—enlarged leg, slight naevoid
staining of skin

Maffucci's syndrome—multiple haemangiomata with dys-
chondroplasia and abnormal growth of long bones

Osler–Rendu–Weber syndrome (p. 364)

Blue bleb syndrome (p. 96)

Disseminated haemangiomatosis—very numerous skin naevi

Linear naevus (sebaceous)—naevi present on face at birth,
linear naevi on body, skull abnormalities, hirsutism,
fits, mental subnormality

Xeroderma pigmentosum

See also telangiectasia (p. 363).

## References

1 Esterly NB, Solomon LM. Pigmentary lesions and hemangiomas. *J Pediatr*
1972; **81:** 1003.
2 Øster J, Nielsen A. Nuchal naevi and interscapular telangiectases. *Acta
Paediatr Scand* 1970; **59:** 416.

## NAIL LESIONS

Numerous conditions affect the nails:

Absence of nails—may be genetic

Hypoplasia of nails

Drugs in pregnancy—phenytoin, anticoagulants, alcohol

Prone sleeping [2]: most infants sleeping in the prone position have one foot drawn up and one extended and rotated. The toes of the foot drawn up are flexed and the toe-nails may be abnormal, hypoplastic or curved

Familial genetic factors are the commonest cause other than the above. Bass [1] described a rare familial condition in which there was absence of the middle phalanges with hypoplasia of nails

Nail–patella syndrome (see p. 268)

Hypoparathyroidism—deformed or atrophic nails

Friable nails

Chondro-ectodermal dysplasia

Fungus infection, juvenile chronic arthritis, hypoparathyroidism

Pitted nails—psoriasis, candidiasis

Hollow nails (koilonychia)

Familial, iron deficiency, hypothyroidism, hyperthyroidism

Yellow—congenital lymphoedema [3]. This syndrome consists of yellow or greenish nails, with accentuated convexity and sometimes cross-ridging, with congenital generalized lymphoedema: the yellow colour of the nails may precede the development of lymphoedema by several years. There may be pleural effusion

Tetracycline in pregnancy

Psoriasis

Red half-moon—heart failure

Red purple—porphyria

Brown—tetracycline in pregnancy

Fungal infection

Chronic renal disease

Adriamycin, arsenic, bleomycin, chloroquine, cyclosphosphamide, demeclocycline, doxorubicin, phenolphthalein, silver

Black—*Pseudomonas* infection
Blue—mepacrine, argyria
  Blue half-moon—Wilson's disease
White—anaemia, cirrhosis, diabetes, heart disease
  White hands—hypoalbuminaemia
For other conditions, see Samman [4] and Zaias [5].

## References

1 Bass HN. Familial absence of middle phalanges and nail dysplasia. *Pediatrics* 1968; **42**: 318.
2 Culley P. Unilateral outward-turning leg in infancy. *Br Med J* 1981; **1**: 1236.
3 Norkild P, Kromann-Andersen H, Struve-Christensen F. Yellow nail syndrome—the triad of yellow nails, lymphedema and pleural effusion. *Acta Med Scand* 1986; **219**: 221.
4 Samman PD. Nail Disorders. In: Rook A, Wilkinson DS, Ebling FJG (eds) *Textbook of dermatology*. Oxford: Blackwell Scientific Publications, 1979.
5 Zaias N. *The nail in health and disease*. Lancaster: MTP Press, 1980.

# Side Effects of Drugs (General)

Almost all drugs have unpleasant side effects, and it was felt that a book concerning the common symptoms of disease would not be complete without a brief account of the side actions of drugs used to treat disease—side effects which are commonly confused with the disease itself. There are several reasons why it is easy to miss the fact that a child's symptoms are the side effect of the drug, and not due to the disease for which the drug is being given [5]: the reaction may be bizarre, the reaction may closely mimic a common disease, the reaction to the drug may be delayed, and the clinical picture may be so complex that the side effects of the drug are not recognized. For further reference concerning side effects of drugs, see the books by Davies [2] and Dukes [3].

At the risk of some over-simplification, one may group the side effects of drugs as follows, according to the tissue predominantly involved:

1 Action on the skin—rashes, erythematous, urticarial, scarlatiniform, morbilliform, erythema multiforme, erythema nodosum,

exfoliative dermatitis, purpura, acne, striae, photosensitivity, pigmentation, hair loss or hypertrichosis, Stevens–Johnson syndrome, disseminated lupus, fixed drug eruptions.

**2** Action on the brain, psychological or otherwise [1, 4]. Advantageous—the patient thinking that he is better, although the drug had no relevant pharmacological action. Disadvantageous—the patient imagining that the drug is causing untoward symptoms. Direct action on the brain—causing confusion or other symptoms.

**3** Action on the eye—causing cataract, optic atrophy, papilloedema, retinal changes, conjunctivitis.

**4** Action on the ear—causing deafness or ataxia.

**5** Action on the heart.

**6** Action on the liver—hepatitis.

**7** Action on the kidney—albuminuria, haematuria, nephrotic syndrome.

**8** Action on the blood.

> Predominantly red cells—haemolysis, megaloblastic anaemia, hypoplastic anaemia.
>
> Predominantly white cells—granulopenia, agranulocytosis.
>
> Predominantly platelets—thrombocytopenic purpura.
>
> Action on several of the blood elements.
>
> Action on clotting mechanisms.
>
> Action on the haemoglobin—methaemoglobinaemia.

**9** Action on the alimentary tract—abdominal pain, ulceration, bleeding, vomiting, diarrhoea, constipation.

**10** Allergic and anaphylactoid reactions. Asthma.

**11** Drug fever.

**12** Collagen disease—disseminated lupus, periarteritis.

**13** Superinfection—especially moniliasis.

**14** Drug resistance and antagonism.

**15** Drug dependence and addiction.

**16** Action on the fetus when drug is taken in pregnancy.

Drug reactions are usually due to over-dosage, intolerance, side effects including secondary effects, idiosyncrasy, hypersensitivity and allergy.

In the section to follow, I have made no attempt to list side effects in order of frequency. This would be impossible. Some of the side effects mentioned are probably rare, but it was felt that a fairly comprehensive list would be useful.

**Some rashes caused by drugs**

Acne—actinomycin D, barbiturates, bromides, chloral, cortico-steroids, ethambutol, ethionamide, iodides, isioniazid, phenytoin, tetracycline, thiouracil and troxidone

Bullous eruptions

Disseminated lupus erythematosus

Erythema multiforme—barbiturates, chloral, codeine, penicillin, phenolphthalein, phenytoin, salicylates, sulphonamides, tetracycline and thiazide diuretics

Erythema nodosum (p. 363)

Exfoliative dermatitis (p. 357)

Eczema

Fixed drug eruptions—anticonvulsants, antihistamines, barbiturates, chlordiazepoxide, iodides, mepacrine, meprobamate, penicillin, phenolphthalein, quinine, salicylates, sulphonamides and tetracycline

Lichen planus—antimalarials, arsenic, gold and PAS

Photosensitivity rashes

Pigmentation

Psoriasis—beta blockers, chloroquine

Purpura

Stevens–Johnson syndrome (p. 175)—anticonvulsant drugs, clindamycin, penicillin, quinine, rifampicin, long acting sulphonamides.

Toxic epidermal necrolysis—barbiturates, nitrofurantoin, penicillin, phenytoin, pyrimethamine with sulfadoxine, sulphonamides

Urticaria

**References**

1 Ashton H. Adverse effects of prolonged benzodiazepine use. *Adverse Drug Reaction Bulletin* 1986; **No. 118:** 440.

2 Davies DM. *Textbook of adverse drug reactions.* Oxford: Oxford University Press, 1981.

3 Dukes MNG (ed.). *Meyler's side effects of drugs.* Amsterdam: Excerpta Medica, 1979.

4 King DJ. Drug-induced psychiatric syndromes. *Prescribers Journal* 1986; **26:** 50.

5 Vere DW. Drug adverse reactions as masqueraders. *Adverse Drug Reaction Bulletin* 1976; **No. 60.**

# Side Effects of Individual Drugs

**Some of the side effects listed are rare. Selected important side effects are in italics.**

Acetazolamide—action on blood, kidney, liver; confusion, depression, diarrhoea, drowsiness, excitement, fever, fits, glycosuria, haematuria, headaches, irritability, melaena, paraesthesiae, polydipsia, rash, renal calculus, taste disturbance, vertigo, vision blurring, vomiting.

Actinomycin D—action on blood, alopecia, deafness, diarrhoea, intestinal ulceration, oral ulcers, rash.

Acyclovir—action on liver, kidney, blood; encephalopathy, urticaria, vomiting, hypersensitivity reaction.

Adrenaline—*fainting, nervousness, pallor, sweating,* tremor.

Aminophylline—*agitation,* anxiety, coma, *death,* dehydration, delirium, fever, fits, haematemesis, haematuria, headache, overventilation, rashes, respiratory paralysis, restlessness, shock, thirst, tremor, vertigo, vomiting.

Amitriptyline—abdominal pain, action on blood and liver; ataxia, blurring of vision, constipation, *drowsiness,* dry mouth, dysuria, excitement, fatigue, fever, fits, hallucinations, headache, ileus, mouth ulcers, myocarditis, myoclonus, nausea, numbness, oedema of face, oliguria, paraesthesiae, photosensitivity, pruritus, rash, sweating, tremors, urine green, urine retention, vertigo, vomiting, weakness.

Amphetamine—aggressiveness, *anorexia, defective physical growth,* depression, drowsiness, *drug dependence,* dry mouth, hallucinations, hyperthermia, *insomnia,* irritability, jaundice, paranoia, pupils dilated, rash, schizoid reactions, sweating, taste and smell changes, tearfulness, tics, tooth-grinding, tremor, weight loss.

Ampicillin—action on blood; anaphylaxis, colitis, rash.

Anabolic steroids—*jaundice,* liver cancer, lower PBI, *premature closure of epiphyses,* raised serum lipoids, virilization.

Anticonvulsants—see Barbiturates, Carbamazepine, Ethosuximide, Phensuximide, Phenytoin, Sulthiame, Valproate.

Antihistamines—action on blood, amblyopia, anorexia, ataxia, concentration poor, confusion, delirium, dental decay, *drowsiness, dry mouth,* dystonia, dysuria, facial spasms, fainting fits, fever, frequency of micturition, gastric disturbance, hallucinations, headache, insomnia, irritability, lassitude, rash, tachycardia, taste and smell changes, tinnitus, trismus, urinary retention, vertigo.

Antithyroid drugs—see Thiouracil.

Aspirin—see Salicylates.

Atropine group—confusion, delirium, dry mouth, fever, visual disturbance.

Azathioprine—*action on blood,* arthralgia, diarrhoea, fever, muscular wasting, pancreatitis, tumour formation.

Bacitracin—action on kidney, anorexia, nausea, pain at site of injection, rash.

Baclofen—confusion, drowsiness, muscle weakness, smell and taste disturbance, vertigo.

Barbiturates—amblyopia, *bad behaviour* (especially in mentally subnormal child), *concentration impaired,* confusion, depression, diplopia, *drowsiness, drug dependence,* fever, hepatosplenomegaly, *insomnia, irritability,* megaloblastic anaemia, nystagmus, optic neuritis, purpura, *rash,* Stevens–Johnson syndrome, tearfulness, yellow vision. Withdrawal symptoms—delirium, fits, tremors.

Becotide—oral thrush.

Bephenium—diarrhoea, nausea, vomiting.

Betamethasone—see Corticosteroids.

Boric acid—death, diarrhoea and vomiting, fits, haemorrhages, meningism, peripheral circulatory failure, red beefy rash.

Bromides—acne, hallucinations, slow thought, *tearfulness.*

Calcium chloride—*gastric irritation.*

Capreomycin—action on kidney, deafness, defective colour vision, hypocalcaemia, hypokalaemia, optic neuritis.

Carbamazepine—abdominal pain, action on blood, amblyopia, alopecia, adenopathy, anorexia, ataxia, blood pressure rise or fall, cataract, conjunctivitis, confusion, diarrhoea, diplopia, disseminated lupus, dizziness, drowsiness, dry mouth, dystonia, fever, fits, frequency of micturition, headache, heart block, hepatosplenomegaly, hyperacousia, insomnia, irritability, jaundice, limb pains, nausea, nystagmus, oliguria, opisthotonos, peripheral neuritis, photosensitivity, pneumonitis, pruritus, purpura, rash, Stevens–Johnson syndrome, syncope, taste and smell changes, tics, tinnitus, vomiting.

Carbenicillin—action on blood, hypokalaemia, purpura. See also penicillin.

Cephalosporins—abdominal discomfort, action on blood, kidney and liver; allergy, anorexia, confusion, diarrhoea, fever, nausea, oedema, parkinsonism, rash, serum-sickness-like symptoms, superinfection, thrombophlebitis at injection site, vomiting, wheezing.

Chloral—rash.

Chlorambucil—cataract.

Chloramphenicol—newborn baby: abdominal distension, cyanosis, death, flaccidity, *grey syndrome,* failure to thrive, hypothermia, irregular respirations, loose stools, optic neuritis, pruritus, rash, vomiting; older children: *action on the blood,* especially granulopenia; action on liver; optic neuritis, peripheral neuritis, enterocolitis.

Chlordiazepoxide—abdominal discomfort, action on blood and liver; anorexia, arthralgia, ataxia, confusion, constipation, depression, drowsiness, excitement, *extrapyramidal symptoms,* hostility, hypotension, mania, memory impaired, mouth dry, muscle cramps, nausea, oedema, over-activity, rashes, salivation, urinary difficulty, vertigo, vomiting. Withdrawal—irritability, tremors.

Chloroquine—accommodation impaired, action on blood and liver; *blurred vision,* burning in epigastrium, burning in mouth, *cataract,* colour vision impaired, deafness, depression, diplopia, fits, hair loss and loss of colour, involuntary movements, myopathy, nausea, peripheral neuritis, photosensitivity, pigmentation, pruritus, rashes, *retinal changes* (may be delayed for 4–5 years), torticollis, vomiting.

Chlorothiazide group—action on blood, allergy, cramps, hyperglycaemia, lassitude, melaena, nausea, pancreatitis, paraesthesiae, *potassium loss,* rashes, vertigo.

Chlorpromazine—see Phenothiazines.

Cimetidine—arthralgia, confusion, constipation, delirium, depression, diarrhoea, granulopenia, gynaecomastia, headache, muscle pain, myopathy, peripheral neuritis, rash, tremors, vertigo.

Ciprofloxacin—arthralgia, rash, confusion, fits, headache.

Clindamycin—enterocolitis, *ulcerative colitis,* Stevens–Johnson syndrome, urticaria.

Clonazepam—aggressiveness, ataxia, concentration defective, diarrhoea, drooling, drowsiness, dysphagia, fatigue, hypotonia, irritability, oedema of face, over-activity, over-eating, parotid swelling, pigmentation, salivary or bronchial hypersecretion, thirst, vertigo.

Clonidine—angioneurotic oedema, depression, dry mouth, insomnia, jaundice, nausea, pruritus, rash, sedation, thirst, vertigo.

Codeine—collapse of lung if cough productive, drying of secretions.

Colistin—*action on kidney, deafness,* muscle weakness, nystagmus, paraesthesiae, vertigo.

Corticosteroids—*acne,* abdominal pain, agranulocytosis, *cataract, Cushing's syndrome, death sudden,* delayed healing, *dermal atrophy, diabetes,* fits, glaucoma, *growth inhibition,* hallucinations, *hypertension, increased severity of chickenpox, muscle pains, muscle weakness, obesity, operative shock, osteoporosis,* pancreatitis, panniculitis, *peptic ulcer,* pigmentation, *purpura, sodium retention, striae, suppression of pain in infection,* thrombocytopenia, thrombo-embolic phenomena.

On discontinuing—increased intracranial pressure.

Skin applications—*acne,* burning sensation, *dermal atrophy,* folliculitis, hypertrichosis, miliaria, pruritus, *striae, telangiectasia.*

Corticotrophin—same as corticosteroids; more tendency to acne, allergy, hirsutism, hypertension, pigmentation: less bruising, less dyspepsia, osteoporosis, striae.

Cotrimoxazole—action on blood, skin, kidney, and liver; alopecia, angioneurotic oedema, deafness, diarrhoea, glossitis, hallucinations, headache, nausea, paraesthesiae, photosensitivity, vertigo, vomiting.

Cromoglycate—allergic granulomatosis, anaphylaxis, angioneurotic oedema, pulmonary eosinophilia, urticaria, wheezing.

Cyclopentolate—*acute psychosis,* ataxia, delirium, dry mouth, diarrhoea, visual hallucinations, ileus, vomiting.

Cyclophosphamide—*action on blood* and *liver; alopecia,* amenorrhea, anorexia, *cystitis, diarrhoea,* glycosuria, headache, intestinal ulceration, lymphoma, malignant disease, myelitis, myocarditis, nail pigmentation, nausea, oral ulcers, pneumonitis, protein-losing enteropathy, pulmonary fibrosis, reduced resistance to virus infections, *sterility,* vomiting.

Cycloserine—action on blood, fits, neurotoxic, psychoses.

Cytotoxic drugs—see Actinomycin D, Azathioprine, Cyclophosphamide, Methotrexate, 6-Mercaptopurine.

Demeclocycline—diarrhoea, facial oedema, *photosensitivity,* polydipsia, polyuria, *staining of teeth,* staining of nails, vomiting.

Diazepam—action on blood and liver; acute excitement, ataxia, blurred vision, cardiac arrhythmia, constipation, depression, diplopia, drowsiness, dry mouth, dysarthria, gynaecomastia, hallucinations, headache, hostility, impaired memory, irritability, nausea, rash, *respiratory depression,* sleep disturbed, temperature fall, tremors, vertigo, weakness. Prenatal—hypotonia.

Diazoxide—cardiac arrhythmia, *hypertrichosis,* involuntary movements.

Dichloralphenazone—pruritus.

Dicyclomine—dyspnoea, rash, salivation, sensitivity reactions, vertigo.

Digoxin—anorexia, *bradycardia, coupling of the beats,* diarrhoea, gynaecomastia, nausea, *oliguria,* scotoma, *vomiting,* xanthopsia.

Dioctyl sulphosuccinate—jaundice.

Diodoquin—optic atrophy.

Diphenoxylate—abdominal distension, areflexia, ataxia, depression, dizziness, drowsiness, fits, hypotonia, insomnia, nausea, nystagmus, pancreatitis, pruritus, pupils small, rash, vomiting.

Ephedrine—headache, *insomnia,* nausea, *nervousness,* pallor, palpitation, sweating, tremor.

Ergotamine—abdominal pain, blurred vision, chilling of extremities, cramps, diarrhoea, *gangrene,* headache, limb pains, nausea, *numbness,* papilloedema, taste disturbance, *tingling,* vomiting.

Erythromycin—abdominal pain, allergy, deafness, diarrhoea, dry mouth, fever, *jaundice* (mainly the estolate), nausea, rash, vomiting, wheezing.

Ethacrynic acid—electrolyte disturbance, deafness, pancreatitis, ventricular fibrillation.

Ethambutol—arthralgia, fever, gastrointestinal symptoms, hair loss, headache, jaundice, loss of colour vision, peripheral neuritis, rash, *reduced visual acuity*, retrobulbar neuritis, taste and smell changes.

Ethamivan—*convulsions*.

Ethionamide—abdominal pain, acne, alopecia, anorexia, diarrhoea, jaundice, mental changes, peripheral neuritis, photosensitivity, rash, salivation, vomiting.

Ethosuximide—abdominal pain, action on blood, kidney and liver; anorexia, confusion, depression, disseminated lupus, drowsiness, facial swelling, fatigue, headache, hiccough, nausea, parkinsonism, photophobia, psychosis, rash, stammer, stomatitis, vaginal bleeding, vertigo, vomiting.

Fenfluramine—alopecia, concentration poor, confusion, depression, diarrhoea, diplopia, drowsiness, dry mouth, dyskinesia, headache, insomnia, lethargy, nightmares, opisthotonos, rash, teeth-grinding, urinary frequency, vertigo, vomiting. Withdrawal—*agitation*.

Flufenamic acid—diarrhoea.

Framycetin—deafness.

Frusemide—bullous skin, deafness, hyperglycaemia, hypokalaemia, pancreatitis, photosensitivity.

Gentamicin—*action on ears* and *kidney*; alopecia, blurred vision, muscle weakness, permanent vestibular damage, psychological disturbance.

Gold—*action on blood, kidney, liver*; colitis, peripheral neuritis, photosensitivity, pruritus, *rashes*, stomatitis.

Griseofulvin—action on blood, kidney, liver, stomach; altered taste and smell, concentration poor, disseminated lupus, gynaecomastia, headache, insomnia, peripheral neuritis, photosensitivity, pigmented genitalia, superinfection, urticaria, vertigo.

Haloperidol—action on liver and skin; aphonia, depression, deterioration in school, drowsiness, dry mouth, dysphagia, fever, hyperthermia, involuntary movement, lethargy, salivation, sweating, tremors, vision blurred, vomiting.

Hyoscine—*atropine-like action*, coma, dryness of mouth, excitement, hallucination.

Ibuprofen—amblyopia, deafness, dyspepsia, jaundice, optic neuritis.

Imipramine—abdominal pain, accommodation impaired, action on blood and liver; aggressiveness, angioneurotic oedema, anxiety, ataxia, cold extremities, concentration impaired, constipation, delirium, dental decay, difficulty in micturition, diplopia, drowsiness, dryness of mucous membranes, dysarthria, dysphagia, dysuria, excitability, fits, giddiness, glossitis, gynaecomastia, headache, hypothermia, ileus, insomnia, irritability, lactorrhoea, lethargy, nausea, nystagmus, ocular palsy, oliguria, over-activity, palpitation, paraesthesiae, parkinsonism, peripheral neuritis, photosensitivity, postural hypotension, pruritus, pulmonary infiltration, rashes, renal damage, retrobulbar neuritis, stomatitis, sudden falls, sweating, tachycardia, taste disturbance, tearfulness, tremors, vertigo, vision blurred.

Indomethacin—abdominal distension, action on blood and liver; anorexia, asthma, ataxia, blurred vision, buccal ulcer, confusion, corneal and retinal changes, deafness, death, depression, diplopia, drowsiness, diarrhoea, fever, hair loss, headache, melaena, nausea, necrotizing enterocolitis, neuropathy, oedema, optic neuritis, pancreatitis, peptic ulcer, pruritus, psychological changes, rash, vertigo, vomiting.

Iodides—*acne, coryza,* fever, gastric disturbances, goitre, oedema of eyelids, swelling of salivary glands, urticaria.

Iron—abdominal discomfort, blackening of teeth and stools, constipation, diarrhoea.

Isoniazid—action on blood, kidney, liver; albuminuria, arthralgia, confusion, cramp, disseminated lupus, drowsiness, dysuria, excitability, fever, fits, gynaecomastia, headache, mouth dry, optic atrophy, optic neuritis, pancreatitis, *peripheral neuritis,* psychological changes, pulmonary eosinophilia, rash, vertigo, vision blurred, vomiting.

Kanamycin—action on blood, ear, kidney, liver; amblyopia, diarrhoea, muscle weakness, paraesthesiae, rash, superinfection, tinnitus, vertigo.

Ketoconazole—jaundice.

Lincomycin—abdominal pain, action on blood and liver; altered taste or smell; diarrhoea, muscle pain, overgrowth of yeasts, pruritus, rashes, superinfection, urticaria, vomiting.

Mefenamic acid—diarrhoea, dyspepsia, haemolysis, leucopenia, rash.

Mepacrine—action on blood, psychosis, rash, *yellow staining of skin.*

Meprobamate—action on blood, agitation, anaphylactoid reaction, anorexia, ataxia, blurred vision, bronchospasm, depression, drowsiness, drug dependence, fever, frequency, gastro-enteritis, lymphadenopathy, parkinsonism, proctitis, rash, stomatitis, thirst, vertigo, vomiting, weakness. Withdrawal—insomnia, tremors, twitching.

6-Mercaptopurine—action on *blood, liver*; anorexia, diarrhoea, intestinal ulceration, lupus disseminated, muscular wasting, oral ulcers, vomiting.

Methicillin—kidney damage, rigors.

Methotrexate—abdominal pain, action on *blood* and *liver*; alopecia, anorexia, diarrhoea, lung infiltration, melaena, nausea, oral ulceration, pulmonary eosinophilia, rash, renal tubular damage, vomiting.

Methylphenidate—*anorexia,* anxiety, depression, dyspepsia, *growth retardation,* headache, insomnia, irritability, lacrymation, mouth dry, palpitation, psychological disturbance, rash, spasmodic torticollis, sweating, tearfulness, tics, tremors.

Metoclopramide—*dysarthria, dysphagia, dystonia, facial grimacing,* lactorrhoea, *oculogyric crises, opisthotonos,* stiff neck, *torticollis,* tremors, *trismus.*

Metronidazole—action on blood, skin; anorexia, abdominal pain, ataxia, convulsions, diarrhoea, drowsiness, fever, gynae-comastia, paraesthesiae, peripheral neuritis, smell and taste disturbance, urine dark, vertigo, vomiting.

Morphia—nausea, vomiting, dry mouth.

Nalidixic acid—anaemia, action on blood, depression, diarrhoea, drowsiness, false positive for urinary reducing substances, fits, glycosuria, haemolysis, headache, hyperglycaemia, hyper-tension, increased intracranial pressure, jaundice, muscle weakness, myalgia, nausea, paraesthesiae, photosensitivity, polyarthritis, pruritus, rash, sixth nerve weakness, squint, vertigo, visual disturbance, vomiting.

Neomycin—action on ear, kidney and liver; muscle weakness, rash, steatorrhoea, wheezing.

Niclosamide—abdominal pain, ataxia, dry mouth, headache, loose stools, nausea, paraesthesiae, rash, sleep disturbed, stomatitis, vomiting.

Nitrazepam—ataxia, *bronchial hypersecretion*, depression, drowsiness, excitement, increased appetite, lachrymation, memory impaired, *salivation*, taste disturbed.

Nitrofurantoin—action on blood, kidney and liver; alopecia, anaphylaxis, angioneurotic oedema, anorexia, chills, cyanosis, eosinophilia, fever, fits, haemolysis in presence of glucose-6-phosphate dehydrogenase deficiency, hallucinations, headache, muscle pains, nausea, paraesthesiae, parotitis, peripheral neuritis, pigmentation, pleural effusion, pulmonary infiltration, rash, teeth discoloured, urine brown, vomiting.

Non-steroidal anti-inflammatory drugs—see ibuprofen, indomethacin, mefenamic acid, phenylbutazone.

Novobiocin—action on blood and liver; rash, yellow staining of skin.

Nystatin—diarrhoea.

Oleandomycin—jaundice.

Oestrogens—gynaecomastia.

PAS (Para-amino salicylic acid)—abdominal pain, action on blood, kidney and liver; diarrhoea, disseminated lupus, drowsiness, fever, gynaecomastia, haemorrhages, hair loss, lymphadenopathy, optic atrophy, optic neuritis, photophobia, pulmonary eosinophilia, pulmonary infiltration, rash, steatorrhoea, thyroid enlargement, vitamin B deficiency, vomiting.

Paracetamol—encephalopathy, granulopenia, haemolysis, hepatitis, pancreatitis. Dextropropoxyphene ('Distalgesic')—abdominal pain, circulatory collapse, coma, convulsions, drowsiness, headache, nausea, visual disturbance, vomiting, weakness. Addiction—psychoses.

Penicillamine—action on blood, action on kidney, diarrhoea, disseminated lupus, fever, loss of taste, myopathy, purpura, rash, vomiting.

Penicillin—*anaphylaxis,* angioneurotic oedema, arthralgia, asthma, conjunctivitis, dermatomyositis, *diarrhoea* when taken by mouth, disseminated lupus, effusion into joints, *haemolysis,* hypertrichosis, increased intracranial pressure, lachrymation, limb pain, myocarditis, periarteritis, polyneuritis, pruritus, pulmonary eosinophilia, rashes, superinfection, visual defect, wheezing.

Pethidine—nausea, vertigo.

Phenacetin—jaundice, action on kidney.

Phenazopyridine—action on blood, yellow urine.

Phenothiazine group of tranquillizers (e.g. Chlorpromazine, Pro chlorperazine)—abdominal pain, action on blood and liver; catatonia, concentration impaired, constipation, *corneal opacities,* constriction of chest, depression, dental decay, diarrhoea, drowsiness, dry mouth, *extrapyramidal symptoms,* facial oedema, fever, fits, gynaecomastia, headache, hirsutism, hyperthermia, hypothermia, inability to sit still, involuntary movements, lactorrhoea, limb pains, muscle rigidity, nasal congestion, neck stiffness, oculogyric crises, oedema, opis thotonos, paralysis of accommodation, photosensitivity, pigmentation of retina and skin, postural hypotension, pruritus, rash, rigidity, stomatitis, sweating, tremors, urine red, urinary retention, vertigo, visual blurring.

Phensuximide—action on blood; ataxia, disseminated lupus, drowsiness, haematuria, hepatosplenomegaly, lymphadenopathy, nausea, rash, vertigo.

Phenylbutazone—action on blood, lymphadenopathy.

Phenytoin—abdominal discomfort, action on blood, kidney and liver; acne, alopecia, amblyopia, anorexia, arthropathy, *ataxia,* choreo-athetosis, concentration defective, conjunctivitis, constipation, decalcification, depression, diplopia, disseminated lupus, drowsiness, dysarthria, fever, *gingivitis,* haematuria, headache, hepatosplenomegaly, *hirsutism,* hyperglycaemia, immunosuppression, interaction with phenobarbitone, phenothiazines, PAS, sulthiame; joint effusion, lymphadenopathy, lymphoma, megaloblastic anaemia, mental slowing, mental deterioration, myocarditis, nausea, nystagmus, over-activity, periarteritis, peripheral neuritis, pigmentation, pruritus, psychological disturbance, rash, rickets, skull thickening, Stevens–Johnson syndrome, striae, taste and smell changes, tremors, vomiting.

Piperazine—abdominal pain, accommodation impaired, allergic purpura, ataxia, blurring of vision, coma, confusion, diarrhoea, hallucinations, hypotonia, incoordination, muscle weakness, paraesthesiae, precipitation of fits in epileptics, rashes, tremors, urticaria, vertigo, vomiting.

Polymyxin—action on kidney; ataxia, circumoral numbness, fever, neurotoxic, paraesthesiae, pruritus, rash, slurred speech, vertigo.

Primidone—abdominal pain, action on blood, alopecia, amblyopia, angioneurotic oedema, ataxia, decalcification, diplopia, disseminated lupus, *drowsiness,* dysarthria, hair loss, *irritability,* lymphadenopathy, megaloblastic anaemia, nausea, *nystagmus,* oedema of eyelids, over-activity, psychoses, rash, vertigo, vomiting.

Propranolol—bronchospasm, depression, hypotension, lassitude, nightmares, psoriasis.

Pyrazinamide—action on liver, limb pains.

Pyrimethamine—action on blood, convulsions.

Quinine—action on blood and skin, deafness, jaundice, tinnitus, visual defect.

Rifampicin—abdominal pain, action on blood, liver and kidney; bone pain, conjunctivitis, deafness, diarrhoea, drowsiness, dyspepsia, dyspnoea, fever, headache, muscle pain, myopathy, nausea, pancreatitis, pruritis, rash, red urine and sputum, red tears; Stevens–Johnson syndrome, vertigo, visual disturbance, vomiting, weakness, wheezing.

Ristocetin—action on blood and kidney; albuminuria, thromboses.

Salbutamol—hallucinations, hyperglycaemia, myopathy, tremors.

Salicylates—*anaemia, angioneurotic oedema, asthma, bleeding* by causing hypoprothrombinaemia or thrombocytopenia, deafness, haematemesis, increase of chronic urticaria, jaundice, nystagmus, *over-ventilation,* pulmonary eosinophilia, Reye's syndrome, *tinnitus,* vertigo, vomiting. Aspirin particles also cause bleeding by direct action on gastric mucosa.

Sodium fusidate—diarrhoea, vomiting.

Streptomycin—action on blood; *ataxia, deafness,* disseminated lupus, fever, jaundice, muscle weakness, myocarditis, optic neuritis, paraesthesiae, peripheral neuritis, pruritus, rash, wheezing, yellow vision.

Sulphasalazine—action on blood, anorexia, arthralgia, fever, headache, lung changes, muscle pain, nausea, pancreatitis, rash, urine retention, vomiting.

Sulphonamides—*action on blood and liver; crystalluria,* diplopia, disseminated lupus, *drug fever,* headache, lymphadenopathy, myopia, nausea, necrotizing angiitis, optic neuritis, pancreatitis, photosensitivity, polyarteritis, polyneuritis, pulmonary infiltration, rash, vertigo, yellow vision.

Long-acting sulphonamides—*Stevens–Johnson syndrome.*

Sulthiame—action on blood and kidney; anorexia, ataxia, blurred vision, confusion, depression, drowsiness, dysarthria, headache, loss of weight, nephrotic syndrome, *over-ventilation,* paraesthesiae, photophobia, psychotic excitement, ptosis, raised blood level of phenytoin, rash, renal calculus, status epilepticus, vertigo, vomiting.

Tartrazine—allergic purpura, amblyopia, angioneurotic oedema, asthma, dyspnoea, epiphora, over-activity, rhinitis.

Theophylline—abdominal pain, confusion, convulsions, depression, headache, insomnia, over-activity, restlessness, vomiting.

Terbutaline—tremors, palpitation.

Testosterone group—acne, jaundice, premature closure of epiphyses, virilization.

Tetanus toxoid—dysarthria, peripheral neuritis, pruritus, sweating, urticaria, wheezing.

Tetracyclines—abdominal pain, action on kidney, anaphylaxis, *bulging fontanelle, diarrhoea,* disseminated lupus, *enamel hypoplasia, enterocolitis,* fever, glossitis, jaundice, myocarditis, myopia, *overgrowth of monilia,* papilloedema, pancreatitis, peptic ulcer, *photosensitivity,* pruritus, rash, thrombocytopenia, *tooth and nail discoloration,* vertigo, *wheezing.*

Old stocks—abnormal amino-aciduria, Fanconi-like syndrome, nausea, oedema, polydipsia, polyuria, vomiting.

Thiabendazole—dyspepsia, headache, hyperglycaemia, leucopenia, numbness, pruritus, tinnitus, vertigo, xanthopsia.

Thiouracil—acne, action on blood and liver; disseminated lupus, fever, lymphadenopathy, rash.

Thyroxine—*heart failure at onset, loss of weight.*

Overdose—*advanced skeletal maturation followed by premature closure of epiphyses, diarrhoea, irritability, tachycardia.*

Tranquillizers and sedatives—see benzodiazepines (e.g. Clonazepam, Diazepam, Nitrazepam), Bromides, Chloral,

Dichloralphenazone, Haloperidol, Meprobamates, Methylphenidate, Paracetamol, Phenothiazines (e.g. Chlordiazepoxide, Chlorpromazine).

Trimeprazine—abdominal pain, depression, drowsiness, dry mouth, headache, nasal stuffiness, rash, vertigo.

Trimethoprim—see Cotrimoxazole.

Troxidone—abdominal pain, acne, *action on blood and liver*; alopecia, angioneurotic oedema, diplopia, disseminated lupus, drowsiness, effusion into joints, grand mal, haematuria, headache, hiccoughs, irritability, lymphadenopathy, *nephrotic syndrome*, photophobia, rash, Stevens–Johnson syndrome, vomiting, white vision.

Valproate sodium—anorexia, drowsiness, elevation of serum barbiturate, extrapyramidal symptoms, hair loss, headache, hepatic damage, hyperammonaemia, nausea, pancreatitis, purpura, vomiting, weight gain.

Vancomycin—action on blood, ears, kidney and liver; fever, paraesthesiae, phlebitis, rash, respiratory arrest, rigor, superinfection, thromboses, urticaria.

Vincristine—abdominal pain, *action on blood; alopecia*, ataxia, constipation, diarrhoea, diplopia, facial palsy, headache, hoarseness, insomnia, jaw pain, myopathy, oral ulcers, pain in fingers, paraesthesiae, peripheral neuritis, pigmentation, pulmonary fibrosis, ptosis, rash, vomiting.

Viomycin—action on ears, kidney and liver; electrolyte disturbances, rashes.

Viprynium—abdominal pain, diarrhoea, nausea, red stools, vomiting.

Vitamin A excess—abdominal pain, anorexia, arthralgia, *bone pain*, brittle nails, diplopia, dry mouth, dry skin, fractures, *hepatosplenomegaly*, hydrocephalus, hypoplastic anaemia, increased intracranial pressure, myalgia, oedema of occiput, papilloedema, *periostitis*, pruritus, sparse hair, *stomatitis*, vomiting.

Vitamin $B_3$ (nicotinamide)—alopecia, arrhythmia, hepatitis, peptic ulcer.

Vitamin $B_6$ (pyridoxine)—dependency, peripheral neuritis.

Vitamin D excess—anorexia, *hypercalcaemia*, hypertension, nephrocalcinosis, polyuria.

Vitamin K excess—*haemolysis, kernicterus*.

# Psychological and Organic

Psychological factors are so commonly associated with organic disease that it is essential to eliminate organic disease before concluding that the cause is entirely psychological. In fact *one should never conclude that a symptom is entirely psychological without positive evidence of a psychological disorder and without eliminating organic disease*. It is then necessary to see the child again in order to make sure that one is right about the absence of organic disease. The difficulty is that organic disease may cause psychological disorders, and psychological disorders may cause somatic symptoms.

Many psychological symptoms are caused by disease. For instance, infections and other diseases which result in a child necessarily or unnecessarily missing school may lead to his worrying about dropping behind others in his class—and may even make it difficult for him to return to school. A common example of this is asthma: many parents keep their asthmatic child away from school when he has the slightest wheeze (or even a cold which might perhaps lead to a wheeze), and as a result the child drops behind in his work, worries, and wheezes all the more, and so is kept away longer still. It is a difficult vicious circle which must be broken. If a mother is over-anxious about the child's health, she makes him neurotic and hypochondriacal.

Many school difficulties which have an organic basis lead to psychological symptoms. Learning disorders commonly present as a behaviour problem such as truancy. Clumsiness of movement commonly leads to unhappiness at school because of the unkindness of the teachers who ascribe the child's bad writing to carelessness and naughtiness. Defects of hearing or seeing lead to troublesome behaviour problems because the child is unable to follow the work of the class. A child who finds the work too much for him, either because of a learning difficulty in a particular subject or because his IQ is lower than that of others in his form or for other reasons, may lose heart, become worried, depressed and insecure.

Epilepsy leads to behaviour difficulties in several ways. The child may be rejected from entry to a school because of the epilepsy, or he may be treated differently from others, being prevented, for example, from swimming. He may live in fear of having a convulsion in the street or in class, especially if he has already experienced such an attack. If he suffers from frequent attacks of petit mal he may so frequently miss what is being said that he drops behind in his class work. He may have temporal lobe epilepsy, which causes bad behaviour, leading, for instance, to outbursts of temper. It is particularly important to remember that drugs given for epilepsy may make him clumsy, drowsy and irritable and may interfere with his concentration. Phenobarbitone is particularly liable to cause undue irritability and bad behaviour.

Over-activity, which is sometimes related to prematurity, events during pregnancy or hypoxia at birth, leads to difficulties at school, poor concentration and punishment.

On p. 1 it is noted that certain diseases which lead to poor physical growth lead to food refusal because of food forcing. For instance, congenital heart disease is commonly associated with defective physical growth. This leads to the mother worrying about the child's small size, and so she tries to make him eat more—and he refuses.

Some bad behaviour is due to hypoglycaemia. Some children (and adults) become bad-tempered when hungry. Others behave badly because they are tired as a result of an infection or anaemia.

Children with an intracranial neoplasm, tuberculous meningitis or chorea may present as a behaviour problem.

Chronic diarrhoea, such as occurs in ulcerative colitis, leads to bad temper and irritability. This may lead some to ascribe the ulcerative colitis to a behaviour problem. Admittedly there are often psychological factors in association with ulcerative colitis. Any chronic handicap, such as diabetes, haemophilia, muscular dystrophy, juvenile chronic arthritis, or defects of vision or hearing, has psychological consequences and interferes with school work.

Several studies have shown that there is a higher incidence of physical handicap in juvenile delinquents than in the normal population.

Other conditions which may present as behaviour problems include thyrotoxicosis, migraine, anorectal stenosis, bladder neck obstruction, and (rarely) phaeochromocytoma or neuroblastoma.

Children may be embarrassed and unhappy because of their ugliness or other aspects of their physical appearance, such as obesity, sexual precocity, delayed puberty, short stature or lipodystrophy.

More than half of all the symptoms discussed in this book, all of which may be due to organic disease, may also be psychological in origin. For instance, one of the three components of asthma is psychological disturbance (the other two being allergy and infection). There may be a psychological component in allergic rhinitis. A cough may be merely a habit or an attention-seeking device.

Numerous somatic symptoms may arise from psychological problems. They include diarrhoea, abdominal pain, vomiting, frequency of micturition, dysuria, dysmenorrhoea, bed-wetting, polydipsia, polyuria, a poor appetite, indigestion and peptic ulcer, obesity, dirt eating, headache and limb or chest pains. There is a psychological component to several skin conditions, such as eczema, urticaria, lichen planus and pruritus. Many other somatic symptoms can be caused by psychological problems.

# Some Symptoms of Importance

At the risk of repetition, I propose in this section to enumerate some symptoms of special importance in children, because failure to take note of them may have disastrous results:

Jaundice on the first day, because it requires urgent treatment: it is due to haemolytic disease until proved otherwise, though this is now rare. Severe jaundice in the newborn period calls for urgent investigation.

Vomitus containing bile in the newborn period, or vomiting with abdominal distension, suggests intestinal obstruction.

Blood in a baby's vomitus after the newborn period, suggests hiatus hernia or reflux, or, in the first month or two, prothrombin deficiency.

Diarrhoea in an infant or young child is important because of the rapidity with which dehydration may occur.

Stridor from birth, even if only inspiratory, should be investigated because treatment may occasionally be necessary. Stridor of acute onset is important because of the rapidity with which it may get worse and cause complete obstruction.

Cough of really sudden onset, without an upper respiratory infection, suggests an inhaled foreign body.

Ear pain, due to otitis media, requires immediate antibiotic treatment (and *not* drops in the ear).

Neck stiffness (in flexion) suggests meningitis. It is essential to have a lumbar puncture carried out before an antibiotic is given, so that if it is due to pyogenic meningitis the organism can be isolated and the appropriate treatment can be given.

Fits with fever in the child are important. Although from the age of about 6 months to 4 to 5 years the most likely diagnosis is a benign febrile convulsion, it could be a fever-precipitated fit in an epileptic, and that would be likely after the age of 4 or 5. At any age it could be due to pyogenic meningitis.

The onset of drowsiness with an infection may represent pyogenic meningitis.

Loss of weight is important because of the many serious causes which could be responsible.

A severe attack of asthma, not responding to the usual treatment.

Poisoning of any kind is important because hospital investigation and treatment are needed. After ingestion of salicylates, especially enteric-coated or sustained-release tablets, or after iron or diphenoxylate ingestion, there is a dangerous latent period between the time of ingestion of the poison and the onset of symptoms. Unexplained abnormal excitement, drowsiness, convulsions or vomiting may be due to an overdose of drugs or poisoning—and may be non-accidental injury.

# Common Diagnostic Difficulties and Pitfalls

After more than 50 years of postgraduate clinical experience, I thought it suitable to list what seem to me to be the commonest or most important diagnostic errors or pitfalls.

The most common diagnostic error, certainly the commonest to have medicolegal consequences, is over-confidence. But often, because of fear of medicolegal consequences, excessive caution in diagnosis leads to unnecessarily expensive, often unpleasant and sometimes dangerous investigations.

Although one is more likely to be right if one ascribes all a child's symptoms to *one* disease, the occasional coexistence of two diseases may cause confusion. For instance, a child with asthma may inhale a foreign body, or may have cystic fibrosis or complicating aspergillosis.

The presence of one major congenital anomaly should alert one to the likelihood that there is a second anomaly. For instance, if there is oesophageal atresia, there is a high risk of an anomaly elsewhere— e.g. in the anus or kidney; and, if there is an imperforate anus, there is a high risk of another anomaly, in the upper gastrointestinal tract or elsewhere. If there is congenital pyloric stenosis, there is a slightly increased risk of an anomaly in the urinary tract. A spontaneous pneumothorax may be associated with renal anomalies. A child with Down's syndrome may have hypothyroidism, and it is very easy to miss it. A child with purpura and a blood disease may suffer non-accidental injury, or vice versa. There are many other important associations, such as those with Wilms' tumour (p. 326).

Non-accidental injury, in its many forms, may present considerable diagnostic difficulties. Sexual abuse is an important cause of behaviour problems, including depression, and a variety of bizarre symptoms. Similarly with the syndrome of Munchausen by proxy, which I have mentioned in many parts of this book; it may present with a wide variety of bizarre symptoms or continuation of symptoms.

Around 90 per cent of all the symptoms discussed in this book could be side effects of drugs, so that no clinical history is complete unless one has made specific enquiries about all drugs taken. One may forget the possibility of the interaction of drugs, when more than one drug at a time is taken. Studies have shown that most mothers take some drug in pregnancy, and many of these drugs may occasionally affect the fetus, causing symptoms in the newborn period and later.

Though a history of drugs taken by the mother in pregnancy or by the child after birth is relevant, it may also be relevant to know what previous surgical or radiotherapeutic treatment the child has had.

One has to remember the possibility of poisoning, or of an overdose of medicine, as in epilepsy, even though the parents stoutly deny its possibility, claiming that the child could not have had access to drugs, or could have taken only a small quantity. The true diagnosis may be non-accidental injury, or carelessness which the parents do not want to admit.

Because there are so many drugs of addiction, and because of the frequent combination of these drugs, the wide variety of symptoms resulting may cause confusion in diagnosis. It is easy to forget the result of a child's exposure to 'passive smoking'—smoking by parents, siblings or others in the home, so that one misses the true cause of a child's respiratory symptoms, such as cough or wheezing.

Foreign bodies in the nose, ear, eye, bronchus, rectum, vagina or bladder can cause confusing symptoms. For instance, the absence of a history of sudden cough or of the possible exposure to the risk of inhalation of a foreign body or the absence of positive X-ray findings does not exclude the possibility of a foreign body in the bronchus.

Referred pain (p. 100) can cause diagnostic errors. The commonest examples are the misdiagnosis of abdominal pain (referred from the chest) or of pain in the knee (referred from the hip).

A common mistake in diagnosis is failure to obtain the history of prenatal factors other than drugs taken in pregnancy. The history should include the history of previous pregnancies, of relative infertility, of illness in pregnancy, of indications of placental insufficiency, and of genetic and familial factors. Failure to do this may lead to the error of ascribing a child's neonatal problems or later handicap to perinatal difficulties, when the true cause lay in the prenatal period.

A mother's real anxiety may be concealed. When she complains of her child's innumerable symptoms, none of them suggesting disease, she may be anxious because the symptoms are similar to those of a neighbour's child or a relative's child who had a fatal disease.

Having taken a detailed history and having examined the child, one should sit and think—*before* proceeding to a series of investigations. Many investigations would be avoided by a little thought before ordering a series of laboratory tests.

There is a special danger of diagnostic error, and of missing organic disease, when the parents are known psychopaths, or when the child is unusually badly behaved, or the parents are aggressive, or belong to a known problem family.

An important omission in a difficult case of infection is failure to elicit a history of a holiday on a farm or abroad.

Below are some common symptoms which are liable to lead to incorrect diagnoses:

Vomiting, crying, green stools or diarrhoea are *not* due to breast milk not suiting the baby. The only exceptions to this are the rare conditions galactosaemia or lactose intolerance. If these are suspected the child should be referred to a paediatrician for the appropriate tests. Green stools in fully breast-fed babies are normal. Green stools passed by a bottle-fed baby are normal unless there is diarrhoea.

Vomiting, crying or diarrhoea are *not* due to the breast milk being too strong for the baby—or not strong enough.

Vomiting, crying or diarrhoea in a full-term breast-fed or bottle-fed baby are *not* due to overfeeding.

Vomiting, crying or diarrhoea are *not* due to the particular dried food or other properly constituted feed not suiting the baby. Nothing will be achieved by changing from one dried food to another. The child may, however, be intolerant of certain carbohydrates. The child with coeliac disease is probably intolerant of gluten. The child with hypercalcaemia is intolerant of ordinary foods and requires a special low-calcium milk. A very occasional baby is sensitive to milk protein.

Infrequent stools in a well breast-fed baby are *not* due to constipation. They are normal.

True constipation in an artificially fed baby is *not* due to insufficiency of roughage in the diet. It may be due to inadequate fluid or other factors. One has several times seen children treated for *diarrhoea* when the diagnosis was constipation with overflow.

Crying at night by a well child is *not* due to indigestion or wind. It is almost certainly due to mismanagement and habit formation.

A poor appetite in a well child is almost certainly *not* due to disease; it is almost certainly due to food-forcing.

When a child has never been dry, bed-wetting after the age of 3 is almost certainly *not* primarily psychological in origin or due to faulty management—though psychological problems can be superimposed on the basic problem of delayed maturation, usually familial.

Constant dribbling incontinence is *not* due to delayed maturation. In the boy it is usually due to urethral valves and in the girl to an ectopic ureter in the vagina or a ureterocele.

Urinary tract infection is commonly diagnosed when it is non-existent, and commonly not diagnosed when it is present. Dysuria in the girl is more likely to be due to soreness around the vulva than to urinary tract infection; and frequency in a toddler is more likely to be an attention-seeking device.

Teething does *not* cause bronchitis, convulsions, fever, rash or diarrhoea.

Delayed walking is *not* a problem for the orthopaedic specialist. It is most unlikely to be due to congenital dislocation of the hip.

Delayed talking is *not* due to tongue-tie, laziness, 'everything being done for him'. It is almost certainly *not* due to jealousy.

Obesity is almost certainly *not* due to Fröhlich's syndrome. I have not yet seen a case.

Mental subnormality is *not* diagnosed on the basis of retardation in one or even two fields of development, and cerebral palsy is *not* diagnosed on the basis of one physical sign; both are diagnosed only on a combination of signs.

Many infants are thought to be blind because of lack of eye-following or deaf because of lack of response to sound, when the true diagnosis is retardation due to mental subnormality.

Symptoms and signs suggesting encephalitis may be due not to encephalitis but to a metabolic disease.

Drowsiness following a head injury may be due not to head injury, but to acute otitis media, urinary tract infection or other disease.

If a child has convulsions and is unwell between fits, or shows deterioration in school work, the diagnosis is almost certainly *not* uncomplicated epilepsy. The symptoms could be due to side effects of drugs, or to cerebral tumour or hypertension.

If a child is thought to have attacks of migraine, but is unwell between the attacks, or there is a change in personality, lethargy or deterioration of school work, the diagnosis is almost certainly something else—such as cerebral tumour, hypertension or drugs.

A normal epicanthic fold is a common cause of a wrong diagnosis of a squint.

*On innumerable occasions one has seen a mother furious because a doctor has told her that she is over-anxious, fussing, worrying about nothing, or that the child is just putting it on, or hysterical, or wants a good smacking, or will grow out of it, when there is serious organic disease. Not only do such mistakes infuriate, but they are liable to have medicolegal consequences.*

# Useful Books

### General textbooks of medicine and surgery

Behrman RE, Vaughan V (eds.). *Nelson's textbook of pediatrics.* Philadelphia: Saunders, 12th edn, 1983.

Forfar JO, Arneil GC. *Textbook of paediatrics.* Edinburgh: Churchill Livingstone, 1983.

Jones PG. *Clinical paediatric surgery.* Oxford: Blackwell Scientific Publications, 1986.

Raffensperger JG. *Swenson's pediatric surgery.* New York: Appleton Century Crofts, 1980.

Rudolph AM. *Pediatrics.* Connecticut: Appleton Century Crofts, 1982.

### Rare diseases and syndromes

Bergsma D. *Birth defects compendium.* London: Macmillan Press, 1979.

El Shafie M, Klippel CH. *Associated congenital anomalies.* Baltimore: Williams Wilkins, 1981.

Salmon M, Lindenbaum R. *Developmental defects and syndromes.* Aylesbury: HM and M Publishers, 1978.

Warkany J. *Congenital malformations.* Chicago: Year Book Publications, 1971.

Wiedmann HR, Grosse K, Dibern H. *The atlas of characteristic syndromes.* London: Wolfe Medical Publications, 1985.

### Other specialized books

Anderson CM, Burke V. *Paediatric gastroenterology.* Oxford: Blackwell Scientific Publications, 1975.

Avery ME, Taeusch HW. *Schaffer's diseases of the newborn.* Philadelphia: Saunders, 1984.

Bakwin H, Bakwin RM. *Clinical management of behavior disorders in children*. Philadelphia: Saunders, 1972.

Bluestone CD, Stool SE. *Pediatric otolaryngology*. Philadelphia: Saunders, 1983.

Brett EM. *Paediatric neurology*. London: Churchill, 1983.

Brook CGD. *Clinical paediatric endocrinology*. Oxford: Blackwell Scientific Publications, 1981.

Caffey J. *Pediatric X-ray diagnosis*. Chicago: Year Book Publications, 1985.

D'Arck P, Griffin J. *Iatrogenic diseases*. London: Oxford University Press, 1983.

Davies DM. *Textbook of adverse drug reactions*. Oxford: Oxford University Press, 1981.

Drillien CM, Drummond MB. *Neurodevelopmental problems in early childhood*. Oxford: Blackwell Scientific Publications, 1977.

Dubowitz V. *Muscle disorders in childhood*. Philadelphia: Saunders, 1978.

Duke-Elder S. *System of ophthalmology*. London: Kimpton, 14 volumes (various dates).

Dukes MNG. *Meyler's side effects of drugs*. Amsterdam: Excerpta Medica, 1984.

Emans SJ, Goldstein D. *Pediatric and adolescent gynecology*. Boston: Little Brown and Co, 1982.

Falkner F, Tanner J. *Human growth*. New York: Plenum, 1986.

Ford FR. *Diseases of the nervous system in infancy, childhood and adolescence*. Springfield: Charles Thomas, 1973.

Gardner LI. *Endocrine and genetic diseases of childhood*. Philadelphia: Saunders, 1977.

Gryboski J, Walker WA. *Gastrointestinal problems in the infant*. Philadelphia: Saunders, 1983.

Harley RD. *Pediatric ophthalmology*. Philadelphia: Saunders, 1983.

Harries JT. *Essentials of paediatric gastroenterology*. London: Churchill Livingstone, 1977.

Hendrickse RG. *Paediatrics in the tropics*. London: Oxford University Press, 1981.

Illingworth RS. *The normal child*. London: Churchill Livingstone, 9th edn, 1987.

Illingworth RS. *Development of the infant and young child, normal and abnormal*. Edinburgh: Churchill Livingstone, 9th edn, 1987.

Jelliffe DB, Stanfield JP. *Diseases of children in the subtropics and tropics.* London: Edward Arnold, 1978.

Krugman S, Katz SL. *Infectious diseases of children.* St Louis: Mosby, 1986.

Lagos JC. *Differential diagnosis in pediatric neurology.* Boston: Little Brown and Co, 1971.

Miller D, Pearson H, Baehner RL, McMillan C. *Smith's blood diseases of infancy and childhood.* St Louis: Mosby, 1984.

Mowat AP. *Liver disorders in childhood.* London: Butterworths, 1979.

Nussbaum E, Galant SP. *Pediatric respiratory disorders.* New York: Grune and Stratton, 1984.

Rook A, Wilkinson DS, Ebling FJG. *Textbook of dermatology.* Oxford: Blackwell Scientific Publications, 1987.

Rosenberg RN. *Neurology.* New York: Grune and Stratton, 1980.

Rutter M, Hersov L. *Child and adolescent psychiatry.* Oxford: Blackwell Scientific Publications, 1985.

Sharrard WJW. *Paediatric orthopaedics and fractures.* Oxford: Blackwell Scientific Publications, 1979.

Sherlock S. *Diseases of the liver and biliary system.* Oxford: Blackwell Scientific Publications, 1985.

Stanbury JB, Wyngaarden JB, Frederickson DS. *The metabolic basis of inherited disease.* New York: McGraw Hill, 1978.

Steiner M. *Essential paediatric radiology.* Oxford: Blackwell Scientific Publications, 1983.

Swaiman KF, Wright PS. *Pediatric neuromuscular diseases.* St Louis: Mosby, 1982.

Tampion J. *Dangerous plants.* London: David and Charles, 1977.

Verbov J. *Paediatric dermatology.* London: Heinemann, 1979.

Verbov J, Morley N. *Colour atlas of paediatric dermatology.* London: MTP Press, 1983.

Vinken PJ, Bruyn GW. *Handbook of clinical neurology.* Amsterdam: North Holland, 1982. 42 volumes.

Walker-Smith Hamilton J, Walker W. *Practical paediatric gastroenterology.* London: Butterworth, 1983.

Walsh FB, Hoyt WF. *Clinical ophthalmology.* Baltimore: Williams and Wilkins, 1982.

Williams DI, Johnston JH. *Paediatric urology.* London: Butterworths, 1982.

# Index

Principal references are given in bold type

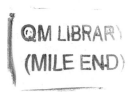